T0348622

Cardiothoracic Anesthesia and Critical Care

Editors

KARSTEN BARTELS
STEFAN J.M. DIELEMAN

ANESTHESIOLOGY CLINICS

www.anesthesiology.theclinics.com

Consulting Editor
LEE A. FLEISHER

December 2019 • Volume 37 • Number 4

ELSEVIER

1600 John F. Kennedy Boulevard • Suite 1800 • Philadelphia, Pennsylvania, 19103-2899

http://www.theclinics.com

ANESTHESIOLOGY CLINICS Volume 37, Number 4
December 2019 ISSN 1932-2275, ISBN-13: 978-0-323-70892-0

Editor: Colleen Dietzler
Developmental Editor: Kristen Helm

Anesthesiology Clinics (ISSN 1932-2275) is published quarterly by Elsevier Inc., 360 Park Avenue South, New York, NY 10010-1710. Months of issue are March, June, September, and December. Periodicals postage paid at New York, NY and at additional mailing offices. Subscription prices are $100.00 per year (US student/resident), $360.00 per year (US individuals), $446.00 per year (Canadian individuals), $693.00 per year (US institutions), $876.00 per year (Canadian institutions), $225.00 per year (Canadian and foreign student/resident), $469.00 per year (foreign individuals), and $876.00 per year (foreign institutions). To receive student and resident rate, orders must be accompanied by name of affiliated institution, date of term, and the *signature* of program/residency coordinator on institutions letterhead. Orders will be billed at individual rate until proof of status is received. Foreign air speed delivery is included in all *Clinics'* subscription prices. All prices are subject to change without notice. POSTMASTER: Send address changes to *Anesthesiology Clinics,* Elsevier Health Sciences Division, Subscription Customer Service, 3251 Riverport Lane, Maryland Heights, MO 63043. Customer Service (orders, claims, online, change of address): Elsevier Health Sciences Division, Subscription Customer Service, 3251 Riverport Lane, Maryland Heights, MO 63043. **Tel:1-800-654-2452 (U.S. and Canada); 314-447-8871 (outside U.S. and Canada). Fax: 314-447-8029. E-mail: journalscustomerservice-usa@elsevier.com (for print support); journalsonlinesupport-usa@elsevier.com (for online support).**

Reprints. For copies of 100 or more of articles in this publication, please contact the Commercial Reprints Department, Elsevier Inc., 360 Park Avenue South, New York, NY 10010-1710. Tel.: 212-633-3874; Fax: 212-633-3820; E-mail: reprints@elsevier.com.

Anesthesiology Clinics, is also published in Spanish by McGraw-Hill Inter-americana Editores S. A., P.O. Box 5-237, 06500 Mexico D. F., Mexico.

Anesthesiology Clinics, is covered in *MEDLINE/PubMed (Index Medicus), Current Contents/Clinical Medicine, Excerpta Medica, ISI/BIOMED*, and *Chemical Abstracts*.

Contributors

CONSULTING EDITOR

LEE A. FLEISHER, MD, FACC, FAHA
Robert D. Dripps Professor and Chair of Anesthesiology and Critical Care, Professor of Medicine, Perelman School of Medicine, University of Pennsylvania, Philadelphia, Pennsylvania, USA

EDITORS

KARSTEN BARTELS, MD, PhD
Associate Professor of Anesthesiology, Psychiatry, Medicine, and Surgery, Department of Anesthesiology, University of Colorado, Aurora, Colorado, USA

STEFAN J.M. DIELEMAN, MD, PhD
Cardiac Anaesthesiologist, Department of Anaesthesia, Westmead Hospital, Westmead, New South Wales, Australia

AUTHORS

DARRYL ABRAMS, MD
Assistant Professor of Medicine, Division of Pulmonary, Allergy, and Critical Care, Columbia University Vagelos College of Physicians and Surgeons, New York, New York, USA

MICHAEL A. ACKERMANN, MD
Department of Anesthesiology and Intensive Care Medicine, Heart Centre Leipzig, Leipzig, Germany

MARCO AGUIRRE, MD
Associate Professor, Department of Anesthesiology and Pain Management, The University of Texas Southwestern Medical Center, Dallas, Texas, USA

STEFAAN BOUCHEZ, MD
Department of Anesthesiology and Perioperative Medicine, Ghent University Hospital, Ghent, Belgium

SUE A. BRAITHWAITE, MBChB
Department of Anesthesiology, University Medical Center Utrecht, Utrecht, The Netherlands

DANIEL BRODIE, MD
Professor of Medicine, Division of Pulmonary, Allergy, and Critical Care, Columbia University Vagelos College of Physicians and Surgeons, New York, New York, USA

WOLFGANG F. BUHRE, MD, PhD
Chair, Department of Anaesthesiology and Pain Medicine, Maastricht University Medical Center, Maastricht, The Netherlands

ANNE D. CHERRY, MD
Assistant Professor, Department of Anesthesiology, Duke University, Durham, North Carolina, USA

SREEKANTH CHERUKU, MD
Assistant Professor, Department of Anesthesiology and Pain Management, The University of Texas Southwestern Medical Center, Dallas, Texas, USA

J. RANDALL CURTIS, MD, MPH
Professor of Medicine, Division of Pulmonary and Critical Care Medicine, Harborview Medical Center, University of Washington, Seattle, Washington, USA

JÖRG K. ENDER, MD
Professor, Department of Anesthesiology and Intensive Care Medicine, Heart Centre Leipzig, Leipzig, Germany

A. RESHAD GARAN, MD
Assistant Professor of Medicine, Division of Cardiology, Columbia University Vagelos College of Physicians and Surgeons, New York, New York, USA

RICHARD HALL, MD, FRCPC
Professor Emeritus, Departments of Anesthesia, Pain Management and Perioperative Medicine, and Critical Care Medicine, Dalhousie University, Department of Anesthesia, Halifax Infirmary Hospital, Halifax, Nova Scotia, Canada

JONATHAN HASTIE, MD
Assistant Professor, Department of Anesthesiology, Columbia University Vagelos College of Physicians and Surgeons, New York, New York, USA

AYMAN HENDY, MB BCh, FRCPC
Assistant Professor of Anesthesia, Department of Anesthesia, Pain Management and Perioperative Medicine, Dalhousie University, Halifax, Nova Scotia, Canada

KIMBERLY HOWARD-QUIJANO, MD, MS
Associate Professor, Department of Anesthesiology and Perioperative Medicine, University of Pittsburgh School of Medicine, Pittsburgh, Pennsylvania, USA

NORMAN HUANG, DO
Assistant Professor, Department of Anesthesiology and Pain Management, The University of Texas Southwestern Medical Center, Dallas, Texas, USA

KIROLOS A. JACOB, MD, PhD
Department of Cardiothoracic Surgery, University Medical Center Utrecht, Utrecht, the Netherlands

YUKI KUWABARA, MD
Department of Anesthesiology and Perioperative Medicine, University of Pittsburgh School of Medicine, Pittsburgh, Pennsylvania, USA

DAVID E. LEAF, MD, MMSc
Division of Renal Medicine, Brigham and Women's Hospital, Boston, Massachusetts, USA

ECKHARD MAUERMANN, MD, MSc
Department of Anesthesiology and Perioperative Medicine, Ghent University Hospital, Ghent, Belgium; Department for Anesthesia, Surgical Intensive Care, Prehospital Emergency Medicine and Pain Therapy, Basel University Hospital, Basel, Switzerland

C. DAVID MAZER, MD, FRCPC
Department of Anesthesia, Li Ka Shing Knowledge Institute of St. Michael's Hospital,
Departments of Anesthesia and Physiology, University of Toronto, Toronto, Ontario,
Canada

MICHAEL ISAÄC MEESTERS, MD, PhD, DESA
Anesthesiologist, Department of Anesthesiology, University Medical Center Utrecht,
Utrecht, the Netherlands

KYLE MEINHARDT, MD
Department of Anesthesiology and Pain Management, The University of Texas
Southwestern Medical Center, Dallas, Texas, USA

KENNETH M. PRAGER, MD
Professor of Medicine, Division of Pulmonary, Allergy, and Critical Care, Columbia
University Vagelos College of Physicians and Surgeons, New York, New York, USA

VALÉRIE M. SMIT-FUN, MD
Department of Anaesthesiology and Pain Medicine, Maastricht University Medical Center,
Maastricht, The Netherlands

JESSICA SPENCE, MD, FRCPC
Departments of Anesthesia and Critical Care and Health Research Methods, Evaluation,
and Impact, McMaster University, Population Health Research Institute (PHRI), C3-7B
David Braley Cardiac, Vascular and Stroke Research Institute (DBCVSRI), Hamilton,
Ontario, Canada

NIELS P. VAN DER KAAIJ, PhD, MD
Department of Cardiothoracic Surgery, University Medical Center Utrecht, Utrecht, The
Netherlands

MICHAEL VANDENHEUVEL, MD
Department of Anesthesiology and Perioperative Medicine, Ghent University Hospital,
Ghent, Belgium

CHRISTIAN VON HEYMANN, MD, PhD, DEAA
Professor of Anaesthesiology and Intensive Care Medicine, Chair, Department of
Anaesthesia, Intensive Care Medicine, Emergency Medicine and Pain Therapy, Vivantes
Klinikum im Friedrichshain, Berlin, Germany

PATRICK WOUTERS, MD, PhD
Department of Anesthesiology and Perioperative Medicine, Ghent University Hospital,
Ghent, Belgium

Contents

Thoracic endovascular aneurysm repair (TEVAR) is fast becoming the primary treatment of thoracic aortic aneurysms, thoracic aortic dissections, acute aortic injuries, and other conditions affecting the thoracic aorta. Patients scheduled for TEVAR tend to have a host of comorbid conditions, including coronary artery disease, diabetes, and chronic obstructive pulmonary disease. Intraoperative management should optimize end-organ perfusion, facilitate neuromonitoring, and adjust hemodynamic management. Complications include spinal cord injury, peripheral vascular injury, contrast-induced nephropathy, postimplantation syndrome, and endoleaks. Patients who undergo TEVAR require care in a postoperative environment where these complications can be rapidly detected and aggressively treated.

Ventricular arrhythmias are associated with significant morbidity and mortality. In the perioperative period, more than 10% of patients undergoing a general anesthetic have an abnormal heart rhythm. Arrhythmia development is a dynamic interplay between an arrhythmogenic substrate, myocardial electrophysiologic properties, modifying factors, and triggering factors. Imbalances in the autonomic nervous system can lead to increased myocardial excitability, which is a major contributor to the pathophysiology of ventricular tachyarrhythmias. Myocardial excitability and ventricular arrhythmogenesis is modulated perioperatively through hemodynamic management, electrolyte balance, anesthetic agents, or regional anesthetic and surgical techniques.

New developments in transcatheter valve technologies including aortic valve replacement and mitral valve and tricuspid valve interventions are described. Recent studies evaluating the success rate, patient outcomes, and anesthesiologic management of the procedures are discussed.

Video content accompanies this article at www.anesthesiology. theclinics.com

Injuries sustained by donor heart and lung allografts during the transplantation process are multiple and cumulative. Optimization of allograft function plays an essential role in short- and long-term outcomes after transplantation. Therapeutic targets to prevent or attenuate injury are present in the donor, the preservation process, during transplantation, and in postoperative management of the recipient. The newest and most promising methods of optimizing donor heart and lung allografts are found in alternative preservation strategies, which enable functional assessment of donor organs and provide a modality to initiate therapies for injured allografts or prevent injury during reperfusion in recipients.

Extracorporeal life support can support patients with severe forms of cardiac and respiratory failure. Uncertainty remains about its optimal use owing in large part to its resource-intensive nature and the high acuity illness in supported patients. Specific issues include the identification of patients most likely to benefit, the appropriate duration of support when prognosis is uncertain, and what to do when patients become dependent on extracorporeal life support but no longer have hope for recovery or transplantation. Careful deliberation of ethical principles and potential dilemmas should be made when considering the use of extracorporeal life support in advanced cardiopulmonary failure.

This article reviews transesophageal echocardiography–based assessment of perioperative right ventricular function and failure, including catheter-based methods, three-dimensional echocardiography, and their combination to make pressure-volume loops. It outlines right ventricular pathophysiology, multiple assessment methods, and their relationship to analogous transthoracic echocardiogram measurements. technologies used and developed for transthoracic or left ventricular assessment show significant limitations when applied to transesophageal assessment of the right ventricle. The article provides an overview of right ventricular assessment modalities that can be used in transesophageal echocardiography. Ultimately, clinicians must know limitations of measurements, synthesize information, and assess it in the clinical context.

An-depth assessment of right ventricular function is important in a many perioperative settings. After exploring 2-dimensional echo-based evaluation, other proposed monitoring modalities are discussed. Pressure-based methods of right ventricular appraisal is discussed. Flow-based assessment is reviewed. An overview of the state of current right ventricular 3-dimensional echocardiography and its potential to construct clinical pressure-volume loops in conjunction with pressure measurements is provided. An overview of right ventricular assessment modalities that do not rely on 2-dimensional echocardiography is discussed. Tailored selection of monitoring modalities can be of great benefit for the perioperative physician. Integrating modalities offers optimal estimations of right ventricular function.

Bleeding and transfusion are common in cardiac surgery and associated with poorer outcome. Bleeding is frequently due to coagulopathy caused by the complex interaction between cardiopulmonary bypass, major surgical trauma, anticoagulation management, and perioperative factors. Patient blood management has emerged to improve outcome by the prediction, prevention, monitoring, and treatment of bleeding and transfusion. Each part of this chain has several individual modalities and when combined leads to result in a better outcome. This article reviews the hemostasis disturbances in cardiac surgery with cardiopulmonary bypass and gives an overview of the most important patient blood management strategies.

Acute kidney injury is a common and often severe postoperative complication after cardiac surgery, and is associated with poor short-term and long-term outcomes. Numerous randomized controlled trials have been conducted to investigate various strategies for prevention of cardiac surgery-associated acute kidney injury. Unfortunately, most trials that have been conducted to date have been negative. However, encouraging results have been demonstrated with preoperative administration of corticosteroids, leukocyte filtration, and administration of inhaled nitric oxide intraoperatively, and implementation of a Kidney Disease: Improving Global Outcomes bundle of care approach postoperatively. These findings require validation in large, multicenter trials.

Adult patients with congenital heart disease are a complex population with a variety of pathophysiologic conditions based on the anatomy and type of surgery or intervention performed, usually during the first years of life. Nowadays, the majority of patients survive childhood and present for a number of noncardiac surgeries or interventions needing appropriate perioperative management. Heart failure is a major contributing factor to perioperative morbidity and mortality. In this review, we present an overview of the most common types of adult patients with congenital heart disease and actual knowledge on therapy and specific risks in this challenging patient population.

Anne D. Cherry

Mitochondria are key to the cellular response to energetic demand, but are also vital to reactive oxygen species signaling, calcium hemostasis, and regulation of cell death. Cardiac surgical patients with diabetes, heart failure, advanced age, or cardiomyopathies may have underlying mitochondrial dysfunction or be more sensitive to perioperative mitochondrial injury. Mitochondrial dysfunction, due to ischemia/reperfusion injury and an increased systemic inflammatory response due to exposure to cardiopulmonary bypass and surgical tissue trauma, impacts myocardial contractility and predisposes to arrhythmias. Strategies for perioperative mitochondrial protection and recovery include both well-established cardioprotective protocols and targeted therapies that remain under investigation.

Ayman Hendy and Richard Hall

Neurologic abnormality after cardiac surgery is common, and neurologic complications after cardiac surgery are among the most devastating problems that can occur in the postoperative period. Disruption of the blood-brain barrier (BBB) plays an important role in these complications. Assessment of the BBB integrity relies on cognitive testing, MRI, and measurement of brain biomarkers. In applying these methods, up to 50% of cardiac patients show some degree of BBB disruption and most of these abnormalities are short lived. To date there is no single test or measure that can predict BBB disruption in cardiac surgery.

Jessica Spence and C. David Mazer

This article provides an overview of knowledge gaps that need to be addressed in cardiac anesthesia, including mitigating the inflammatory effects of cardiopulmonary bypass, defining myocardial infarction after cardiac surgery, improving perioperative neurologic outcomes, and the optimal management of patients undergoing valve replacement. In addition, emerging approaches to research conduct are discussed, including the use of new analytical techniques like machine learning, pragmatic trials, and adaptive designs.

ANESTHESIOLOGY CLINICS

Foreword

Cardiac Anesthesia and Critical Care: New Procedures and Dilemmas Inside and Outside Our Operating Rooms

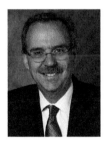

Lee A. Fleisher, MD, FACC, FAHA
Consulting Editor

Cardiac anesthesia as a practice has evolved over the past 50 years. With the advent and increasing use of transesophageal echocardiography, its practitioners acquired a unique skill that required specialty training and eventually certification. Cardiac critical care evolved out of cardiac anesthesia in addition to critical care. Because of the large number of similar procedures with high rates of adverse events, clinical trials could be performed to advance the evidence base for the field. With this long history of focused attention on the field, some would ask about how much advancement would be seen? This issue of *Anesthesiology Clinics* demonstrates that cardiac anesthesia and critical care are alive and exciting. The editors have invited authors to write articles on advances both inside and outside the operating room, from the question of large-scale clinical trials to the new ethical dilemmas in the field. They created a great source of new information that will educate all of those caring for patients undergoing cardiac surgery, but also those with cardiovascular disease undergoing both surgical and other invasive procedures.

When looking for coeditors for this issue, I turned to 2 rising stars in the field. Karsten Bartels, MD, PhD is Associate Professor of Anesthesiology at the University of Colorado and is Board Certified in anesthesiology, critical care medicine, pain medicine, and advanced perioperative transesophageal echocardiography. He has NIH funding and numerous publications. Stefan Dieleman, MD, PhD is Staff Specialist and Clinical Researcher in the Department of Anaesthesia and Perioperative Medicine at the Westmead Hospital in Sydney and Adjunct Senior Lecturer in the Department of Anaesthesia and Perioperative Medicine at the Alfred

Anesthesiology Clin 37 (2019) xiii–xiv
https://doi.org/10.1016/j.anclin.2019.08.013
1932-2275/19/© 2019 Published by Elsevier Inc.

anesthesiology.theclinics.com

Hospital/Monash University in Melbourne. He focuses his research on clinical trials in cardiac anesthesia. Together, they have created an important monograph for all to learn from.

Lee A. Fleisher, MD, FACC, FAHA
Perelman School of Medicine
University of Pennsylvania
3400 Spruce Street, Dulles 680
Philadelphia, PA 19104, USA

E-mail address:
Lee.Fleisher@uphs.upenn.edu

Preface

Cardiothoracic Anesthesia and Critical Care: An Ever-Changing (and Evolving) Field

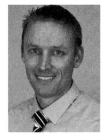 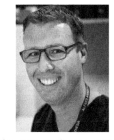

Karsten Bartels, MD, PhD   Stefan J.M. Dieleman, MD, PhD
Editors

Perioperative care for patients undergoing cardiothoracic surgery has evolved significantly since the first open-heart procedures were performed in the 1950s. Nowadays, the majority of cardiac surgical procedures are considered "routine" operations that, given the presence of significant comorbid disease in most of these patients, come with a rather acceptable risk of major perioperative complications. As a result, long-term outcomes for most patients are usually very good, too.

Inevitably, having consistently good results leads to further advancements in the field. Patients who would (or could) not be considered for cardiac surgery 10 to 20 years ago because of severe comorbid disease, advanced age, or congenital defects, are now presenting to our operating rooms. Also, several new interventional techniques have emerged that present the anesthesiologist with the challenge to further evolve their practice in order to provide state-of-the-art perioperative care for these patients. However, despite the great potential of all these advancements, it also requires an increased awareness of the ethical aspects of such developments. While it may be technically possible to provide certain interventions to an increasingly sick patient population, careful consideration should be given to patient selection.

This issue of *Anesthesiology Clinics* focuses on several aspects of the recent developments in the area of cardiothoracic anesthesiology and critical care. Multiple experts from several fields have contributed to a variety of articles to provide an update on several exciting developments in techniques, optimization of clinical care, as well as basic science. Evolving techniques that are discussed include endovascular approaches to thoracic aortic repair,[1] modulation of ventricular excitability,[2] catheter-based cardiac valve procedures,[3] and ex vivo optimization of donor hearts and lungs,[4]

Anesthesiology Clin 37 (2019) xv–xvii
https://doi.org/10.1016/j.anclin.2019.08.012
1932-2275/19/© 2019 Published by Elsevier Inc.

respectively. In a separate article, the ethical dilemmas of the increasing technical possibilities in the field of mechanical circulatory support are considered.[5] The articles on optimization of clinical care encompass a review of both echocardiographic[6] and catheter-based intraoperative assessment of right ventricular function,[7] optimization of coagulation and blood transfusion management,[8] prevention of perioperative acute kidney injury,[9] as well as an overview of the aspects of perioperative management of adult patients with congenital heart disease.[10] Two articles focused on emerging basic science will outline the effects of cardiac surgery on mitochondrial[11] and blood-brain barrier function,[12] respectively. Finally, an update is provided on recent, upcoming, and highly needed clinical trials,[13] in order to make cardiac anesthesiology an even more evidence-based field.

While we cannot claim that this issue of *Anesthesiology Clinics* provides an all-encompassing picture of developments in the field of cardiothoracic anesthesiology and critical care, we believe that the authors offer a thought-provoking summary of exciting insights driven by leaders in our field. We would like to sincerely thank the authors of this issue for providing their valuable time to share this progress with our readers, and we hope readers will enjoy their contributions as much as we did.

Karsten Bartels, MD, PhD
Department of Anesthesiology
University of Colorado
12401 East 17th Avenue, MS B-113
Aurora, CO 80045, USA

Stefan J.M. Dieleman, MD, PhD
Department of Anaesthesia
Westmead Hospital
CNR Hawkesbury Road/Darcy Road
Westmead, NSW 2145, Australia

E-mail addresses:
karsten.bartels@cuanschutz.edu (K. Bartels)
stefandieleman@me.com (S.J.M. Dieleman)

REFERENCES

1. Cheruku S, Huang N, Meinhardt K, et al. Anesthetic management for endovascular repair of the thoracic aorta. Anesthesiol Clin 2019;37(4):593–607.

2. Howard-Quijano K, Kuwabara Y. Modulating perioperative ventricular excitability. Anesthesiol Clin 2019;37(4):609–19.

3. Ackermann MA, Ender JK. Recent developments in catheter-based cardiac procedures. Anesthesiol Clin 2019;37(4):621–38.

4. Braithwaite SA, van der Kaaij NP. New techniques for optimization of donor lungs/hearts. Anesthesiol Clin 2019;37(4):639–60.

5. Abrams D, Curtis JR, Prager KM, et al. Ethical considerations for mechanical support. Anesthesiol Clin 2019;37(4):661–73.

6. Vandenheuvel M, Bouchez S, Wouters P, et al. Assessing right ventricular function in the perioperative setting, Part I: echo-based measurements. Anesthesiol Clin 2019;37(4):675–95.

7. Vandenheuvel M, Bouchez S, Wouters P, et al. Assessing right ventricular function in the perioperative setting, part II—what about catheters? Anesthesiol Clin 2019;37(4):697–712.

8. Meesters MI, von Heymann C. Optimizing perioperative blood and coagulation management during cardiac surgery. Anesthesiol Clin 2019;37(4):713–28.
9. Jacob KA, Leaf DE. Prevention of cardiac surgery-associated acute kidney injury: a review of current strategies. Anesthesiol Clin 2019;37(4):729–49.
10. Smit-Fun VM, Buhre WF. Heart failure in adult patients with congenital heart disease. Anesthesiol Clin 2019;37(4):751–68.
11. Cherry AD. Mitochondrial dysfunction in cardiac surgery. Anesthesiol Clin 2019; 37(4):769–85.
12. Hendy A, Hall R. Cardiac surgery and the blood-brain barrier. Anesthesiol Clin 2019;37(4):787–800.
13. Spence J, Mazer CD. The future directions of research in cardiac anesthesiology. Anesthesiol Clin 2019;37(4):801–13.

Anesthetic Management for Endovascular Repair of the Thoracic Aorta

Sreekanth Cheruku, MD*, Norman Huang, DO,
Kyle Meinhardt, MD, Marco Aguirre, MD

KEYWORDS

- Thoracic aortic aneurysm • Thoracic endovascular aortic repair • Aortic dissection
- Penetrating atherosclerotic ulcer • Endoleak • Spinal cord protection • Paraplegia

KEY POINTS

- Thoracic endovascular aneurysm repair (TEVAR) has become the treatment of choice for acute type B dissections, complex thoracic aneurysm repair, and acute traumatic injuries of the thoracic aorta.
- General anesthesia is currently the most popular anesthetic technique for TEVAR because it provides a secure airway with controlled ventilation, facilitates transesophageal echocardiography monitoring, and ensures immobility.
- Evoked potential monitoring is used to test the integrity of spinal cord pathways and both motor-evoked potentials and somatosensory-evoked potentials are sensitive monitors for spinal cord ischemia (SCI) in patients undergoing TEVAR.
- SCI is a devastating complication that can result in transient or permanent paraplegia after TEVAR. Strategies to prevent TEVAR include increasing mean arterial pressure and cerebrospinal fluid drainage to optimize spinal cord perfusion pressure.
- Endoleaks are relatively common complications following TEVAR; require lifetime surveillance; and, when indicated, aggressive intervention.

INTRODUCTION

Aneurysmal disease of the thoracic aorta has an incidence of 6 to 10 per 100,000 person-years and contributes significantly to morbidity and mortality in the United States. Of thoracic aortic aneurysms (TAAs), 60% affect the ascending aorta and aortic arch, whereas 40% involve the descending thoracic aorta.[1] The Crawford classification can be used to categorize TAAs by the extent of the aneurysm (**Fig. 1**).

Disclosure Statement: No disclosures (S. Cheruku, N. Huang, K. Meinhardt, M. Aguirre).
Department of Anesthesiology and Pain Management, UT Southwestern Medical Center, Mail Code 9068, 5323 Harry Hines Boulevard, Dallas, TX 75390, USA
* Corresponding author.
E-mail address: Sreekanth.Cheruku@UTSouthwestern.edu

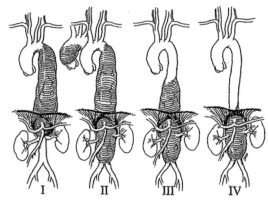

Fig. 1. Crawford classification of thoracoabdominal aortic aneurysms. Extent I aneurysms begin in the descending thoracic aorta and do not extend beyond the renal arteries. Extent II aneurysms begin in the descending thoracic aorta and extend to the infrarenal aorta. Extent III aneurysms begin at or below the sixth intercostal space and extent IV aneurysms begin below the diaphragm. (*From* Coselli JS, LeMaire SA, Köksoy C. Thoracic Aortic Anastomoses. Operative Techniques in Thoracic and Cardiovascular Surgery 2000;5(4):260; with permission.)

Thoracic endovascular aneurysm repair (TEVAR) is a minimally invasive approach to repair thoracic and thoracoabdominal diseases using endovascular stent grafts, or endografts. Originally developed for poor surgical candidates who could not tolerate open repair, it has become the preferred approach for the treatment of TAAs, as well as traumatic aortic injuries, complicated type B aortic dissections, and penetrating atherosclerotic ulcers (PAUs). Recent advances in endograft technology resulting in better procedural success and fewer complications have expanded their use in younger patients and for uncomplicated dissections.

Risk Factors

Common risk factors for the development of TAAs include a family history of aneurysmal disease, advanced age, hypertension, and tobacco use. Although atherosclerosis was once thought to play an etiologic role in the development of aneurysmal disease, recent studies have shown the relationship between the 2 to be mediated by multiple genetic and environmental factors.[2,3] Collagen vascular diseases, such as Marfan syndrome, Ehlers-Danlos syndrome, and Loeys-Dietz syndrome, can weaken the aortic wall, rendering it more susceptible to aneurysm formation. Rarely, infections such as syphilis and inflammatory conditions such as Takayasu arteritis can result in TAAs.

Pathophysiology

The pathophysiology of aneurysmal disease involves the degeneration of the connective tissue components of the vessel wall through mechanical stress, as well as inflammatory and autoimmune mechanisms. Increased wall tension within the aneurysm predicted by the Laplace law results in progressive growth until a critical dimension is reached, after which the aneurysm dissects or ruptures. In aortic dissection, a tear in the intimal layer results in pressure-induced dissection of the media, resulting in the formation of a false lumen. This dissection can extend both proximally and distally to impair perfusion to aortic branch vessels, and cause aortic valve insufficiency and cardiac tamponade. Rupture of the false lumen can result in cata-strophic bleeding and death.

PAUs, distinct from aneurysmal disease, are focal atherosclerotic lesions that erode through the aortic intima, resulting in hematoma formation in the media. PAUs measuring 20 mm in diameter or 10 mm in depth have a high likelihood of progression and require intervention.[4] Aortic intramural hematomas (IMHs) are also independent entities and result from rupture of the vasa vasorum, resulting in aortic wall bleeding. Patients with an IMH affecting the descending thoracic aorta associated with chest pain, an expanding hematoma, or an aortic leak are candidates for TEVAR.[5]

SURGICAL CONSIDERATIONS
Diagnosis

Most patients with TAAs are asymptomatic and are diagnosed incidentally while be-ing evaluated for another condition. Patients with a family history of aneurysmal dis-ease or genetic syndromes predisposing them to aneurysms are often diagnosed during scheduled surveillance examinations. Symptomatic patients often present with larger aneurysms and the symptoms are often related to compression of organs, nerves, and vascular structures. Severe chest and back pain are common presenting symptoms from descending TAAs, whereas aneurysms of the ascending aorta and arch may can present with hoarseness, orthopnea, wheezing, dysphagia, and dys-pnea due to compression of the esophagus, the tracheobronchial tree, and cardiac structures.

The diagnostic evaluation of patients with TAAs begins with a history and physical examination; however, physical examination alone is unreliable for diagnosing these aneurysms.[6] A chest radiograph is often the next diagnostic step in patients who pre-sent with sudden chest or back pain. The presence of a wide mediastinum with a shadow extending from the cardiac silhouette should arouse suspicion and prompt further evaluation using computed tomography (CT) or MRI. Both CT and MRI provide accurate information regarding the anatomy of the aortic lumen, branch vessels, thrombus burden, and calcification. A contrasted CT scan is often the first test ordered to make a diagnosis in a symptomatic patient because it more readily available and can quickly distinguish among acute aortic syndromes, including acute aortic dissec-tion and a PAU. MRI imaging is used for serial surveillance of asymptomatic patients at risk of TAA owing to its avoidance of nephrotoxic contrast agents. MRI can also be used to evaluate aortic valve and ventricular function. Three-dimensional reconstruc-tion of CT images can be used to make precise anatomic measurements (**Fig. 2**). Transthoracic echocardiography (TTE) is a low-cost, noninvasive bedside test that can be used to evaluate cardiac function in addition to the thoracic aorta. It is often used to screen for aortic pathologic conditions, such as bicuspid aortic valve and aortic insufficiency in patients with TAAs. Transesophageal echocardiography (TEE) can be used to examine the thoracic aorta in emergent situations when the patient is too unstable to be transferred for CT scan. TEE is limited by its inability to visualize the distal ascending aorta and a small segment of the aortic arch, which are obscured by tracheobronchial air.

Indications

The 2010 American College of Cardiology Foundation (ACCF) and American Heart As-sociation (AHA) *"Guidelines for the Management of Patients with Thoracic Aortic Dis-ease,"* endorsed by 10 professional societies, including the American Society of Anesthesiologists (ASA), strongly recommends TEVAR for acute traumatic injury to

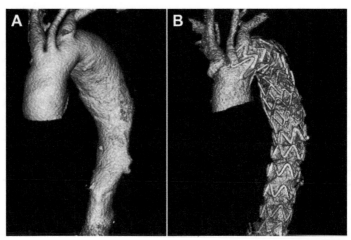

Fig. 2. Three-dimensional reconstruction of CT angiography showing a TAA (*A*) before and (*B*) after TEVAR.

the descending aorta and acute type B dissection with ischemia (class I recommendation).[7] TEVAR is also indicated for TAAs measuring more than 5.5 cm with significant comorbidities (class IIa recommendation) and without comorbidities (class IIb recommendation). In patients with uncomplicated type B dissections and those with subacute and chronic dissections, TEVAR is also recommended (class IIb recommendation). The guidelines do not recommend TEVAR for patients with connective tissue disorders owing to problems with the endograft landing zones and the potential that new aortic dilation after graft deployment will result in a leak around the graft.[7]

Endovascular Procedure

In patients who are candidates for TEVAR, a detailed evaluation of peripheral vascular and aortic anatomy is necessary to determine if their pathologic condition is amenable to endovascular repair (EVAR). To allow access to the diseased aorta, the iliac arterial system must be wide enough to accommodate the graft-introducer system, which can be as large as 24 F in diameter. In patients with stenotic iliac vessels, balloon angioplasty or stenting can be performed to increase the diameter of the artery. Additionally, an iliac conduit can be created to accommodate the endograft apparatus. An iliac conduit is a Dacron graft that is anastomosed end-to-side with the common iliac artery. When accessing the iliac system is not possible, the endograft can also be delivered through the abdominal aorta.

CT angiography is used to determine the dimensions of diseased aorta and endograft landing zones: the regions of the aorta where the proximal and distal ends of the endograft are seated. In general, a 2-cm length of histologically normal aortic tissue is required at both the proximal and distal landing zones of the endograft. This ensures an adequate seal and prevents displacement of the graft after it is deployed. If the proximal landing zone includes the takeoff of the left subclavian artery, the Society of Vascular Surgery guidelines recommend revascularizing the artery before elective TEVAR procedures.[8] This is most commonly accomplished through a left common carotid-left subclavian bypass. When the proximal landing zones are more proximal, complicated bypass and hybrid debranching procedures are required. The diameter of the endograft is selected to be 10% to 20% larger than the diameter of the aorta at the proximal landing zone to allow a tight seal and it should have enough length to exclude the pathologic condition. In TEVAR performed for aortic dissection, the endograft should extend 2 to 4 cm in either direction of the dissection flap. If an endograft has insufficient length, coverage can be extended by deploying additional endografts.

The TEVAR procedure begins with ultrasound-guided femoral arterial access and percutaneous suture placement. After systemic heparinization, the initial series of access catheters and guidewires are then advanced under fluoroscopic guidance into the thoracic aorta. Contrast angiography is then used to confirm the anatomy of the aorta and branch vessels (**Fig. 3**A). Intravascular ultrasound (IVUS), combined with fluoroscopy, is also used to confirm anatomic landmarks (**Fig. 4**). Once the target landing zones have been identified, the graft-deployment system is advanced into position and angiography is performed, confirming landmarks for deployment (**Fig. 3**B, C). The endograft is then deployed (**Fig. 3**D). Balloon dilation of the graft overlaps (if multiple components are used) and distal seal zone is performed to achieve a tight seal. Angiography is then used to evaluate for endoleaks and confirm the integrity of the arterial system from the aorta to the iliac artery. Balloon dilation of the proximal seal zone may be a source of embolic stroke, so it is avoided except in cases in which a type 1a endoleak is seen on completion angiogram. At completion of the operation, the introducer is removed and the femoral artery access site is closed percutaneously.

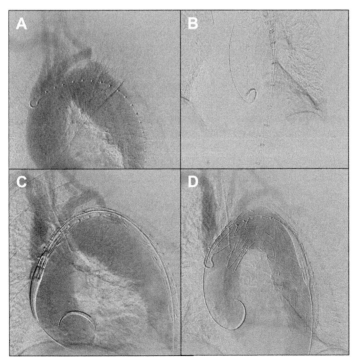

Fig. 3. TEVAR under contrast angiography. (*A*) Aortogram of TAA. (*B*) Celiac angiogram of endograft delivery device. (*C*) Predeployment aortogram of endograft in position. (*D*) Post-deployment aortogram with endograft in position.

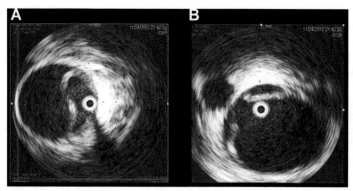

Fig. 4. IVUS used to guide TEVAR. (*A*) IVUS used to place wire in the true lumen. (*B*) IVUS used to identify the primary intimal tear. (*From* Leshnower BG, Chen EP. TEVAR for Acute Complicated Type B Aortic Dissection. Operative Techniques in Thoracic and Cardiovascular Surgery: A Comparative Atlas 2018;23(1):24; with permission.)

ANESTHETIC CONSIDERATIONS
Preoperative Evaluation

Because the indications for TEVAR have increased in recent years, a diverse population of patients now undergoes the procedure for a multitude of aortic pathologic conditions. One large series of subjects who underwent TEVAR found that a significant number had hypertension (87%), coronary artery disease (29%), chronic obstructive pulmonary disease (COPD; 27%), chronic kidney disease (26%), and diabetes (15%).[9] The preoperative evaluation should be as comprehensive as one that is performed for patients undergoing open aortic surgery and should address the presenting disease, comorbid conditions, procedural considerations, and potential complications.

Cardiovascular

Because vascular and cardiac diseases share common risk factors, it is not surprising that the cohort of patients scheduled for TEVAR tend to have significant cardiac comorbidities. An evaluation of functional capacity and a screening electrocardiogram (ECG) are required for all patients presenting for elective TEVAR. TTE is part of the recommended diagnostic evaluation for patients presenting with thoracic aortic disease,[10] and the results should be reviewed as part of the preoperative evaluation. Stress testing should be limited to patients with abnormal findings on ECG or TTE. Patients with inducible ischemia on stress testing may require coronary angiography and revascularization (**Fig. 5**).

Pulmonary

Patients presenting for TEVAR can exhibit a variety of respiratory symptoms due to proximity of the thoracic aorta to the tracheobronchial tree. Wheezing, dyspnea, and cough can occur due to compression of the airway by a large aneurysm. These symptoms are important to monitor during the preoperative evaluation because they can worsen with a rapidly growing aneurysm. Because every patient undergoing TEVAR will have CT or MRI examinations required for preprocedure planning, these should be used to evaluate the anatomic relationship between the thoracic aorta, the airway, and pulmonary structures. The contribution of COPD to aneurysmal disease is poorly understood but it is thought that the chronic inflammation and

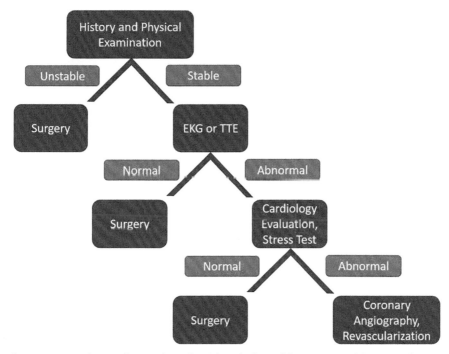

Fig. 5. Preoperative cardiac workup algorithm. (*Adapted from* Ganapathi AM, Englum BR, Schechter MA, et al. Role of cardiac evaluation before thoracic endovascular aortic repair. J Vasc Surg 2014;60(5):1198; with permission.)

hypoxemia seen in patients with COPD may result in local hypoperfusion in the aorta.[11] Pulmonary function testing should be obtained in patients with known or suspected COPD to guide preoperative optimization, intraoperative ventilation strategies, and postoperative rehabilitation. If warranted, a pulmonary medicine consultation may be necessary to initiate preoperative steroid or bronchodilator therapies.

Neurologic

A thorough neurologic examination should be performed to document any preoperative sensory or motor deficits. Given the relatively high incidence of stroke and paraplegia with TEVAR, this baseline examination can be used to detect subtle neurologic deficits. Patients at heightened risk for postoperative paraplegia should be identified during the preoperative visit. Risk factors for paraplegia include advanced age, hypertension, COPD, renal failure,[12] a history of abdominal aortic aneurysm (AAA) or concomitant AAA repair,[13,14] and the extent of graft coverage required.[15] High-risk patients may also benefit from a prophylactic cerebrospinal fluid (CSF) drain, though there is little evidence regarding the timing of placement.

Renal

The patient's volume status and renal function should be determined from physical examination and laboratory tests. Acid-base disturbances should be evaluated and corrected. Before TEVAR, patients should be adequately hydrated to decrease the risk of contrast-induced nephropathy (CIN). Nephrotoxic agents, such as metformin, aminoglycoside antibiotics, and high-dose loop diuretics, should be discontinued several days before the surgical procedure.[16] Identifying patients at risk for postoperative acute kidney injury (AKI) enables risk-stratification and allows the institution of preventive measures, such as maintaining a higher intraoperative mean arterial pressure (MAP). The potential need for postoperative dialysis should be discussed with patients whose preoperative glomerular filtration rate is less than 30 mL/min/1.73 m².

Intraoperative Management

Choice of anesthetic

Most TEVARs are performed under general anesthesia (GA) but the procedure can also be safely managed with regional and local anesthetic techniques. Patient factors such as preoperative comorbidities and hemodynamic stability, as well as procedural factors such as procedure time, expected blood loss, and the need for TEE, should influence the choice of anesthetic technique. Regardless of the technique selected, the intraoperative plan should optimize patient safety and comfort while mitigating the risk of complications. The authors envision that faster procedural time and improvements in endograft technology will result in decreased utilization of GA in the future.

General anesthesia

GA is currently the most popular anesthetic technique for TEVAR because it provides a secure airway with controlled ventilation, facilitates TEE monitoring, and ensures immobility. In complex cases with longer procedure times, more bleeding, and a higher risk of conversion to open aortic repair, GA provides a controlled perioperative environment. Immobility and controlled ventilation under GA improves intraoperative angiographic imaging and provides stability during endograft deployment. GA should also be used when significant back pain, anxiety, or patient comorbidities prevent them from lying flat for a prolonged period of time. Disadvantages of GA include the prolonged need for mechanical ventilation due to alteration of pulmonary mechanics and greater hemodynamic lability.

Regional anesthesia

Regional anesthesia (RA) for TEVAR includes spinal, epidural, and combined spinal-epidural approaches. The benefits of RA include avoidance of GA with its pulmonary complications and postoperative pain management with continuous epidural catheters. Interestingly, 1 large multicenter database review of more than 6000 abdominal EVAR procedures demonstrated decreased pulmonary morbidity with spinal but not epidural anesthesia when compared with GA.[17] Outcomes data comparing RA to GA for EVAR have also demonstrated a decreased length of stay in the hospital, improved hemodynamics,[18] and decreased mortality.[19] However, these studies evaluated only EVAR procedures, which are less complex than TEVARs, and the results may be influenced by selection bias. Disadvantages of RA include the potential for hemodynamic instability from sympathetic blockade and neuraxial hematoma with concurrent anticoagulation. Hypotension after neuraxial blockade should be treated aggressively to prevent ischemia. Patients on preoperative anticoagulants should have their therapy discontinued and reinitiated based on the current American Society of Regional Anesthesia guidelines.[20]

Local anesthesia

Local anesthetic infiltration of the femoral access site allows for an arousable patient with an intact sympathetic nervous system who can follow commands (eg, to hold their breath or demonstrate motor function) and exhibit symptoms (eg, chest pain consistent with aneurysm rupture). Local anesthesia can be supplemented with short-acting sedatives, such as propofol and dexmedetomidine, or with peripheral nerve blocks. Compared with GA, local anesthesia for EVAR was associated with fewer pulmonary complications,[17] a lower fluid requirement, less vasopressor support, and a shorter hospital length of stay.[18] Disadvantages of local anesthesia for TEVAR include patient movement during critical portions of the procedure and the potential for conversion to open aneurysm repair.

Intraoperative Management

Hemodynamic monitors

All patients undergoing TEVAR should have standard ASA monitors applied. A 5-lead ECG is necessary to monitor for arrhythmias, which can occur due to the primary aortic pathologic condition and due to cardiac irritation by aortic wires and catheters. Although invasive arterial line monitoring is required, the location of the arterial line should be discussed with the vascular surgeon. Coverage of the left subclavian arterial takeoff by the endograft or surgical placement of an angiography catheter into the left brachial artery may necessitate right radial arterial cannulation.[21] If measurement of arterial pressure distal to the endograft is necessary, femoral arterial access is typically established by the surgical team and should be transduced simultaneously with the radial arterial line to allow a comparison of pressures.

The authors recommend the routine use of central venous access in patients undergoing TEVAR to facilitate the rapid transfusion of intravenous fluids and blood products, to monitor central venous pressure, and to allow the use of vasopressors and inotropes.

Transesophageal echocardiography

In patients undergoing TEVAR under GA, TEE can be used to directly visualize cardiac function, assess aortic pathologic conditions, guide endograft positioning, and evaluate endoleaks after graft deployment. TEE should be used to evaluate ventricular function and the structure and function of the aortic valve because TAAs and dissections can grow rapidly to involve the aortic valve. A comprehensive evaluation of the thoracic aorta is necessary to evaluate for the primary disease, as well as for atheromas and other pathologic conditions.

TEE can also be used to guide vascular access by visualizing the placement of wires in the descending aorta. During endograft placement, TEE can be used to ensure that the graft covers the aortic pathologic condition. After the endograft is deployed, TEE can also be used to ensure that the aortic pathologic condition is excluded and to ensure that retrograde dissection has not occurred.[22] Color Doppler can be used to evaluate for endoleaks, which are leaks between the endograft and aortic wall. Lowering the color Doppler aliasing velocity to 20 to 30 cm per second may be necessary to detect lower flow endoleaks.[23] In a study of 42 subjects undergoing endovascular thoracic aortic repairs for descending dissection, TEE allowed visualization of endoleaks in 13 subjects (compared with 6 detected by angiography) and new intimal tears in 7 subjects (compared with 2 detected by angiography). In these cases, endoleaks were treated by balloon dilation and intimal tears were treated by placing additional stents.[24]

Neuromonitoring

Spinal cord ischemia (SCI) is a devastating complication that can result in transient or permanent paraplegia after TEVAR. Though the incidence of SCI after TEVAR is comparatively lower than open TAA repair (3%–6% vs 14%), it remains significant enough to warrant aggressive perioperative monitoring and treatment. Evoked potential monitoring is used to test the integrity of spinal cord pathways and both motor-evoked potentials (MEPs) and somatosensory-evoked potentials (SSEPs) are sensitive monitors for SCI in patients undergoing TEVAR. MEPs are conducted through the anterior corticospinal tract, whereas SSEPs ascend the lateral and posterior columns of the spinal cord. Monitoring both MEPs and SSEPs together, therefore, allows continuous assessment of global spinal cord perfusion.

Volatile anesthetics significantly decrease the amplitude and increase the latency of evoked potentials, whereas propofol and opioids have milder effects. In patients undergoing evoked potential monitoring, the authors recommend limiting the volatile anesthetic concentration to 0.5 minimum alveolar concentration (MAC) and avoiding paralytics after the initial dose required for intubation because they interfere with measurement of the electromyography response to stimulation. Significant changes to the anesthetic plan during the case should be discussed with the electrophysiologist in order to provide context for changes in the amplitude or latency of evoked potentials.

Near-infrared spectroscopy (NIRS) is another minimally invasive modality that can be used to monitor cerebral and spinal cord tissue oxygenation, which is thought to correlate with perfusion. Most commercially available NIRS monitors are designed for forehead placement and monitor perfusion originating from the anterior and middle cerebral arteries. In this configuration, a bilateral decrease in regional oxygenation represents global hypoperfusion, whereas a unilateral decrease represents a focal event such as embolic stroke. The placement of NIRS optodes over the thoracolumbar paraspinous muscles to measure the oxygenation of tissue supplied by spinal cord collateral network vessels has also been reported in the literature.[25,26] In these small studies, events associated with spinal cord hypoperfusion, such as application of the cross-clamp or deployment of the endograft, were associated with decreased lumbar tissue oxygenation. Larger, prospective studies are necessary to support the routine monitoring of spinal cord perfusion using NIRS.

Kidney protection

AKI after TEVAR is mediated by multiple hemodynamic, vascular, and medication-induced mechanisms. Impaired renal perfusion due to aortic pathologic conditions, as well as embolic events, can result in preoperative AKI. The use of intravenous contrast agents can precipitate CIN due to several poorly understood mechanisms, including renal medullary hypoxia, free radical toxicity, and renal cell apoptosis.[27] Strategies to reduce the risk of AKI include maintaining both kidney perfusion pressure and intravascular volume, avoiding nephrotoxic agents, and minimizing the use of intravenous contrast. Patients who present to the procedure in a volume-depleted state should undergo gentle intravenous hydration. Studies evaluating sodium bicarbonate and N-acetylcysteine infusions as free radical scavengers to reduce the development of postoperative AKI have yielded mixed results. In patients at risk for postoperative AKI, contrast angiography should be minimized and supplemented as much as possible with IVUS.

Cerebrospinal fluid drainage

SCI during TEVAR is thought to occur from decreased spinal cord perfusion pressure (SCPP), resulting in hypoperfusion of the spinal cord collateral blood vessels.[28] The mathematical expression of SCPP is

SCPP = MAP – CSF pressure

As a result, perioperative strategies for reducing the incidence of SCI are focused on optimizing this relationship by increasing MAP and CSF drainage to reduce CSF pressure. CSF drainage requires the placement of an intrathecal catheter through a lumbar interspace. Though CSF drainage has been shown to improve outcomes after open thoracic aneurysm repair, there are insufficient data supporting their routine use in TEVAR. The 2010 ACCF/AHA *"Guidelines for the Management of Patients with Thoracic Aortic Disease"* strongly recommends the use of CSF drains for patients undergoing TEVAR who are at high risk for SCI (class I).[7] This include patients with a history of aortic repair, those with extent I to III thoracoabdominal aneurysms, and those who require graft coverage of large areas of the aorta.[29] There is controversy over whether CSF drains should be placed prophylactically in lower-risk elective TEVARs. The authors' experience has been that the potential for complications associated with CSF drains, ranging from CSF leak to spinal hematoma (**Table 1**), outweighs the benefits of preoperative placement in low-risk patients. The authors advocate the placement of spinal drains in this cohort only if evoked potential monitoring suggests SCI or if the patient develops postoperative motor weakness.

Anesthetic management
Induction of GA should be performed with short-acting sedative hypnotics, such as propofol or etomidate, along with small doses of opioids, to blunt the sympathetic response to intubation. Paralytics can be used to facilitate intubation but should be reversed before obtaining baseline evoked potential measurements. Maintenance of anesthesia can be achieved with 0.5 MAC of volatile anesthetics supplemented with opioids or a total intravenous anesthesia technique.

Before the graft-introducer is inserted into to the arterial system, systemic anticoagulation with heparin is required. 100 U/mL of heparin is typically administered to achieve a target activated clotting time (ACT) of 200 seconds. The target ACT should be maintained throughout the procedure until the graft is deployed and the introducer is removed.

Hemodynamic goals should be discussed with the surgical team; however, it is reasonable to maintain the MAP close to baseline for elective TEVARs. When there is a concern for aneurysm rupture or extension of an acute dissection, a lower blood pressure goal may be selected. Both vasoconstrictors and vasodilators should be readily available to allow precise titration of blood pressure. Immediately before deployment of the endograft, the blood pressure should be lowered to prevent distal migration of the graft. After graft deployment, a higher blood pressure is required to optimize SCPP and collateral blood flow to other organs.

After the procedure is complete, hemodynamically stable patients should be routinely extubated to facilitate neurologic examination. Short-acting opioids or dexmedetomidine can be used to blunt the sympathetic stimulation associated with

Table 1
Complications occurring during thoracic endovascular aneurysm repair

Surgical Complications	Medical Complications	CSF Drain Complications
Access-site hematoma	SCI, paraplegia	Bloody tap
Pseudoaneurysm	AKI	Epidural hematoma
Endograft migration	Contrast nephropathy	Intracerebral hemorrhage
Endoleak	Stroke	CSF leak
Aneurysm rupture	Mesenteric ischemia	Postdural puncture headache
	Arrhythmias	Fractured catheter
	Postimplantation syndrome	Meningitis

extubation. In the authors' experience, a low-dose infusion of dexmedetomidine (0.2–0.7 mcg/kg/h), running throughout the intraoperative period and continued postoperatively, provides excellent analgesia and enables a patient to lie flat for a prolonged period after surgery, if necessary.

POSTOPERATIVE CARE

Patients who undergo TEVAR should be transferred to an intensive care unit or similar environment where frequent vital sign, neurologic, and neurovascular monitoring can be performed. **Table 1** lists the spectrum of perioperative complications associated with TEVAR. The postoperative care should be directed by clinicians and nursing staff who are familiar with the procedure and associated complications. In the immediate postoperative period, complications related to the vascular access, such as hematomas and pseudoaneurysms, are most common. The femoral introducer site should be inspected for hematoma formation. If an expanding hematoma is detected, proximal pressure should be applied while surgical consultation is obtained.

The hemodynamic management of TEVAR includes maintenance of MAP at the higher end of the autoregulation range. Hypotension can result in impaired perfusion to the spinal cord, kidney, and other organs. However, excessive hypertension should be avoided because it can result in bleeding and downstream migration of the endograft. Motor deficits after TEVAR can manifest hours or days after the procedure, and the postoperative care should focus on detecting these symptoms early so that prompt treatment can be initiated. Serial measurement of the straight leg raise test (a patient's ability to lift their extended straight leg off the bed) is 1 tool that can be used to measure lower extremity motor strength.[30]

New or worsening lower extremity motor weakness should prompt aggressive measures to improve spinal cord perfusion. The MAP target should be raised, and fluids and vasoconstrictors should be administered, to meet this goal. In patients who do not improve with blood pressure management, a CSF drain should be placed. Though institutional standards for the management of CSF drains vary, the CSF pressure is generally maintained at or below 10 mm Hg. To prevent excessive drainage of CSF, which can result in subdural hematoma, the authors recommend that the drain be set to continuously monitor CSF pressure and intermittently drain CSF. Additionally, standing orders for nursing staff should limit the hourly drainage of CSF to 10 mL and any further drainage should be guided by intensive care physicians.

Postimplantation syndrome is a variant of systemic inflammatory response syndrome, which has been reported after endograft placement. It is characterized by fever, leukocytosis, and elevated levels of biomarkers associated with inflammation.[31] The proposed pathophysiology includes interaction of endograft components with the aortic endothelium, tissue injury, and consequent production of inflammatory mediators. The syndrome is generally short-lived and managed conservatively with nonsteroidal antiinflammatory drugs.[7]

Up to 38% of TEVARs performed to repair TAAs are complicated by endoleaks, which are defined as blood flow within the aneurysm sac external to the endograft.[32] Endoleaks are classified by their location and cause (**Fig. 6**). Endoleaks can be diagnosed intraoperatively after graft deployment, during the postoperative CT angiogram, or much later on surveillance imaging. Type I and III endoleaks represent a failure to exclude the aneurysm sac from the systemic circulation and are generally treated at the time of diagnosis using balloon dilation of the existing graft or placement of a new stent. Type II endoleaks are managed conservatively and treated if they result in aneurysm sac expansion. Type IV endoleaks generally seal spontaneously after

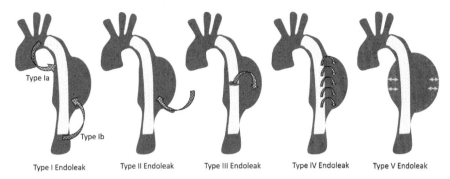

Type Ia

Type Ib

Type I Endoleak   Type II Endoleak   Type III Endoleak   Type IV Endoleak   Type V Endoleak

Fig. 6. Classification of endoleaks. Type I endoleaks are leaks into the aneurysm sac from the proximal or distal ends of the endograft. Type II endoleaks are leaks from collateral blood vessels. Type III endoleaks are leaks between overlapping endografts or through defects in the endograft. Type IV endoleaks are temporary, self-limited leaks through the endograft fabric. Type V endoleaks are not true leaks, but the category is used for aneurysm sac expansion in the absence of a leak.

intraoperative anticoagulation is reversed. Type V endoleaks are treated either with placement of a new endograft or with open repair.[32] Lifelong surveillance for endoleaks is mandatory for all patients who undergo TEVAR.

SUMMARY

TEVAR is fast becoming the primary treatment of TAAs, thoracic aortic dissections, acute aortic injuries, and other pathologic conditions affecting the thoracic aorta. Patients who are scheduled for TEVAR tend to have a host of comorbid conditions, including coronary artery disease, diabetes, and COPD. The anesthetic plan should address these comorbidities, as well as the surgical plan and the potential for complications. GA is the most commonly used technique for TEVAR; however, regional and local anesthesia are increasingly used owing to a greater number of healthier patients presenting for elective procedures. Regardless of the anesthetic modality, the intraoperative management should optimize end-organ perfusion, facilitate neuromonitoring, and adjust hemodynamic management as the procedure progresses. Paraplegia is a devastating complication of TEVAR and prevention requires a collaborative approach with the electrophysiologist, surgeon, and intensive care team. Increasing SCPP by raising MAP and decreasing CSF pressure through drainage of CSF are effective strategies in treating paraplegia. Other complications associated with TEVAR include peripheral vascular injury, CIN, postimplantation syndrome, and endoleaks. Patients who undergo TEVAR require care in a postoperative environment where these complications can be rapidly detected and aggressively treated.

ACKNOWLEDGMENTS

The authors would like to acknowledge the contributions of Lisa Bennett, MD, MSCS, Department of Vascular Surgery, UT Southwestern Medical Center, for comments that greatly improved the article.

REFERENCES

1. Kuzmik GA, Sang AX, Elefteriades JA. Natural history of thoracic aortic aneurysms. J Vasc Surg 2012;56(2):565–71.

2. Shimizu K, Mitchell RN, Libby P. Inflammation and cellular immune responses in abdominal aortic aneurysms. Arterioscler Thromb Vasc Biol 2006;26(5):987–94.
3. Brophy CM, Reilly JM, Smith GW, et al. The role of inflammation in nonspecific abdominal aortic aneurysm disease. Ann Vasc Surg 1991;5(3):229–33.
4. Ganaha F, Miller DC, Sugimoto K, et al. Prognosis of aortic intramural hematoma with and without penetrating atherosclerotic ulcer: a clinical and radiological analysis. Circulation 2002;106(3):342–8.
5. Svensson LG, Kouchoukos NT, Miller DC, et al. Expert consensus document on the treatment of descending thoracic aortic disease using endovascular stent-grafts. Ann Thorac Surg 2008;85(1):S1–41.
6. Isselbacher EM. Thoracic and abdominal aortic aneurysms. Circulation 2005; 111(6):816–28.
7. Hiratzka LF, Bakris GL, Beckman JA, et al. 2010 ACCF/AHA/AATS/ACR/ASA/ SCA/SCAI/SIR/STS/SVM guidelines for the diagnosis and management of patients with thoracic aortic disease. J Am Coll Cardiol 2010;55(14):e27–129.
8. Matsumura JS, Lee WA, Mitchell RS, et al. The Society for Vascular Surgery Practice Guidelines: management of the left subclavian artery with thoracic endovascular aortic repair. J Vasc Surg 2009;50(5):1155–8.
9. Ganapathi AM, Englum BR, Schechter MA, et al. Role of cardiac evaluation before thoracic endovascular aortic repair. J Vasc Surg 2014;60(5):1196–203.
10. Grabenwöger M, Alfonso F, Bachet J, et al. Thoracic Endovascular Aortic Repair (TEVAR) for the treatment of aortic diseases: a position statement from the European Association for Cardio-Thoracic Surgery (EACTS) and the European Society of Cardiology (ESC), in collaboration with the European Association of Percutaneous Cardiovascular Interventions (EAPCI). Eur Heart J 2012;33(13):1558–63.
11. Ando K, Kaneko N, Doi T, et al. Prevalence and risk factors of aortic aneurysm in patients with chronic obstructive pulmonary disease. J Thorac Dis 2014;6(10): 1388.
12. Scali ST, Wang SK, Feezor RJ, et al. Preoperative prediction of spinal cord ischemia after thoracic endovascular aortic repair. J Vasc Surg 2014;60(6): 1481–90.e1.
13. Schlösser FJ, Verhagen HJ, Lin PH, et al. TEVAR following prior abdominal aortic aneurysm surgery: increased risk of neurological deficit. J Vasc Surg 2009;49(2): 308–14.
14. Baril DT, Cho JS, Chaer RA, et al. Thoracic aortic aneurysms and dissections: endovascular treatment. Mt Sinai J Med 2010;77(3):256–69.
15. Feezor RJ, Lee WA. Strategies for detection and prevention of spinal cord ischemia during TEVAR. Semin Vasc Surg 2009;22(3):187–92.
16. McCullough PA. Contrast-induced acute kidney injury. J Am Coll Cardiol 2008; 51(15):1419–28.
17. Edwards MS, Andrews JS, Edwards AF, et al. Results of endovascular aortic aneurysm repair with general, regional, and local/monitored anesthesia care in the American College of Surgeons National Surgical Quality Improvement Program database. J Vasc Surg 2011;54(5):1273–82.
18. Bettex D, Lachat M, Pfammatter T, et al. To compare general, epidural and local anaesthesia for endovascular aneurysm repair (EVAR). Eur J Vasc Endovasc Surg 2001;21(2):179–84.
19. Walschot LH, Laheij RJ, Verbeek AL. Outcome after endovascular abdominal aortic aneurysm repair: a meta-analysis. J Endovasc Ther 2002;9(1):82–9.
20. Horlocker TT, Wedel DJ, Rowlingson JC, et al. Regional anesthesia in the patient receiving antithrombotic or thrombolytic therapy: American Society of Regional

Anesthesia and Pain Medicine Evidence-Based Guidelines. Reg Anesth Pain Med 2010;35(1):64–101.

21. Nicolaou G, Ismail M, Cheng D. Thoracic endovascular aortic repair: update on indications and guidelines. Anesthesiol Clin 2013;31(2):451–78.

22. Hughes GC, Andersen ND, McCann RL. Management of acute type B aortic dissection. J Thorac Cardiovasc Surg 2013;145(3S):S202–7.

23. Swaminathan M, Lineberger CK, McCann RL, et al. The importance of intraoperative transesophageal echocardiography in endovascular repair of thoracic aortic aneurysms. Anesth Analg 2003;97(6):1566–72.

24. Rocchi G, Lofiego C, Biagini E, et al. Transesophageal echocardiography–guided algorithm for stent-graft implantation in aortic dissection. J Vasc Surg 2004;40(5):880–5.

25. Etz C, von Aspern K, Gudehus S, et al. Near-infrared spectroscopy monitoring of the collateral network prior to, during, and after thoracoabdominal aortic repair: a pilot study. Eur J Vasc Endovasc Surg 2013;46(6):651–6.

26. Badner NH, Nicolaou G, Clarke CF, et al. Use of spinal near-infrared spectroscopy for monitoring spinal cord perfusion during endovascular thoracic aortic repairs. J Cardiothorac Vasc Anesth 2011;25(2):316–9.

27. Mohammed NM, Mahfouz A, Achkar K, et al. Contrast-induced nephropathy. Heart Views 2013;14(3):106.

28. Awad H, Ramadan ME, El Sayed HF, et al. Spinal cord injury after thoracic endovascular aortic aneurysm repair Lésion de la moelle épinière après réparation endovasculaire d'un anévrisme de l'aorte thoracique. Can J Anaesth 2017;64(12): 1218–35.

29. Hanna JM, Andersen ND, Aziz H, et al. Results with selective preoperative lumbar drain placement for thoracic endovascular aortic repair. Ann Thorac Surg 2013; 95(6):1968–75.

30. Svensson LG, Hess KR, D'Agostino RS, et al. Reduction of neurologic injury after high-risk thoracoabdominal aortic operation1. Ann Thorac Surg 1998;66(1): 132–8.

31. Arnaoutoglou E, Kouvelos G, Milionis H, et al. Post-implantation syndrome following endovascular abdominal aortic aneurysm repair: preliminary data. Interact Cardiovasc Thorac Surg 2011;12(4):609–14.

32. Ricotta JJ. Endoleak management and postoperative surveillance following endovascular repair of thoracic aortic aneurysms. J Vasc Surg 2010;52(4):91S–9S.

Modulating Perioperative Ventricular Excitability

Kimberly Howard-Quijano, MD, MS*, Yuki Kuwabara, MD

KEYWORDS

- Perioperative • Ventricular arrhythmias • Myocardial excitability
- Autonomic nervous system • Regional anesthesia • Thoracic epidural anesthesia
- Stellate ganglion block

KEY POINTS

- Cardiac arrhythmias are associated with significant morbidity and mortality. Myocardial hyperexcitability is a major contributor to the pathophysiology of ventricular tachyarrhythmias.
- The primary myocardial mechanisms underlying ventricular tachyarrhythmias are abnormal automaticity, triggered activity, and reentry.
- Arrhythmia development is a dynamic interplay among an arrhythmogenic substrate, myocardial electrophysiologic properties, modifying factors, and triggering factors.
- Ventricular arrhythmias are modulated perioperatively through hemodynamic and physiologic management, anesthetic agents, or regional anesthetic and surgical techniques.

INTRODUCTION

Cardiac arrhythmias are associated with significant morbidity and mortality.[1] In the United States alone, sudden cardiac death claims more than 350,000 lives per year[2,3] and nearly 11% of patients undergoing a general anesthetic have an abnormal heart rhythm in the perioperative period.[4,5] Ventricular arrhythmias are the leading cause of sudden cardiac death and are associated with a wide range of pathophysiologic mechanisms.[1,3,6,7] A strong link has been demonstrated between the autonomic nervous system and ventricular arrhythmogenesis.[8,9] Imbalances in the autonomic nervous system, namely excessive sympathetic stimulation, can lead to increased myocardial excitability, which is a major contributor to the pathophysiology of ventricular tachyarrhythmias (VTs).[8,10–12]

Although ventricular arrhythmias are often associated with patients having a history of ischemic cardiomyopathy or structural heart disease, this only represents a portion of the population at risk for ventricular arrhythmias. Other patients at risk include those

Disclosures: None.

Department of Anesthesiology and Perioperative Medicine, University of Pittsburgh School of Medicine, Biomedical Science Tower W1401, 200 Lothrop Street, Pittsburgh, PA 15213, USA

* Corresponding author.

E-mail address: khq@pitt.edu

Anesthesiology Clin 37 (2019) 609–619

https://doi.org/10.1016/j.anclin.2019.08.002

1932-2275/19/© 2019 Elsevier Inc. All rights reserved.

with channelopathies or idiopathic ventricular arrhythmias.[3] It has been demonstrated that the number of sudden cardiac death cases per year are actually higher in the general population, than it is in patients with identifiable and known risk factors.[7,13] Therefore, the possibility of developing ventricular arrhythmias in the perioperative period is not just isolated to the cases with known elevated risk, such as cardiac surgery, electrophysiology laboratory procedures, or patients with history of arrhythmias. The scope of perioperative cardiac arrhythmias is far reaching and requires a thorough understanding of the mechanisms underlying myocardial excitability and arrhythmogenesis to diagnose and treat life-threatening ventricular arrhythmias in a timely manner.

VENTRICULAR ARRHYTHMIA CLASSIFICATION AND DEFINITIONS

Cardiac arrhythmias represent abnormal myocardial electrophysiologic activation that leads to perturbations in heart rhythms that are either abnormally fast (tachyarrhythmias) or abnormally slow (bradyarrhythmias). The most worrisome and potentially malignant of these arrhythmias are the VTs. The clinical sequelae of ventricular arrhythmias can range from asymptomatic premature ventricular complexes (PVC) to ventricular fibrillation (VF) (**Box 1**). The clinical impact of any arrhythmia depends on the patient's underlying ventricular function, ventricular response rate, duration, and other comorbid conditions.[14]

Premature Ventricular Complexes

PVCs are the most common ventricular arrhythmia, especially in the perioperative period, because they are often associated with metabolic and electrolyte perturbations.[3,14] Isolated PVCs, in patients with normal ventricular function, are usually benign and not associated with increased risk of more serious arrhythmia development.[15,16] Frequent PVCs (>30/hour) can reduce ventricular function and cardiac output causing hemodynamic instability during important intraoperative and postoperative periods.[14] PVCs in patients with reduced ventricular function may be associated with increased postoperative mortality. A study looking at nearly 130 patients who underwent cardiac surgery found that postoperative complex PVCs were not a predictor of long-term mortality unless patients had reduced ejection fraction of less than 40%.[15] This study demonstrates the close relationship between ventricular arrhythmias, underlying ventricular function, and perioperative outcomes.

Box 1
Ventricular arrhythmia classification

Premature ventricular complexes
  Isolated PVC
  Frequent PVC (>30/hour)

Ventricular tachyarrhythmias
  Duration
    Nonsustained (VT <30 seconds, resolves spontaneously)
    Sustained (VT ≥30 seconds, requiring intervention)
    VT storm (three or more separate episodes of sustained VT within 24 hours)
  Morphology
    Monomorphic (similar QRS configuration)
    Polymorphic (QRS changing continuously)
    Pleomorphic (>1 QRS morphology)

Ventricular fibrillation

Ventricular Tachycardia

VT is defined as three or more consecutive QRS complexes at a rate of 100 beats per minute or greater. VT type is classified by duration or morphology (see **Box 1**). As defined by duration, sustained VT is defined as VT lasting greater than 30 seconds and requiring therapeutic intervention because of hemodynamic instability. Nonsustained VT terminates spontaneously in less than 30 seconds with no intervention. VT storm is defined as three or more separate episodes of sustained VT, requiring intervention, within 24 hours. VT can also be classified by morphology; monomorphic (similar beat to beat QRS morphology), polymorphic (continuously changing QRS morphology), or pleomorphic (more than one QRS morphology but not continuous change).

Sustained ventricular arrhythmias (VT or VF) are infrequent in the perioperative period, with a reported incidence of less than 1.4% after cardiac surgery.[17,18] The pathophysiology of VTs is multifactorial and several commonly encountered perioperative risk factors have been implicated including hemodynamic instability, hypovolemia, hypoxia, myocardial ischemia, and electrolyte imbalances.[15] The clinical consequences of VT are related to the type of VT and the degree of underlying heart disease. Patients with sustained postoperative ventricular arrhythmias have an in-hospital mortality rate of nearly 50%.[16,19] Among the patients who survive to discharge 40% may have a reoccurrence and 20% die from cardiac-related causes within 2 years after surgery.

PATHOPHYSIOLOGY OF VENTRICULAR ARRHYTHMIA GENERATION

The development of ventricular arrhythmias, or ventricular arrhythmogenesis, is a complex interplay between intrinsic myocardial properties and external factors. Arrhythmia development involves: (1) an arrhythmogenic substrate (myocardial scar, channelopathies); (2) myocardial electrophysiologic properties; (3) modifying factors (increased sympathetic activity, ischemia); and (4) triggering factors (electrolyte imbalances, hypoxemia, PVCs), which can increase or decrease arrhythmia risk (**Box 2**). There are three basic mechanisms underlying the pathogenesis of all cardiac arrhythmias:

- Abnormal automaticity: automaticity is an intrinsic property of all myocytes. Abnormal automaticity occurs when myocardial cells pacemaker function is either suppressed of enhanced by insults, such as scarring, ischemia, acid base disorders, or enhanced sympathetic tone.
- Triggered activity: occurs after early or delayed depolarizations, which if they reach a certain threshold, can initiate spontaneous multiple depolarizations thus precipitating VT. Examples include digitalis toxicity and prolonged QT syndromes.
- Reentry: is one of the most common mechanisms of ventricular arrhythmogenesis. Reentry arises when there is a unidirectional block in the myocardium, which leads to bidirectional conduction. Microreentry arises from conduction around scarred myocardium, whereas macroreentry is often associated with conduction through accessory pathways, such as Wolff-Parkinson-White syndrome.

MODULATION OF VENTRICULAR ARRHYTHMIAS

Although some of the risk factors for ventricular arrhythmias are static, such as myocardial scars and decreased ventricular function, there are several other modifying and triggering factors that are dynamic (see **Box 2**), thus allowing modulation

---

Box 2
Pathogenesis of ventricular arrhythmias

Arrhythmogenic substrate

- Myocardial scar
- Structural heart disease
- Genetic channelopathies

Electrophysiologic myocardial properties

- Electrical activation
- Impulse propagation

Modifying factors

- Autonomic dysregulation, increased sympathetic activity
- Ongoing ischemia
- Heart failure

Triggering factors

- Electrolyte imbalance
- Increased heart rate
- PVC

---

of myocardial excitability and ventricular arrhythmogenesis in the perioperative period. Ventricular arrhythmogenesis is modulated perioperatively through hemodynamic management, electrolyte balance, and anesthetic agents, whereas autonomic dysregulation/increased sympathetic tone are modulated via regional anesthetic and surgical techniques.

Hemodynamic and Physiologic Management

Hemodynamic instability can increase the risk of ventricular arrhythmogenesis. Severe hypotension and hypoxemia decrease myocardial perfusion and oxygen delivery, which can lead to cardiac ischemia, ectopic activity, or conduction abnormalities. These effects are more dramatic in patients with reduced ventricular systolic function or diastolic dysfunction. Severe hypertension can also precipitate ischemia and ventricular arrhythmias by increasing left ventricular afterload. Maintenance of normal heart rate is of importance, because profound bradycardia can reduce cardiac output and perfusion pressure, whereas severe tachycardia is a trigger for ventricular arrhythmias.

Normal electrolyte balance is paramount in reducing cardiac arrhythmogenesis. Hyperkalemia and hypokalemia have been associated with ventricular ectopic beats, VT, and even VF.[20] Hypomagnesemia has been associated with torsades de pointes, whereas hypocalcemia can prolong the QT interval, both of which are associated with increased risk of ventricular arrhythmias.[21] Electrolytes are altered in the perioperative period because of fasting, medications, bleeding, and surgical stress. When ventricular arrhythmias occur, electrolytes should be checked and corrected rapidly to reduce further risk.

Anesthetics

Arrhythmogenicity of anesthetic medications is typically evaluated in terms of their effect on action potential duration and most commonly the QT interval length.

Prolongation of cardiac repolarization, which is measured by the QT interval, has been associated with torsades de pointes and ventricular arrhythmias. Although multiple anesthetics have been shown to prolong the QT interval, the risk of malignant ventricular arrhythmias does not seem to be increased with the possible exceptions of methadone and droperidol[22-25]:

- No change in QT interval: no increase in arrhythmogenesis
  Propofol,[26,27] fentanyl,[28] alfentanil,[29] remifentanil,[30,31] local anesthetics (lidocaine, bupivacaine, ropivacaine),[32,33] neuromuscular blocking agents (succinylcholine, rocuronium, vecuronium),[34] and suggamadex[35]
- Prolongation of QT interval: no increase in arrhythmogenesis
  Volatile anesthetics,[36,37] ketamine,[38] sufentanil,[31] mizadolam,[27,39] ondanesetron,[24,25] and dexmedetomidine[40]
- Prolongation of QT interval: possible increase in arrhythmogenesis
  Droperidol[24,25] and methadone[22,23]

Neuromodulation for Ventricular Arrhythmias

Increased sympathetic activity has been implicated in several cardiac disease processes, in the pathophysiology of ventricular arrhythmias, and is associated with worsening prognoses.[1,12] Given the intricate role that the autonomic nervous system plays in cardiac arrhythmogenesis and sudden cardiac death, multiple therapies aimed at neuromodulation of the autonomic nervous system have emerged.[10,41] Neuromodulation therapies include regional anesthetic techniques, such as thoracic epidural anesthesia (TEA) and stellate ganglion blocks (SGB), and surgical interventions including spinal cord stimulation (SCS) and thoracic sympathectomy. Each neuromodulatory technique aims to rebalance the autonomic nervous system through attenuation of cardiac sympathetic activity and reduction in efferent sympathetic signaling to the heart (**Fig. 1**).

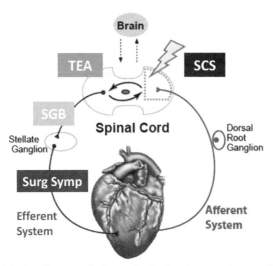

Fig. 1. Neuromodulation for ventricular arrhythmias. Increased sympathetic activity has been implicated in the pathophysiology of ventricular arrhythmias. Each neuromodulatory technique aims to rebalance the autonomic nervous system through attenuation of cardiac sympathetic activity or reduction in efferent sympathetic signaling to the heart. Neuromodulation therapies include TEA, SGB, SCS, and thoracic surgical sympathectomy (Surg Symp).

Thoracic epidural anesthesia

In human and animal studies, TEA has been demonstrated to be an effective technique to reduce myocardial sympathoexcitation and malignant VT.[11,42,43] TEA decreases sympathetic signaling to the heart through blockade of neural activity of the spinal nerve rootlets via local anesthetics administered in the thoracic epidural space.[11,44,45] The resultant sympathectomy from thoracic spinal levels T1-T5 decreases ventricular arrhythmogenic potential through prolongation of the repolarization and refractory periods, thus decreasing myocardial excitability.[11,46] In a recent case series, greater than 50% of patients diagnosed with ischemic cardiomyopathy, nonischemic cardiomyopathy, or hypertrophic cardiomyopathy and VT storm responded to TEA and had a reduction in their number of ventricular arrhythmias.[47]

Stellate ganglion block

Another regional anesthetic technique to reduce cardiac sympathoexcitation is percutaneous SGB. SGB was first studied in animal models when it was found that myocardial ischemia induced neuronal remodeling of the stellate ganglia with resultant increased synaptic density and sympathetic output to the heart.[48,49] In a rabbit model of myocardial infarction, left SGB reduced VF threshold through prolongation of the action potential duration and reduced heterogeneity of repolarization.[50] Recently the clinical efficacy of SGB for reducing ventricular arrhythmias has been investigated in a systematic review and meta-analysis, and it was found that SGB is an effective treatment of acute malignant ventricular arrhythmias.[51,52] SGB was found to reduce the number of ventricular arrhythmia events independent of the subtype of ventricular arrhythmia, the degree of left ventricular dysfunction, or the type of cardiomyopathy.[51] In fact, 24 of the 38 patients had complete arrhythmia suppression following SGB, whereas the other 14 patients had partial resolution. However, these results are based on small sample sizes and larger randomized controlled studies are needed to better understand the therapeutic potential of SGB.

Both TEA and SGB are acute procedures that can be performed in the perioperative period to modulate myocardial excitability and decrease ventricular arrhythmias. Although their effects are only temporary, there have been some reports of prolonged utilization. Case studies have demonstrated serial SGB to reduce implantable cardioverter-defibrillator shocks in patients with refractory VT and VF, and continuous SGB to test patients' surgical candidacy for sympathetic denervation.[53-55] Longer term modulation therapies include surgical sympathectomy and SCS.

Sympathectomy

Surgical cardiac sympathectomy reduces ventricular arrhythmias by permanently severing sympathetic efferent innervation to the heart. Most commonly, the lower third of the left stellate ganglion and part of the sympathetic chain from thoracic levels T2-T4 are surgically removed.[43] Nademanee and colleagues[56] demonstrated that surgical sympathectomy was superior to standard pharmacologic therapy with 82% versus 22% survival. Surgical sympathectomy is performed for ventricular arrhythmias associated with ischemic cardiomyopathy and long QT syndrome and other arrhythmic disorders.[52] Unilateral sympathetic denervation is usually attempted first. However, because of anatomic variation in cardiac innervation and possible bilateral sympathetic ganglion remodeling postcardiac injury, this may not always be sufficient and bilateral cardiac denervation may be needed.[57-59] In a large multicenter trial, 50% of patients had freedom from sustained VT, implantable cardioverter-defibrillator shocks, and death at 1 year following either left or bilateral cardiac sympathetic denervation operations.[60]

Spinal cord stimulation

SCS of the upper thoracic spinal segments was originally used as a treatment of refractory angina. However, it has more recently been suggested to also have myocardial antiarrhythmic effects.[11,61–64] SCS is a bioelectric therapy that is postulated to act on spinothalamic tract neurons in the dorsal column of the spinal cord and thus reduce cardiac sympathetic efferent activity.[65–67] Although the efficacy of thoracic SCS to decrease ventricular arrhythmias in animal models has been well demonstrated, the results in clinical trials have been varied.[11,62,68,69] Of note, the primary outcomes of the clinical trials to date investigating SCS in cardiomyopathy patients have been improvement in heart failure symptoms and left ventricular function, not reduction of ventricular arrhythmias. The SCS HEART (Spinal Cord Stimulation for Heart Failure) trial was a small nonrandomized open label trial that demonstrated improvement in greater than four of the six efficacy parameters evaluated and evidence for potential antiarrhythmic effects.[70] However, a larger follow-up randomized trial (DEFEAT-HF) did not find any difference in cardiac arrhythmias between those heart failure patients with SCS as compared with control subjects.[48] Thus, although early studies show promise, further clinical trials are needed to determine the translatability and clinical efficacy of thoracic SCS in modulating ventricular arrhythmogenesis.

SUMMARY

Cardiac arrhythmias are associated with significant morbidity and mortality. Ventricular arrhythmogenesis is a dynamic interplay among an arrhythmogenic substrate, myocardial electrophysiologic properties, modifying factors, and triggering factors. Imbalances in the autonomic nervous system can lead to increased myocardial excitability, which is a major contributor to the pathophysiology of VT. Myocardial excitability and ventricular arrhythmogenesis are modulated perioperatively through hemodynamic and physiologic management, anesthetic agents, or regional anesthetic and surgical techniques.

REFERENCES

1. Chugh SS, Reinier K, Teodorescu C, et al. Epidemiology of sudden cardiac death: clinical and research implications. Prog Cardiovasc Dis 2008;51(3):213–28.
2. Go AS, Mozaffarian D, Roger VL, et al. Heart disease and stroke statistics–2014 update: a report from the American Heart Association. Circulation 2014;129(3): e28–292.
3. Batul SA, Olshansky B, Fisher JD, et al. Recent advances in the management of ventricular tachyarrhythmias. F1000Res 2017;6:1027.
4. Forrest JB, Cahalan MK, Rehder K, et al. Multicenter study of general anesthesia. II. Results. Anesthesiology 1990;72:262–8.
5. Forrest JB, Rehder K, Cahalan MK, et al. Multicenter study of general anesthesia. III. Predictors of severe perioperative adverse outcomes. Anesthesiology 1992; 76:3–15.
6. Chugh SS, Havmoeller R, Narayanan K, et al. Worldwide epidemiology of atrial fibrillation: a Global Burden of Disease 2010 Study. Circulation 2014;129(8): 837–47.
7. Proietti R, Joza J, Essebag V. Therapy for ventricular arrhythmias in structural heart disease: a multifaceted challenge. J Physiol 2016;594(9):2431–43.
8. Shivkumar K, Ajijola OA, Anand I, et al. Clinical neurocardiology defining the value of neuroscience-based cardiovascular therapeutics. J Physiol 2016; 594(14):3911–54.

9. Ardell JL, Andresen MC, Armour JA, et al. Translational neurocardiology: preclinical models and cardioneural integrative aspects. J Physiol 2016;594(14): 3877–909.

10. Vaseghi M, Shivkumar K. The role of the autonomic nervous system in sudden cardiac death. Prog Cardiovasc Dis 2008;50(6):404–19.

11. Howard-Quijano K, Takamiya T, Dale EA, et al. Effect of thoracic epidural anesthesia on ventricular excitability in a porcine model. Anesthesiology 2017; 126(6):1096–106.

12. Shen MJ, Zipes DP. Role of the autonomic nervous system in modulating cardiac arrhythmias. Circ Res 2014;114(6):1004–21.

13. Myerburg RJ, Kessler KM, Castellanos A. Sudden cardiac death: epidemiology, transient risk, and intervention assessment. Ann Intern Med 1993;119(12): 1187–97.

14. Peretto G, Durante A, Limite LR, et al. Postoperative arrhythmias after cardiac surgery: incidence, risk factors, and therapeutic management. Cardiol Res Pract 2014;2014:615987.

15. Huikuri HV, Yli-Mayry S, Korhonen UR, et al. Prevalence and prognostic significance of complex ventricular arrhythmias after coronary arterial bypass graft surgery. Int J Cardiol 1990;27(3):333–9.

16. Smith RC, Leung JM, Keith FM, et al. Ventricular dysrhythmias in patients undergoing coronary artery bypass graft surgery: incidence, characteristics, and prognostic importance. Study of Perioperative Ischemia (SPI) Research Group. Am Heart J 1992;123(1):73–81.

17. Topol EJ, Lerman BB, Baughman KL, et al. De novo refractory ventricular tachyarrhythmias after coronary revascularization. Am J Cardiol 1986;57(1):57–9.

18. Sapin PM, Woelfel AK, Foster JR. Unexpected ventricular tachyarrhythmias soon after cardiac surgery. Am J Cardiol 1991;68(10):1099–100.

19. Pinto RP, Romerill DB, Nasser WK, et al. Prognosis of patients with frequent premature ventricular complexes and nonsustained ventricular tachycardia after coronary artery bypass graft surgery. Clin Cardiol 1996;19(4):321–4.

20. Mattu A, Brady WJ, Robinson DA. Electrocardiographic manifestations of hyperkalemia. Am J Emerg Med 2000;18(6):721–9.

21. Khan AM, Lubitz SA, Sullivan LM, et al. Low serum magnesium and the development of atrial fibrillation in the community: the Framingham Heart Study. Circulation 2013;127(1):33–8.

22. Pearson EC, Woosley RL. QT prolongation and torsades de pointes among methadone users: reports to the FDA spontaneous reporting system. Pharmacoepidemiol Drug Saf 2005;14(11):747–53.

23. Mayet S, Gossop M, Lintzeris N, et al. Methadone maintenance, QTc and torsade de pointes: who needs an electrocardiogram and what is the prevalence of QTc prolongation? Drug Alcohol Rev 2011;30(4):388–96.

24. Charbit B, Albaladejo P, Funck-Brentano C, et al. Prolongation of QTc interval after postoperative nausea and vomiting treatment by droperidol or ondansetron. Anesthesiology 2005;102(6):1094–100.

25. Charbit B, Alvarez JC, Dasque E, et al. Droperidol and ondansetron-induced QT interval prolongation: a clinical drug interaction study. Anesthesiology 2008; 109(2):206–12.

26. Erdil F, Demirbilek S, Begec Z, et al. Effects of propofol or etomidate on QT interval during electroconvulsive therapy. J ECT 2009;25(3):174–7.

27. Michaloudis DG, Kanakoudis FS, Petrou AM, et al. The effects of midazolam or propofol followed by suxamethonium on the QT interval in humans. Eur J Anaesthesiol 1996;13(4):364–8.
28. Chang DJ, Kweon TD, Nam SB, et al. Effects of fentanyl pretreatment on the QTc interval during propofol induction. Anaesthesia 2008;63(10):1056–60.
29. Korpinen R, Saarnivaara L, Siren K. QT interval of the ECG, heart rate and arterial pressure during anaesthetic induction: comparative effects of alfentanil and esmolol. Acta Anaesthesiol Scand 1995;39(6):809–13.
30. Blair JR, Pruett JK, Crumrine RS, et al. Prolongation of QT interval in association with the administration of large doses of opiates. Anesthesiology 1987;67(3):442–3.
31. Blair JR, Pruett JK, Introna RP, et al. Cardiac electrophysiologic effects of fentanyl and sufentanil in canine cardiac Purkinje fibers. Anesthesiology 1989;71(4):565–70.
32. Knudsen K, Beckman Suurkula M, Blomberg S, et al. Central nervous and cardiovascular effects of i.v. infusions of ropivacaine, bupivacaine and placebo in volunteers. Br J Anaesth 1997;78(5):507–14.
33. Owczuk R, Wujtewicz MA, Sawicka W, et al. The effect of intravenous lidocaine on QT changes during tracheal intubation. Anaesthesia 2008;63(9):924–31.
34. Saarnivaara L, Klemola UM, Lindgren L. QT interval of the ECG, heart rate and arterial pressure using five non-depolarizing muscle relaxants for intubation. Acta Anaesthesiol Scand 1988;32(8):623–8.
35. de Kam PJ, van Kuijk J, Smeets J, et al. Sugammadex is not associated with QT/QTc prolongation: methodology aspects of an intravenous moxifloxacin-controlled thorough QT study. Int J Clin Pharmacol Ther 2012;50(8):595–604.
36. Schmeling WT, Warltier DC, McDonald DJ, et al. Prolongation of the QT interval by enflurane, isoflurane, and halothane in humans. Anesth Analg 1991;72(2):137–44.
37. Lischke V, Wilke HJ, Probst S, et al. Prolongation of the QT-interval during induction of anesthesia in patients with coronary artery disease. Acta Anaesthesiol Scand 1994;38(2):144–8.
38. Mitchell GF, Jeron A, Koren G. Measurement of heart rate and Q-T interval in the conscious mouse. Am J Physiol 1998;274(3 Pt 2):H747–51.
39. Saarnivaara L, Klemola UM, Lindgren L, et al. QT interval of the ECG, heart rate and arterial pressure using propofol, methohexital or midazolam for induction of anaesthesia. Acta Anaesthesiol Scand 1990;34(4):276–81.
40. Hammer GB, Drover DR, Cao H, et al. The effects of dexmedetomidine on cardiac electrophysiology in children. Anesth Analg 2008;106(1):79–83.
41. Schwartz PJ. Cardiac sympathetic denervation to prevent life-threatening arrhythmias. Nat Rev Cardiol 2014;11(6):346–53.
42. Mahajan A, Moore J, Cesario DA, et al. Use of thoracic epidural anesthesia for management of electrical storm: a case report. Heart Rhythm 2005;2(12):1359–62.
43. Bourke T, Vaseghi M, Michowitz Y, et al. Neuraxial modulation for refractory ventricular arrhythmias: value of thoracic epidural anesthesia and surgical left cardiac sympathetic denervation. Circulation 2010;121(21):2255–62.
44. Bromage P. Mechanism of action of extradural analgesia. Br J Anaesth 1975;47:199–211.
45. Kamibayashi T, Hayashi Y, Mammoto T, et al. Thoracic epidural anesthesia attenuates halothane-induced myocardial sensitization to dysrhythmogenic effect of epinephrine in dogs. Anesthesiology 1995;82(1):129–34.

46. Meissner A, Eckardt L, Kirchhof P, et al. Effects of thoracic epidural anesthesia with and without autonomic nervous system blockade on cardiac monophasic action potentials and effective refractoriness in awake dogs. Anesthesiology 2001; 95(1):132–8.

47. Do DH, Bradfield J, Ajijola OA, et al. Thoracic epidural anesthesia can be effective for the short-term management of ventricular tachycardia storm. J Am Heart Assoc 2017;6(11) [pii:e007080].

48. Zipes DP, Neuzil P, Theres H, et al. Determining the feasibility of spinal cord neuromodulation for the treatment of chronic systolic heart failure: the DEFEAT-HF study. JACC Heart Fail 2016;4(2):129–36.

49. Zipes DP. Influence of myocardial ischemia and infarction on autonomic innervation of heart. Circulation 1990;82:1095–105.

50. Gu Y, Wang L, Wang X, et al. Assessment of ventricular electrophysiological characteristics at periinfarct zone of postmyocardial infarction in rabbits following stellate ganglion block. J Cardiovasc Electrophysiol 2012;23:S29–35.

51. Meng L, Tseng CH, Shivkumar K, et al. Efficacy of stellate ganglion blockade in managing electrical storm: a systematic review. JACC Clin Electrophysiol 2017; 3(9):942–9.

52. Fudim M, Boortz-Marx R, Ganesh A, et al. Stellate ganglion blockade for the treatment of refractory ventricular arrhythmias: a systematic review and meta-analysis. J Cardiovasc Electrophysiol 2017;28(12):1460–7.

53. Hayase J, Patel J, Narayan SM, et al. Percutaneous stellate ganglion block suppressing VT and VF in a patient refractory to VT ablation. J Cardiovasc Electrophysiol 2013;24(8):926–8.

54. Smith DI, Jones C, Morris GK, et al. Trial ultrasound-guided continuous left stellate ganglion blockade before surgical gangliolysis in a patient with a left ventricular assist device and intractable ventricular tachycardia: a pain control application to a complex hemodynamic condition. ASAIO J 2015;61:104–6.

55. Loyalka P, Hariharan R, Gholkar G, et al. Left stellate ganglion block for continuous ventricular arrhythmias during percutaneous left ventricular assist device support. Tex Heart Inst J 2011;38:409–11.

56. Nademanee K, Taylor R, Bailey WE, et al. Treating electrical storm: sympathetic blockade versus advanced cardiac life support-guided therapy. Circulation 2000;102(7):742–7.

57. Ajijola OA, Lellouche N, Bourke T, et al. Bilateral cardiac sympathetic denervation for the management of electrical storm. J Am Coll Cardiol 2012;59(1):91–2.

58. Han S, Kobayashi K, Joung B, et al. Electroanatomic remodeling of the left stellate ganglion after myocardial infarction. J Am Coll Cardiol 2012;59(10):954–61.

59. Puddu PE, Jouve R, Langlet F, et al. Prevention of postischemic ventricular fibrillation late after right or left stellate ganglionectomy in dogs. Circulation 1988; 77(4):935–46.

60. Vaseghi M, Barwad P, Malavassi Corrales FJ, et al. Cardiac sympathetic denervation for refractory ventricular arrhythmias. J Am Coll Cardiol 2017;69(25): 3070–80.

61. Kingma JG Jr, Linderoth B, Ardell JL, et al. Neuromodulation therapy does not influence blood flow distribution or left-ventricular dynamics during acute myocardial ischemia. Auton Neurosci 2001;13:47–54.

62. Lopshire JC, Zhou X, Dusa C, et al. Spinal cord stimulation improves ventricular function and reduces ventricular arrhythmias in a canine postinfarction heart failure model. Circulation 2009;120(4):286–94.

63. Southerland EM, Milhorn DM, Foreman RD, et al. Preemptive, but not reactive, spinal cord stimulation mitigates transient ischemia-induced myocardial infarction via cardiac adrenergic neurons. AM J Physiol Heart Circ Physiol 2007;292: H311–7.
64. Murray S, Carson KG, Ewings PD, et al. Spinal cord stimulation significantly decreases the need for acute hospital admission for chest pain in patients with refractory angina pectoris. Heart 1999;82:89–92.
65. Foreman RD, Linderoth B, Ardell JL, et al. Modulation of intrinsic cardiac neurons by spinal cord stimulation: implications for its therapeutic use in angina pectoris. Cardiovasc Res 2000;47:367–75.
66. Chandler MJ, Brennan TJ, Garrison DW, Kim KS, et al. A mechanism of cardiac pain suppression by spinal cord stimulation: implications for patients with angina pectoris. Eur Heart J 1993;14:96–105.
67. Ardell JL, Cardinal R, Vermeulen M, et al. Dorsal spinal cord stimulation obtunds the capacity of intrathoracic extracardiac neurons to transduce myocardial ischemia. Am J Physiol Regul Integr Comp Physiol 2009;297(2):R470–7.
68. Issa ZF, Zhou X, Ujhelyi MR, et al. Thoracic spinal cord stimulation reduces the risk of ischemic ventricular arrhythmias in a postinfarction heart failure canine model. Circulation 2005;111(24):3217–20.
69. Odenstedt J, Linderoth B, Bergfeldt L, et al. Spinal cord stimulation effects on myocardial ischemia, infarct size, ventricular arrhythmia, and noninvasive electrophysiology in a porcine ischemia-reperfusion model. Heart Rhythm 2011;8(6): 892–8.
70. Tse HF, Turner S, Sanders P, et al. Thoracic Spinal Cord Stimulation for Heart Failure as a Restorative Treatment (SCS HEART study): first-in-man experience. Heart Rhythm 2015;12(3):588–95.

Recent Developments in Catheter-Based Cardiac Procedures

Michael A. Ackermann, MD, Jörg K. Ender, MD*

KEYWORDS

- Transcatheter procedures • Aortic valve • Mitral valve • Tricuspid valve

KEY POINTS

- Transcatheter aortic valve replacement is noninferior to surgical aortic valve replacement in patients with a high and moderate risk profile.
- Transcatheter aortic valve replacement can be done under general anesthesia or with monitored anesthesia care.
- Transcatheter mitral and tricuspid valve interventions should be performed under general anesthesia.

INTRODUCTION

Since the first transcatheter aortic valve implantation in 2002,[1] the number of catheter-based cardiac procedures has increased tremendously. Meanwhile, not only have transcatheter techniques for the aortic valve been refined, but procedures for the mitral and tricuspid valve have also been developed. This overview gives a short description of devices and procedures that are either CE-mark or US Food and Drug Administration-approved or are currently under clinical investigation.

AORTIC VALVE

The number of transcatheter aortic valve replacement (TAVR) procedures is steadily increasing worldwide and has overtaken the number of isolated surgical aortic valve procedures in Germany.[2]

The devices have become less complex owing to smaller sheath sizes, allowing progression from a surgical cut-down to a percutaneous needle puncture.[3] The development of recapturable and repositionable valves, a decreased need for balloon

Disclosure Statement: The authors have nothing to disclose.
Department of Anesthesiology and Intensive Care Medicine, Heart Centre Leipzig, Struempellstr 39, Leipzig 04289, Germany
* Corresponding author.
E-mail address: Joerg.ender@medizin.uni-leipzig.de

valvuloplasty, and rapid ventricular pacing together with an increase in procedural experience[4] have played a major role therein. Different valve types and their fluoroscopic appearance are shown in **Table 1** and **Fig. 1**.

Valves

A recent meta-analysis including more than 10,822 patients evaluated acute (<30 days) outcomes in patients who underwent TAVR with so-called second-generation devices. The pooled success rate was 94.2%. Postprocedural aortic regurgitation graded more than mild was seen in 1.6% of patients. The pooled estimate for all cause 30-day mortality was 2.2% with a cardiovascular 30-day mortality rate of 1.6%. The complication rates for major disabling stroke (1.1%) and major vascular complications (4.5%) were very low. The need for permanent pacemaker implantation (16%) remains an unresolved issue for both balloon- and self-expandable valves. The low rate for pacemaker implantation for the first generation balloon-expandable valves was not confirmed in the second-generation Sapien 3 valves (Edwards Lifesciences, Irvine, CA).[5]

Specific Patient Subgroups: Controversies

The long-term efficacy of TAVR in high-risk patients has been established.[6] Factors such as frailty, the risks for cognitive impairment and delirium, the presence of a porcelain aorta, and other specific anatomic features are not factored into traditional risk scores. In intermediate risk patients, TAVR was similar to surgical aortic valve replacement (SAVR) with respect to the primary end point of death or disabling stroke.[7]

In a recent meta-analysis, the 30-day mortality in the transfemoral TAVR group was significantly lower compared with the SAVR group. The 12-month mortality, however, was similar between the TAVR and SAVR groups. In the TAVR group, a significantly higher rate of aortic valve regurgitation and permanent pacemaker implantation was seen.[8] Reardon and colleagues[9] also reported higher rates for residual aortic valve regurgitation and need for pacemaker implantation in intermediate risk patients, but lower rates of acute kidney injury, atrial fibrillation, and transfusion requirements, compared with patients who underwent SAVR. The rate of death from any cause and disabling stroke was similar between the procedures at 2 years. TAVR resulted in better postoperative valve hemodynamics on echocardiography as evidenced by lower mean gradients and larger valve areas compared with SAVR.

The challenge, therefore, remains to identify the specific subgroup of patients falling into the intermediate risk group, who would benefit most from a transcatheter procedure.

Transcatheter aortic valve replacement procedures in patients with low surgical risk
More recently, it was shown that the rate of the composite end point of death, stroke, or rehospitalization at 1 year was significantly lower with TAVR than with SAVR in patients with severe aortic stenosis and low surgical risk in whom a balloon-expandable valve was placed. There were no significant differences in major vascular complications, new permanent pacemaker insertion, or moderate or severe paravalvular regurgitation between the TAVR and SAVR groups.[10] In another study using self-expanding valves, TAVR was not inferior to SAVR with regard to the primary end point, which was a composite of death or disabling stroke at 24 months. At 30 days, the incidence of moderate to severe aortic regurgitation (3.5% vs 0.5%) and pacemaker implantation (17.4% vs 6.1%) was higher in the TAVR group compared with the SAVR group.[11]

Table 1
Examples of transcatheter heart valves commercially available or in trials

Transcatheter Valve Name (Manufacturer)	Features	Procedural/Imaging Nuances
SAPIEN 3 (Edwards Lifesciences), commercially available	Cobalt chromium frame Bovine pericardial leaflets PET cuff Balloon-expandable, typically deployed during rapid pacing	Shortens from skirt end Positioning by echocardiography ensures that the aortic end is below the sinotubular junction and covers the native leaflets May be ideal for high risk for coronary obstruction and distorted aortic anatomy May be appropriate for bicuspid aortic valve
EvolutPro (Medtronic), commercially available	Supra-annular valve position Porcine pericardial leaflets External PET wrap Self-expanding frame Repositionable Rapid pacing not required	Ideal position of the ventricular end once deployed should be 2–4 mm below the native annulus (and not ≥ 6 mm) May be more difficult to accurately position with a horizontal aorta or annular/STJ distortion May be ideal for preexisting mitral bioprostheses Has been used for primary AR
Lotus Edge (Boston Scientific, Natick, MA), investigational device	Mechanical expansion of device Repositionable before release Adaptive seal skirt Rapid pacing not required	Relies on fluoroscopic positioning with assistance from echocardiography for paravalvular leak assessment and need for repositioning May be appropriate for bicuspid aortic valve
ACURATE neo (Boston Scientific), investigational device	Supra-annular valve Self-expanding Partially recapturable Three stabilizing arches Rapid pacing not required	Echocardiographic positioning of the ventricular end below the annulus Has been used for primary AR
JennaValve (JenaValve, Munich, Germany), investigational device	Feeler-guided anatomic positioning JenaClip anchoring to native leaflets Retrievable and repositionable Rapid pacing not required	Echocardiographic guidance of anatomic positioning to align clips and commissures Treats primary AS and primary AR
Centera (Edwards Lifesciences), investigational device	Self-expandable, nitinol stent with bovine pericardial tissue valve Annular position PET fabric Motorized deployment Repositionable and retrievable	Echocardiography for paravalvular leak assessment and need for repositioning

Abbreviations: AR, aortic regurgitation; AS, aortic stenosis; PET, Polyethylene Terephthalate; STJ, sinu-tubular Junction.

Adapted from Hahn RT, Nicoara A, Kapadia S, et al. Echocardiographic Imaging for Transcatheter Aortic Valve Replacement. J Am Soc Echocardiogr 2018;31(4):413; with permission.

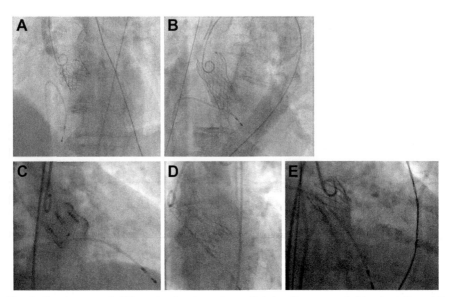

Fig. 1. Fluoroscopy of different valve types immediately after successful implantation. (*A*) Sapien 3, Edwards Lifesciences. (*B*) EvolutPro, Medtronic. (*C*) Lotus Edge, Boston Scientific. (*D*) Acurate Neo, Boston Scientific. (*E*) Centera, Edwards Lifesciences. ([*A, E*] Edwards Lifesciences Corporation, Irvine, CA; and [*B*] *Courtesy of* Medtronic; and [*C, D*] Boston Scientific Corporation, Marlborough, MA.)

Interestingly, the mean patient age decreased along with predicted and observed 30-day mortality in patients undergoing SAVR, but not in those undergoing TAVR (ie, higher age regardless of the risk score).[12] It is well-documented that age remains an important factor for surgical refusal and referral for TAVR. Despite the absence of an absolute age cut-off in the inclusion criteria, patients included in all major recent and on-going TAVR-trials remain octogenarians.[13]

Complications Specific to Transcatheter Aortic Valve Replacement Procedures

Stroke and the role of cerebral protection devices

The rate of disabling stroke after TAVR and SAVR in intermediate risk patients is similar.[7] In a meta-analysis looking for an association between stroke and 30-day mortality, a 12.7% stroke-related mortality was described.[14] Roughly 50% of strokes occur in the first 48 hours. Procedural factors mainly account for these strokes. Embolic protection devices have been developed to either deflect or capture intraprocedural emboli. When filters were used, debris was found in nearly 100% of cases. More than 80% of the debris were 150 to 500 µm in size with fewer than 5% being larger than 1000 µm. The debris consisted of fibrin, endothelium, collagen, valvular tissue, myocardium, and calcium.[15,16]

The question is not only if these devices can decrease the number and size of new lesions on imaging, but also if these can lead to improved clinical neurologic outcome. Because the use of TAVR is also being expanded to patient groups with lower risk, measures to mitigate neurologic risk are warranted.[17]

Different devices investigated are briefly discussed below.

Claret Sentinel Device The Claret Sentinel Device (Claret Medical Inc., Santa Rosa, CA) has a 140-µm pore polyurethane filter with the proximal part positioned in the brachiocephalic trunk and the distal part in the left carotid artery. The device is placed via the right radial or brachial artery (**Fig. 2**). The predecessor of this system was investigated in the CLEAN-TAVI trial, a randomized single-center study. Although most patients in both the study and control groups had new lesions on diffusion-weighted (DW) MRI on days 2 and 7 after the procedure, the amount and the size of these lesions were significantly reduced in the group where the device was used.[18] In the MISTRAL-C trial, patients in whom the Claret Sentinel Device was placed not only had numerically fewer lesions as measured by DW MRI, but also had a smaller total lesion volume.[16] Finally, it could be shown that, in patients undergoing TAVR with cerebral embolic protection devices, the incidence of disabling and nondisabling stroke was significantly reduced, with stroke free survival being more common in the protected group (2.1% vs 6.8%).[19]

Triguard HDH system The Triguard HDH system (Keystone Heart Ltd., Caesarea, IL) has a biocompatible filter with pore size of 130 μm and antithrombotic coating. It is placed via the femoral artery and covers the brachiocephalic trunk, left carotid artery, and left subclavian artery. Cerebral blood flow is maintained with large emboli being diverted to the descending aorta.[20,21]

In a feasibility and safety study, the Triguard HDH System could be successfully deployed in all patients without device-related complications. New ischemic lesions could be demonstrated in 83% of patients who underwent DW MRI imaging, with no change in neurocognitive testing over time.[20]

In a study by Lansky and colleagues,[21] device deployment and retrieval was successful in 89% of patients. Complete freedom from ischemic brain lesions was greater and the lesion volume lower in the Triguard group. They also had fewer neurologic deficits and improvement in neurologic function in some domains at discharge and 30 days compared with the control group. The system seems to be more effective when used in conjunction with the steerable balloon-expandable Sapien XT/3 systems, compared with the nonsteerable self-expandable CoreValve platform.

Embrella Embolic Deflector system Embrella Embolic Deflector (EED) system (Edwards Life-sciences, Irvine, CA) system has an oval-shaped nitinol frame covered with a polyurethane membrane with a pore size of 100 μm. It is placed via the right radial or brachial artery and covers the ostia of the brachiocephalic trunk and left carotid artery. In the PROTAVI-C Pilot study, the EED system did not prevent the occurrence of cerebral microemboli during TAVR. New ischemic lesions were seen in all

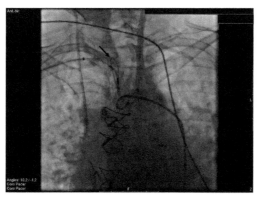

Fig. 2. Periprocedural radiograph with the Claret Device positioned. The black arrow indicates the proximal part in the truncus brachiocephalicus. The red arrow indicates the distal part in the left carotid artery. (Claret Medical Inc., Santa Rosa, CA.)

patients as measured by DW MRI imaging, with more lesions per patient in the EED group, but the lesion volume was reduced in the EED group compared with controls. The burden of procedural cerebral microemboli was higher in the patients in whom the device was deployed. Three neurologic events occurred in the EED group; these were, however, not associated with the device.[22]

Neurologic outcomes Studies have failed to show a correlation between lesions (number and volume) and cognitive decline. However, the baseline lesion burden seems to have a measurable impact in high-risk patients,[20] suggesting the mechanism for the relatively small impact the devices have on TAVR-associated microembolism.[23]

In a systematic review and meta-analysis by Giustino and colleagues,[17] the use of these devices was associated with lower total lesion volume ($P = .002$) and a smaller number of new ischemic lesions ($P = .003$). The risks for overt stroke and all-cause mortality were lower (nonsignificant) in the group where the devices were used.

Anesthetic Technique: Monitored Anesthetic Care and Conscious Sedation, Versus General Anesthesia

General anesthesia is the preferred technique for TAVR using the nontransfemoral (eg, transapical or transaortic) access.[24] There is still debate with regard to which technique is best when it comes to transfemoral TAVR. The specific technique is influenced by practice location, procedure experience, and surgical preference.[24–26] A worldwide survey found that general anesthesia is used in 60% of transfemoral TAVR cases, with conscious sedation being used by the remaining 40%.[27] Although most patients are being treated with general anesthesia, conscious sedation is growing in popularity in managing patients during transfemoral TAVR.[3]

In a large recent meta-analysis that included 26 studies and 10,572 patients by Villablanca and colleagues,[28] the use of local anesthesia/conscious sedation was associated with lower overall 30-day mortality (relative risk, 0.73). This differs from previous meta-analyses, which showed similar mortality rates. Interesting, the rate for cardiovascular death and stroke was similar between the local anesthesia and general anesthesia groups. They postulated noncardiac causes, such as life-threatening infections, as a cause for the higher mortality rate in the general anesthesia group.

Other positive findings include a decrease in the use of inotropes or vasopressors, a shorter intensive care unit and hospital length of stay, as well as shorter procedural and fluoroscopy times in the local anesthesia group. Significant negative findings were similar rates for stroke, cardiovascular mortality, myocardial infarction, permanent pacemaker implantation, acute kidney injury, paravalvular leak, major bleeding, vascular complications, annular rupture, and conduction abnormalities.

Also of note was the similar procedural success rate between the local anesthesia and general anesthesia groups. The conversion rate from local anesthesia to general anesthesia was 7.9%.[28]

These findings echo the results of a large study by Hyman and colleagues[3] consisting of 10,997 patients. In their study. however (although high in both groups), the adjusted intraprocedural success rate was higher for general anesthesia than for conscious sedation. One does need to keep in mind that the association between anesthetic technique and outcome is multifactorial and a definitive association between conscious sedation and decreased mortality cannot be determined. Other factors such as patient selection, variability in technique, evolving technology, and improvement in skill and experience may also have influenced the findings.[3] The direct causal relationship between monitored anesthesia care and improved outcomes is therefore difficult to prove and is discussed in various editorials.[4,29] The conversion rate from monitored anesthesia care/local anesthesia to general anesthesia ranging between 5.9% and 7.9% is also not negligible.[3,4,28]

An important difference compared with earlier studies was the absence of a higher rate for paravalvular leaks and permanent pacemaker implantation in the non-general anesthesia group.[25,28,30,31]

When it comes to monitored anesthesia care, there is a big variability with regard to the anesthetic agents used. Chen and colleagues[32] mainly compared a group who received propofol only for monitored anesthesia care with a group who received propofol and dexmedetomidine and found no association between a specific agent and perioperative outcome or conversion rate to general anesthesia.

At the TCT Meeting 2018 in San Diego the results of the SOLVE TAVI trial, a multi-center randomized trial comparing general versus local anesthesia in TAVR, were presented. Local anesthesia was equivalent to general anesthesia regarding 30-day mortality (2.8% vs 2.3%), stroke (2.4% vs 2.8%), myocardial infarction (0.5% vs 0.5%) and acute kidney injury (8.9% vs 9.2%). Also in secondary end points such as device time (61 minutes vs 65 minutes), total procedural time (116 minutes vs 119 minutes), hospital stay (9 days vs 9 days) and intensive care unit stay (51 hours vs 47 hours) the use of local anesthesia was equivalent to general anesthesia.[33]

One has to emphasize that, in all patients, a team consisting of cardiologists, cardiac surgeons and anesthesiologists, were involved, who were all well-experienced in these procedures. The result of this prospective study challenges the previous results mainly based on retrospective studies or registries not focused on anesthesia management.

The Role of Transesophageal and Transthoracic Echocardiography

The impact of monitored anesthesia care/conscious sedation on the use of transesophageal echocardiography (TEE) is unclear. With the impact of TEE on fluoroscopy times (and amount of contrast used) and the incidence of paravalvular leaks, this is important to keep in mind.[3]

Hayek and colleagues[34] investigated the role of TEE and transthoracic echocardiography (TTE) with regard to the incidence and severity of paravalvular leaks in patients who received a balloon-expandable valve via the transfemoral approach. The group guided by TTE was done under local anesthesia and sedation, whereas the group where the procedure was guided by TEE received a general anesthesia with endotracheal intubation. Patients in the TTE group were more likely to require a balloon after dilation and insertion of a second valve at the time of the procedure compared with the TEE TAVR. After adjustment for covariates, TTE TAVR was found to be a predictor for paravalvular regurgitation related events.

How to perform state of the art echocardiographic imaging for TAVR (TTE and TEE) was published recently.[35]

Intracardiac echocardiography has been used for the procedural guidance for structural heart disease. Although the use of volumetric intracardiac echocardiography as sole image guidance for the TAVR has been described, this modality is rarely reported in the literature.[36]

MITRAL VALVE
Mitral Valve Repair Technologies

Multiple transcatheter mitral valve repair technologies do exist addressing the different anatomic areas of the mitral valve apparatus. For a complete overview of different technologies see **Fig. 3**; not all of these devices are discussed in this article.[37]

Targeting the leaflet

A percutaneous edge-to-edge procedure to the mitral valve may be considered for symptomatic patients deemed to be inoperable or at high surgical risk, with a class IIb recommendation and B or C level of evidence[38,39]

MitraClip The MitraClip device (Abbott Vascular, Santa Clara, CA) is by far the most used transcatheter mitral valve repair technique. When compared with medical therapy alone, percutaneous mitral valve repair using the MitraClip System, in combination with medical therapy, showed a statistically significant relative risk reduction of death from any cause in patients with predominantly functional mitral valve regurgitation and advanced cardiac failure (for appearance in chest radiographs, see **Fig. 3**A). Likewise, the survival free of readmission owing to cardiac disease favored the MitraClip group in patients with functional mitral valve regurgitation significantly, except in patients with an ischemic etiology.[40] Chiarito and colleagues[41] compared the efficacy and safety end points for primary (degenerative) and secondary (functional) mitral valve regurgitation. They found similar 1-year survival rates and percentages for patients with regurgitation grade of 2 or lower, between these 2 groups. Patients with functional regurgitation however, had a significantly lower rate for reintervention at 1 year compared with the degenerative group.

The MITRA-FR randomly assigned patients with severe secondary mitral regurgitation to percutaneous mitral repair or medical treatment. The rate of death and unplanned hospitalization for heart failure did not differ between the groups.[42] In contrast, the COAPT trial found a significant decrease in the annualized rate of all hospitalizations for heart failure within 24 months in patients who had the MitraClip placed

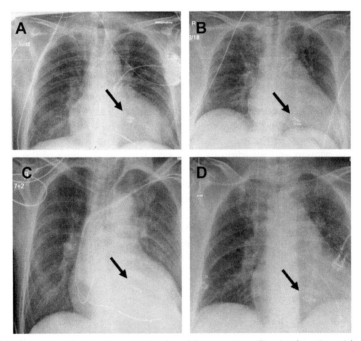

Fig. 3. (*A*) Two MitraClips in the mitral valve. (*B*) Two MitraClips in the tricuspid valve. (*C*) Pascal device in the mitral valve. (*D*) Pascal device in TV. ([*A, B*] © Abbott Medical GmbH, 2019; and [*C, D*] Edwards Lifesciences Corporation, Irvine, CA.)

in combination with medical therapy compared with medical therapy alone. Likewise, the rate of death from any cause was significantly decreased in the device group compared with the control group.[43] The different results of the MITRA-FR and the COAPT trials clearly demonstrate that the prognostic benefit of the MitraClip therapy in heart failure patients is observed if the therapy is performed early.

PASCAL System The width of the PASCAL implant (Edwards Lifesciences) is one and a half times larger than that of the MitraClip implant. In contrast with the MitraClip device, it is possible to grasp each of the mitral valve leaflets separately (see **Fig. 2**). The spring-loaded paddles have a width of 25 mm and the clasps are 10 mm long, allowing for load distribution across the surface area of the inserted leaflets.

In the first in-human study, technical success with residual mitral valve regurgitation of 2+ or less was achieved in 22 of 23 patients (96%). Periprocedural complications were infrequent and occurred in 2 of the 23 patients (9%). Despite the large size of the implant, the gradient across the mitral valve was not increased after implantation.[44] The primary completion date of the CLASP Study (NCT03170349), evaluating the safety, performance and clinical outcomes of the PASCAL System is estimated to be in December of 2019.

Targeting the annulus
Cardioband Mitral Valve Reconstruction System The Cardioband (Edwards Lifesciences) is a polyester sleeve with radiopaque markers spaced 8 mm apart. It contains a premounted contraction wire. The device is delivered into the left atrium via a transseptal puncture. According to the annular size and length of the device, 12 to 17 anchors are implanted starting as anterior as possible to the lateral commissure, progressively moving to posterior to the medial commissure. The close proximity to the circumflex artery is of utmost importance with angiographic control recommended.

The immediate and midterm results of a single-arm prospective multicenter trial of reported technical success in 58 of 60 patients (98%). The device failed to contract in 2 patients. Device success was reported for 43 of the 60 patients (72%) and procedural success for 41 of 60 patients (68%). Fifty-eight patients left the hospital alive. Although there were no procedural deaths, 1 patient had an immediate postprocedural stroke, 1 suffered a myocardial infarction owing to device related circumflex artery occlusion, 1 patient developed cardiac tamponade, and 1 patient had a cardiac arrest owing to rhythm disturbances related to distal circumflex artery occlusion. Partial anchor disengagement was noted in 10 patients, resulting in device inefficacy in 5 patients, albeit with no device migration or embolization. These disengagements occurred early in the study, whereafter several improvements were made. The anchor length was increased by 2 mm and an additional anchor was placed in the lateral commissure. The functional status, quality of life, and the exercise capacity improved significantly, with the observed 1-year mortality one-half of that normally observed with such a high-risk population.[45]

With regard to the Cardioband, the result of the MiBand (NCT03600688) and Active studies (NCT03016975) are expected in 2022 and 2024, respectively.

Carillon Mitral Contour System The Carillon Mitral Contour System (Cardiac Dimensions Inc, Kirkland, WA) is delivered via the right internal jugular vein, into the coronary sinus. It has 2 self-expanding nitinol anchors that are connected with a curvilinear nitinol segment. The distal anchor is unsheathed first and locked into position. After the delivery system is pulled back, the proximal anchor is released. The length of the coronary sinus, as well as that of the device, determines the amount of tension applied to the posterior mitral valve annulus.[46]

In up to one-half of the patients enrolled in studies, the Carillon system could not be implanted or had to be removed owing to compression of the circumflex artery. In patients where implantation was successful, the decrease in functional regurgitation was associated with inverse left ventricular remodeling with reduction in left ventricular volumes, improvement of functional class, and other parameters such as the 6 minute-walk-test and quality of life.[47]

Arto System The mechanism of the Arto System (MVRx Inc., San Mateo, CA) relies on tension applied to a suture connecting 2 anchors, one in the intra atrial septum and the other in the coronary sinus. By shortening the suture, the anteroposterior diameter of the mitral annulus is decrease and thereby leaflet coaptation is improved. In the first 11 patients in whom this system was implanted, there were no procedural adverse events. A reduction in the effective regurgitant orifice area and regurgitant volume was noted with an improvement in the left ventricular end-diastolic and systolic volume indices, as well as functional status.[48]

The Millipede IRIS Annuloplasty Ring The Millipede IRIS Annuloplasty Ring (Millipede, Inc., Santa Rosa, CA) consists of a complete semirigid nitinol frame. Eight stainless steel anchors are attached to the base of the device. Eight sliding collars are located at the upper portion of the device, which can be individually advanced or retracted. When advanced, these collars bring 2 adjacent anchors closer together. The procedural steps have been described elsewhere.[49]

Targeting the chordae
NeoChord device The NeoChord DS 1000 device (NeoChord, Inc., Minneapolis, MN) entails the implantation of polytetrafluoroethylene sutures with a transapical approach as an off-pump beating heart procedure. After grasping of the leaflet with grippers, piercing of the leaflet and fixation of the neochords is performed with a special needle. Thereafter, the free ends of the suture are fixed to the ventricular apex at a defined length ensuring correction of the prolapsing posterior leaflet.[50]

The reported results are as follows: procedural success rate 96.7%, 1-year survival 98%, freedom of residual regurgitation of more than a moderate degree was 92%.[51]

TSD device The TSD-device (Harpoon Medical Inc., Baltimore, MD) is a shafted instrument 3 mm in diameter used to anchor polytetrafluoroethylene artificial cords to an isolated prolapsing posterior mitral valve leaflet via a transapical approach. This procedure is performed through a small left lateral thoracotomy as on off-pump beating heart procedure. In the first in-human study, a 100% success rate was achieved. At 30 days, the severity of regurgitation could be reduced from severe to moderate in 2 of 11 patients (with 1 patient eventually requiring surgical correction of a progressive P2 prolapse), and to mild, trace, or none in 9 of the 11 patients.[52]

In a prospective multicenter trial including 30 patients, the procedural success rate was 90% and severe mitral regurgitation after 6 months occurred in 8%.[53]

Mitral Valve Replacement Technologies

The anatomy specific to the mitral valve making transcatheter replacement difficult includes a asymmetrical annulus, irregular leaflet geometry, large dimensions, the absence of calcified structures, and the presence of the subvalvular apparatus.[54]

Valve in valve
Transcatheter implantation of a balloon-expandable aortic valve (Sapien XT or Sapien 3, Edwards Lifesciences) in the mitral valve position, is usually used for patient with

failed mitral valve bioprosthesis (valve in valve) or annuloplasty rings (valve in ring), or patients who have primary mitral valve disease with severe annular calcification (covering $\geq$180° of the annulus).[55] The Edwards Sapien 3 valve is the only US Food and Drug Administration-approved transcatheter valve for the mitral valve position.[56] The default route for device delivery is via a transseptal puncture (done in 92.3% of cases), with the other being a transapical approach.

Technical procedural success was achieved in 84.6% of patients. The all-cause mortality rates at 1 and 2 years were 21.0% and 35.7%, respectively. Independent predictors of all-cause mortality were procedures done for the group who had severe annular calcification, tricuspid valve regurgitation greater than 2 at baseline and EuroSCORE-2. The presence of tricuspid regurgitation greater than 2 (hazard ratio, 2.73; 95% confidence interval, 1.23–1.07; $P = .014$) at baseline and the EuroSCORE-2 (hazard ratio, 1.04; 95% confidence interval, 1.01–1.07; $P = .009$) were independent predictors of all-cause cumulative mortality after transcatheter mitral valve implantation.[55] Transcatheter mitral valve technologies for native mitral valve diseases are currently under clinical investigation and were described recently by Regueiro and colleagues[54] (**Table 2**).

Anesthesia for Transcatheter Mitral Valve Procedures

Patients coming for transcatheter procedures to the mitral valve usually have a high and prohibitive surgical risk. The anesthetic management of these patients is not that well-described.

Owing to the need for intraprocedural guidance by means of TEE, general anesthesia is usually preferred, although not an absolute prerequisite.[57,58] An arterial line should be placed before induction of general anesthesia. Large bore venous access is usually established. Catheterization of the internal jugular vein should be dictated by whether a venous catheter is placed in the femoral vein or not and whether a pulmonary artery catheter is required. The use of regional anesthesia for transcatheter procedures to the mitral valve is not that well-described in the literature. When being considered for patients in whom a transapical approach is planned, one needs to keep in mind that some of these patients are taking antiplatelet medication or other anticoagulants.[56] Heparin should be administered to achieve a goal activated clotting time of 300 seconds. Measurements should be done at least every 30 minutes. Rapid ventricular pacing is usually used in cases where transcatheter implantation of a balloon-expandable valve is implanted in the mitral valve position.

With regard to guidance by means of TEE, the puncture site in the interatrial septum is of utmost importance. For the MitraClip procedure, this puncture should be made at least 4 cm above the annular plane, typically superior and posterior on the interatrial septum.[56] Multiplane imaging is essential during the MitraClip procedure, with real-time 3-dimensional imaging allowing for rapid imaging of clip arm orientation above and below the leaflets. A simple breath hold may decrease medial to lateral movement and hence aid leaflet capture. Should a 2-clip strategy be planned, the first grasp may be performed adjacent to the largest coaptation gap. This maneuver approximates the leaflets and facilitates grasping of the second clip.[59–61]

In the absence of complications, patients who have undergone a transcatheter procedure to the mitral valve can usually be extubated at the end of the procedure. The level postoperative observation, be it in the intensive care unit, intermediate care, or general ward, is usually dictated by the institutional protocol.[56] For chest radiograph appearance of the MitraClip and the Pascal device in mitral valve position see **Fig. 3**A and C.

Table 2
Transcatheter mitral valve replacement technologies

	CardiAQ-Edwards	Neovasc Tiara	Tendyne	Intrepid Transcatheter Repair of the Mitral Valve
Valve shape	Circular	D-shaped	D-shaped (outer stent) Circular (inner frame)	Circular
Frame	Nitinol, self-expandable	Nitinol, self-expandable	Nitinol, double frame; self-expandable	Nitinol, double stent; self-expandable
Anchoring mechanism	Mitral annulus capture with native leaflet engagement	Fibrous trigone capture with native leaflet engagement	Apical tether	Radial force and subannular cleats
Leaflets	Trileaflet Bovine pericardium	Trileaflet Bovine pericardium	Trileaflet Porcine pericardium	Trileaflet Bovine pericardium
Valve position	Supra-annular	Intra-annular	Intra-annular	Intra-annular
Access	Transapical, transseptal	Transapical	Transapical	Transapical
Delivery system size	33F	32F	36F	35F
Recapture	No	No	Fully recapturable system after complete deployment	No
Valve size(s)	30 mm	35 mm and 40 mm	Outer frame ranges from 30 to 43 mm in the SL dimension and 34 to 50 mm in the IC dimension	27 mm with 3 outer stent sizes (43, 46, and 50 mm)
Additional features	Supra-annular position intra-annular sealing skirt, tapered outflow	2 anterior and 1 posterior anchoring structures	Single inner valve size; Multiple outer frame sizes	Dual stent design; outer frame provides fixation and isolates the inner stent

	Caisson	HighLife TMVR	MValve System	NCSI NaviGate Mitral
Valve shape	D-shape	Circular	—	Circular
Frame	2 components (anchor and valve); nitinol, self-expandable	2 components (ring and valve); nitinol, self-expandable	Dock system to be used with commercially available valves	Nitinol, self-expandable; xenogeneic pericardium
Anchoring mechanism	External anchor; mitral annulus capture with engagement at subannular fibrous groove	External anchor; valve in subannular mitral ring	External anchor; mitral annulus capture	Annular winglets
Leaflets	Trileaflet Porcine pericardium	Trileaflet Bovine pericardium	—	Trileaflet
Valve position	Supra-annular	—	—	—
Access	Transseptal	Transapical (transfemoral artery for loop placement)	Transapical	Transapical, transatrial, or transfemoral
Delivery system size	31F	NA	32F	30F
Recapture	Fully recapturable and retrievable	No	Fully retrievable	NA
Valve size(s)	35–40 mm	31 mm	NA	Inflow/outflow: 30 mm/36 mm; 30 mm/40 mm; 33 mm/44 mm
Additional features	SAM management feature 1 delivery catheter for each system (anchor and valve)	NA	Universal dock system	NA

Abbreviations: IC, intercommissural; NA, not available; SAM, systolic anterior motion of the mitral valve; SL, septal-lateral; TMVR, transcatheter mitral valve replacement.

From Regueiro A, Granada JF, Dagenais F, et al. Transcatheter Mitral Valve Replacement: Insights From Early Clinical Experience and Future Challenges. J Am Coll Cardiol 2017;69(17):2181; with permission.

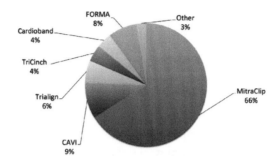

Fig. 4. Transcatheter tricuspid valve repair techniques. (*Adapted from* Taramasso M, Alessandrini H, Latib A, et al. Outcomes After Current Transcatheter Tricuspid Valve Intervention: Mid-Term Results From the International TriValve Registry. JACC Cardiovasc Interv 2019;12(2):157; with permission.)

TRICUSPID VALVE

The different transcatheter tricuspid valve repair techniques are depicted in **Table 2**. Edge-to-edge tricuspid valve repair using the Mitraclip system, is by far the most commonly used percutaneous interventional therapy for the tricuspid valve[62] (**Fig. 4**). Nickening and colleagues described a 97% success rate by using the Mitra-Clip system for compassionate use in patients with severe tricuspid regurgitation. No procedural death or severe complications occurred in the 64 included preselected patients who were deemed unsuitable for surgery. The tricuspid regurgitation could be reduced by at least 1 grade in 91% of patients.[63]

Besler and colleagues[64] defined procedural success of transcatheter tricuspid valve repair as a decrease in the grade of tricuspid valve regurgitation by 1 grade or more, as assessed by TTE within the 30 days after the procedure. Procedural success was most likely in patients with a central or anteroseptal main tricuspid valve regurgitation jet with a coaptation gap of less than 7.2 mm.[64]

In a study evaluating patients with mitral and tricuspid valve regurgitation, the benefit of combined transcatheter repair of the mitral and tricuspid valves (TMTVR), compared with isolated transcatheter repair of the mitral valve was investigated.[65,66] Mitral regurgitation was reduced in all patients. Tricuspid valve regurgitation was significantly reduced in the TMTVR group in contrast with the transcatheter repair of the mitral valve group. Patients in the TMTVR group had a significantly greater improvement in New York Heart Association functional class, compared with the transcatheter repair of the mitral valve group. Although both groups displayed improved results on the 6-minute walk test, this improvement was only statistically significant in the TMTVR group. This finding also translated into significantly fewer hospitalizations for heart failure, as well as longer survival free of hospitalization for heart failure, albeit with similar death rates between the groups.

For chest radiographic appearance of the MitraClip and the Pascal device in tricuspid valve position, see **Fig. 3**B and D.

SUMMARY

TAVR has become a commonly performed procedure in patients with intermediate and high surgical risk. Mortality and stroke rate is comparable with SAVR. The Mitra-Clip device is by far the most used transcatheter repair technique for mitral valve regurgitation. Transcatheter mitral valve replacement techniques are under clinical investigation. Percutaneous tricuspid valve repair is promising but experience is limited. General anesthesia, local anesthesia or monitored anesthesia care is used for TAVR, whereas general anesthesia is preferred for percutaneous mitral and tricuspid valve interventions.

REFERENCES

1. Cribier A, Eltchaninoff H, Bash A, et al. Percutaneous transcatheter implantation of an aortic valve prosthesis for calcific aortic stenosis: first human case description. Circulation 2002;106:3006–8.
2. Beckmann A, Meyer R, Lewandowski J, et al. German Heart Surgery Report 2017: the Annual Updated Registry of the German Society for Thoracic and Cardiovascular Surgery. Thorac Cardiovasc Surg 2018;66:608–21.
3. Hyman MC, Vemulapalli S, Szeto WY, et al. Conscious sedation versus general anesthesia for transcatheter aortic valve replacement: insights from the National Cardiovascular Data Registry Society of Thoracic Surgeons/American College of Cardiology Transcatheter Valve Therapy Registry. Circulation 2017;136:2132–40.
4. Brown CHT, Hasan RK, Brady MB. Is less really more? Conscious sedation or general anesthesia for transcatheter aortic valve replacement. Circulation 2017; 136:2141–3.
5. Barbanti M, Webb JG, Gilard M, et al. Transcatheter aortic valve implantation in 2017: state of the art. EuroIntervention 2017;13:AA11–21.
6. Didier R, Eltchaninoff H, Donzeau-Gouge P, et al. Five-year clinical outcome and valve durability after transcatheter aortic valve replacement in high-risk patients. Circulation 2018;138:2597–607.
7. Leon MB, Smith CR, Mack MJ, et al. Transcatheter or surgical aortic-valve replacement in intermediate-risk patients. N Engl J Med 2016;374:1609–20.
8. Singh K, Carson K, Rashid MK, et al. Transcatheter aortic valve implantation in intermediate surgical risk patients with severe aortic stenosis: a systematic review and meta-analysis. Heart Lung Circ 2018;27:227–34.
9. Reardon MJ, Van Mieghem NM, Popma JJ. Surgical or transcatheter aortic-valve replacement. N Engl J Med 2017;377:197–8.
10. Mack MJ, Leon MB, Thourani VH, et al. Transcatheter aortic-valve replacement with a balloon-expandable valve in low-risk patients. N Engl J Med 2019; 380(18):1695–705.
11. Popma JJ, Deeb GM, Yakubov SJ, et al. Transcatheter aortic-valve replacement with a self-expanding valve in low-risk patients. N Engl J Med 2019;380(18): 1706–15.
12. Prendergast BD, Baumgartner H, Delgado V, et al. Transcatheter heart valve interventions: where are we? Where are we going? Eur Heart J 2019;40:422–40.
13. Tarantini G, Nai Fovino L, Gersh BJ. Transcatheter aortic valve implantation in lower-risk patients: what is the perspective? Eur Heart J 2018;39:658–66.
14. Muralidharan A, Thiagarajan K, Van Ham R, et al. Meta-analysis of perioperative stroke and mortality in transcatheter aortic valve implantation. Am J Cardiol 2016; 118:1031–45.
15. Kapadia SR, Kodali S, Makkar R, et al. Protection against cerebral embolism during transcatheter aortic valve replacement. J Am Coll Cardiol 2017;69:367–77.
16. Van Mieghem NM, van Gils L, Ahmad H, et al. Filter-based cerebral embolic protection with transcatheter aortic valve implantation: the randomised MISTRAL-C trial. EuroIntervention 2016;12:499–507.
17. Giustino G, Mehran R, Veltkamp R, et al. Neurological outcomes with embolic protection devices in patients undergoing transcatheter aortic valve replacement:

a systematic review and meta-analysis of randomized controlled trials. JACC Cardiovasc Interv 2016;9:2124–33.

18. Haussig S, Mangner N, Dwyer MG, et al. Effect of a cerebral protection device on brain lesions following transcatheter aortic valve implantation in patients with severe aortic stenosis: the CLEAN-TAVI Randomized Clinical Trial. JAMA 2016;316: 592–601.

19. Seeger J, Gonska B, Otto M, et al. Cerebral embolic protection during transcatheter aortic valve replacement significantly reduces death and stroke compared with unprotected procedures. JACC Cardiovasc Interv 2017;10:2297–303.

20. Campelo-Parada F, Regueiro A, Dumont E, et al. Embolic protection in patients undergoing transaortic transcatheter aortic valve replacement: initial experience with the TriGuard HDH embolic deflection device. J Card Surg 2016;31:617–22.

21. Lansky AJ, Schofer J, Tchetche D, et al. A prospective randomized evaluation of the TriGuard HDH embolic DEFLECTion device during transcatheter aortic valve implantation: results from the DEFLECT III trial. Eur Heart J 2015;36:2070–8.

22. Rodes-Cabau J, Kahlert P, Neumann FJ, et al. Feasibility and exploratory efficacy evaluation of the Embrella Embolic Deflector system for the prevention of cerebral emboli in patients undergoing transcatheter aortic valve replacement: the PROTAVI-C pilot study. JACC Cardiovasc Interv 2014;7:1146–55.

23. Lazar RM, Pavol MA, Bormann T, et al. Neurocognition and cerebral lesion burden in high-risk patients before undergoing transcatheter aortic valve replacement: insights from the SENTINEL trial. JACC Cardiovasc Interv 2018;11:384–92.

24. Maldonado Y, Baisden J, Villablanca PA, et al. General anesthesia versus conscious sedation for transcatheter aortic valve replacement-an analysis of current outcome data. J Cardiothorac Vasc Anesth 2018;32:1081–6.

25. Brecker SJ, Bleiziffer S, Bosmans J, et al. Impact of anesthesia type on outcomes of transcatheter aortic valve implantation (from the multicenter ADVANCE study). Am J Cardiol 2016;117:1332–8.

26. Patel PA, Ackermann AM, Augoustides JGT, et al. Anesthetic evolution in transcatheter aortic valve replacement: expert perspectives from high-volume academic centers in Europe and the United States. J Cardiothorac Vasc Anesth 2017;31:777–90.

27. Cerrato E, Nombela-Franco L, Nazif TM, et al. Evaluation of current practices in transcatheter aortic valve implantation: the WRITTEN (WoRldwIde TAVI ExperieNce) survey. Int J Cardiol 2017;228:640–7.

28. Villablanca PA, Mohananey D, Nikolic K, et al. Comparison of local versus general anesthesia in patients undergoing transcatheter aortic valve replacement: a meta-analysis. Catheter Cardiovasc Interv 2018;91:330–42.

29. Neuburger PJ, Patel PA, Williams MR. Anesthetic technique for TAVR: more than just "tube" or "no tube". J Cardiothorac Vasc Anesth 2018;32:672–4.

30. Pani S, Cagino J, Feustel P, et al. Patient selection and outcomes of transfemoral transcatheter aortic valve replacement performed with monitored anesthesia care versus general anesthesia. J Cardiothorac Vasc Anesth 2017;31:2049–54.

31. D'Errigo P, Ranucci M, Covello RD, et al. Outcome after general anesthesia versus monitored anesthesia care in transfemoral transcatheter aortic valve replacement. J Cardiothorac Vasc Anesth 2016;30(5):1238–43.

32. Chen EY, Sukumar N, Dai F, et al. A pilot analysis of the association between types of monitored anesthesia care drugs and outcomes in transfemoral aortic valve replacement performed without general anesthesia. J Cardiothorac Vasc Anesth 2018;32:666–71.

33. Thiele H. SOLVE TAVI trial. Available at: https://www.tctmd.com/news/solve-tavi-tavr-equally-safe-balloon-self-expanding-valves-and-general-local-anesthesia 2018.
34. Hayek SS, Corrigan FE 3rd, Condado JF, et al. Paravalvular regurgitation after transcatheter aortic valve replacement: comparing transthoracic versus transesophageal echocardiographic guidance. J Am Soc Echocardiogr 2017;30: 533–40.
35. Hahn RT, Nicoara A, Kapadia S, et al. Echocardiographic imaging for transcatheter aortic valve replacement. J Am Soc Echocardiogr 2018;31:405–33.
36. Kadakia MB, Silvestry FE, Herrmann HC. Intracardiac echocardiography-guided transcatheter aortic valve replacement. Catheter Cardiovasc Interv 2015;85: 497–501.
37. Testa L, Latib A, Montone RA, et al. Transcatheter mitral valve regurgitation treatment: state of the art and a glimpse to the future. J Thorac Cardiovasc Surg 2016; 152:319–27.
38. Baumgartner H, Falk V, Bax JJ, et al. 2017 ESC/EACTS guidelines for the management of valvular heart disease: the Task Force for the Management of Valvular Heart Disease of the European Society of Cardiology (ESC) and the European Association for Cardio-Thoracic Surgery (EACTS). Eur Heart J 2017;38(36): 2739–91.
39. Nishimura RA, Otto CM, Bonow RO, et al. 2017 AHA/ACC focused update of the 2014 AHA/ACC guideline for the management of patients with valvular heart disease: a report of the American College of Cardiology/American Heart Association Task Force on Clinical Practice Guidelines. Circulation 2017;135:e1159–95.
40. Giannini C, D'Ascenzo F, Fiorelli F, et al. A meta-analysis of MitraClip combined with medical therapy vs. medical therapy alone for treatment of mitral regurgitation in heart failure patients. ESC Heart Fail 2018;5:1150–8.
41. Chiarito M, Pagnesi M, Martino EA, et al. Outcome after percutaneous edge-to-edge mitral repair for functional and degenerative mitral regurgitation: a systematic review and meta-analysis. Heart 2018;104:306–12.
42. Obadia JF, Messika-Zeitoun D, Leurent G, et al. Percutaneous repair or medical treatment for secondary mitral regurgitation. N Engl J Med 2018;379:2297–306.
43. Stone GW, Lindenfeld J, Abraham WT, et al. Transcatheter mitral-valve repair in patients with heart failure. N Engl J Med 2018;379(24):2307–18.
44. Praz F, Spargias K, Chrissoheris M, et al. Compassionate use of the PASCAL transcatheter mitral valve repair system for patients with severe mitral regurgitation: a multicentre, prospective, observational, first-in-man study. Lancet 2017; 390:773–80.
45. Messika-Zeitoun D, Nickenig G, Latib A, et al. Transcatheter mitral valve repair for functional mitral regurgitation using the Cardioband system: 1 year outcomes. Eur Heart J 2019;40:466–72.
46. Goldberg SL, Meredith I, Marwick T, et al. A randomized double-blind trial of an interventional device treatment of functional mitral regurgitation in patients with symptomatic congestive heart failure-Trial design of the REDUCE FMR study. Am Heart J 2017;188:167–74.
47. Bail DH. Treatment of functional mitral regurgitation by percutaneous annuloplasty using the Carillon Mitral Contour System-Currently available data state. J Interv Cardiol 2017;30:156–62.
48. Rogers JH, Thomas M, Morice MC, et al. Treatment of heart failure with associated functional mitral regurgitation using the ARTO system: initial results of the first-in-human MAVERIC trial (mitral valve repair clinical trial). JACC Cardiovasc Interv 2015;8:1095–104.

49. Rogers JH, Boyd WD, Smith TW, et al. Early experience with Millipede IRIS transcatheter mitral annuloplasty. Ann Cardiothorac Surg 2018;7:780–6.

50. Seeburger J, Rinaldi M, Nielsen SL, et al. Off-pump transapical implantation of artificial neo-chordae to correct mitral regurgitation: the TACT Trial (Transapical Artificial Chordae Tendinae) proof of concept. J Am Coll Cardiol 2014;63:914–9.

51. Colli A, Manzan E, Aidietis A, et al. An early European experience with transapical off-pump mitral valve repair with NeoChord implantation. Eur J Cardiothorac Surg 2018;54:460–6.

52. Gammie JS, Wilson P, Bartus K, et al. Transapical beating-heart mitral valve repair with an expanded polytetrafluoroethylene chordal implantation device: initial clinical experience. Circulation 2016;134:189–97.

53. Gammie JS, Bartus K, Gackowski A, et al. Beating-heart mitral valve repair using a novel ePTFE Cordal implantation device: a prospective trial. J Am Coll Cardiol 2018;71:25–36.

54. Regueiro A, Granada JF, Dagenais F, et al. Transcatheter mitral valve replacement: insights from early clinical experience and future challenges. J Am Coll Cardiol 2017;69:2175–92.

55. Urena M, Brochet E, Lecomte M, et al. Clinical and haemodynamic outcomes of balloon-expandable transcatheter mitral valve implantation: a 7-year experience. Eur Heart J 2018;39:2679–89.

56. Gregory SH, Sodhi N, Zoller JK, et al. Anesthetic considerations for the transcatheter management of mitral valve disease. J Cardiothorac Vasc Anesth 2019;33: 796–807.

57. de Waha S, Seeburger J, Ender J, et al. Deep sedation versus general anesthesia in percutaneous edge-to-edge mitral valve reconstruction using the MitraClip system. Clin Res Cardiol 2016;105:535–43.

58. Rassaf T, Balzer J, Rammos C, et al. Influence of percutaneous mitral valve repair using the MitraClip(R) system on renal function in patients with severe mitral regurgitation. Catheter Cardiovasc Interv 2015;85:899–903.

59. Hahn RT. Transcatheter valve replacement and valve repair: review of procedures and intraprocedural echocardiographic imaging. Circ Res 2016;119:341–56.

60. Mankad SV, Aldea GS, Ho NM, et al. Transcatheter mitral valve implantation in degenerated bioprosthetic valves. J Am Soc Echocardiogr 2018;31:845–59.

61. Wunderlich NC, Beigel R, Ho SY, et al. Imaging for mitral interventions: methods and efficacy. JACC Cardiovasc Imaging 2018;11:872–901.

62. Taramasso M, Alessandrini H, Latib A, et al. Outcomes after current transcatheter tricuspid valve intervention: mid-term results From the International TriValve Registry. JACC Cardiovasc Interv 2019;12(2):155–65.

63. Nickenig G, Kowalski M, Hausleiter J, et al. Transcatheter treatment of severe tricuspid regurgitation with the edge-to-edge MitraClip technique. Circulation 2017;135:1802–14.

64. Besler C, Orban M, Rommel KP, et al. Predictors of procedural and clinical outcomes in patients with symptomatic tricuspid regurgitation undergoing transcatheter edge-to-edge repair. JACC Cardiovasc Interv 2018;11:1119–28.

65. Besler C, Blazek S, Rommel KP, et al. Combined mitral and tricuspid versus isolated mitral valve transcatheter edge-to-edge repair in patients with symptomatic valve regurgitation at high surgical risk. JACC Cardiovasc Interv 2018;11: 1142–51.

66. Hahn RT, Leipsic J, Douglas PS, et al. Comprehensive echocardiographic assessment of normal transcatheter valve function. JACC Cardiovasc Imaging 2019;12:25–34.

New Techniques for Optimization of Donor Lungs/Hearts

Sue A. Braithwaite, MBChB[a],*, Niels P. van der Kaaij, PhD, MD[b]

KEYWORDS

- Optimization of heart and lung allografts • Lung transplantation
- Heart transplantation • EVLP • EVHP • Primary graft dysfunction • Novel therapies

KEY POINTS

- Primary graft dysfunction of both heart and lung allografts can have a disastrous effect on outcomes after transplantation.
- The injuries occurring in donor heart and lung allograft span the entire transplant process and are multiple and cumulative in nature. Donor, recipient, and preservation issues play a role.
- Marginal lung or heart allografts are more vulnerable to injury incurred during preservation and transplantation.
- Techniques to optimize donor heart and lung allograft preservation and function have a role in improving outcomes of transplantation and expanding the donor pool.
- There is great potential for future research into novel therapies to optimize donor heart and lung allografts. Ex vivo perfusion can play a vital role.

 Video content accompanies this article at www.anesthesiology.theclinics.com.

INTRODUCTION: CLINICAL RELEVANCE OF HEART AND LUNG TRANSPLANTATION

Lung transplantation is at present the only life-prolonging therapy for end-stage lung failure or end-stage vascular lung disease. A wide range of pathologic lung conditions can progress with varying speed to a situation whereby lung function can no longer support life. Affected patients benefit from lung transplantation, the use of lung allografts from deceased patients to replaced diseased lung(s) in the recipient.

Owing to advances in surgical technique, perioperative support, and immunosuppressive therapies, lung transplantation is now an accepted and widely used

Disclosure Statement: Both authors have no disclosures.
[a] Department of Anesthesiology, University Medical Center Utrecht, Mail Stop Q04.2.317, Postbus 85500, Utrecht 3508 GA, The Netherlands; [b] Department of Cardiothoracic Surgery, University Medical Center Utrecht, Room E03.511, Heidelberglaan 100, Utrecht 3584 CX, The Netherlands
* Corresponding author.
E-mail address: s.a.braithwaite@umcutrecht.nl

https://doi.org/10.1016/j.anclin.2019.08.010
1932-2275/19/© 2019 The Authors. Published by Elsevier Inc. This is an open access article under the CC BY license (http://creativecommons.org/licenses/by/4.0/).
anesthesiology.theclinics.com

procedure. Annually, approximately 4100 lung transplants are performed worldwide[1] (**Fig. 1**, survival demonstrated in **Fig. 2**), a number that has stagnated in recent years because of a limit in the number of available donor lungs.

In contrast to end-stage respiratory failure, most patients with terminal heart failure have an alternative to heart transplant for the medium or long term in the form of mechanical circulatory support (MCS). One of the major indications for long-term MCS is to "bridge" the wait to transplantation for otherwise terminal heart-failure patients, offering the opportunity for clinical improvement and preventing worsening secondary end-organ damage. However, for younger patients, or patients who poorly tolerate MCS (eg, biventricular failure, or issues with MCS such as drive-line infections or gastrointestinal bleeding), heart transplant remains the preferred therapy. Annually, approximately 5000 heart transplants are performed worldwide (**Fig. 3**, with survival according to preoperative MCS support shown in **Fig. 4**).

The common themes dominating heart and lung transplantation are the shortage of standard donor organs (**Box 1**, **Table 1**) and an increasingly complex recipient population, both factors that adversely affect waiting-list and transplant outcomes. Fortunately, new techniques are being developed to optimize donor heart and lung allograft function to both improve outcome and quality of life after transplant and to expand the donor pool by using "nonstandard" or marginal allografts. This review explores the clinical relevance of donor heart and lung allograft injury, mechanisms of injury, and ways in which to optimize donor heart and lung allograft function.

CLINICAL RELEVANCE OF PRIMARY GRAFT DYSFUNCTION/FAILURE IN HEART TRANSPLANTATION

In 2011 a definition of primary graft failure (PGF) after heart transplantation (HTx) was proposed based on a retrospective analysis of 621 consecutive heart transplants,[2] resulting in 4 criteria:

1. Significant impairment of systolic graft function affecting right, left or both ventricles during HTx or shortly thereafter

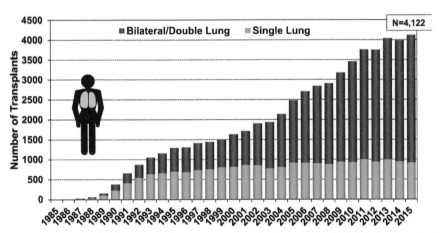

Fig. 1. Number of adult lung transplants reported to the International Society for Heart and Lung Transplantation Registry by year and procedure type. (*From* Chambers DC, Yusen RD, Cherikh WS, et al. The registry of the International Society for Heart and Lung Transplantation: Thirty-fourth Adult Lung And Heart-Lung Transplantation Report-2017; Focus Theme: Allograft ischemic time. J Heart Lung Transplant 2017;36(10):1048; with permission.)

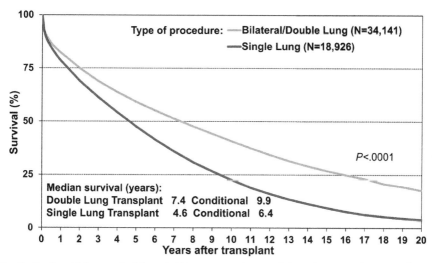

Fig. 2. Kaplan-Meier survival for adult lung transplant recipients by procedure type (transplants: 1990 to June 2015). Conditional median survival is the estimated time to 50% survival for the subset of recipients alive at 1 year after transplantation (*P*<.0001 by log-rank test statistic). (*From* Chambers DC, Yusen RD, Cherikh WS, et al. The registry of the International Society for Heart and Lung Transplantation: Thirty-fourth Adult Lung And Heart-Lung Transplantation Report-2017; Focus Theme: Allograft ischemic time. J Heart Lung Transplant 2017;36(10):1048; with permission.)

2. Severe hemodynamic compromise lasting greater than 1 hour manifested as hypotension (systolic blood pressure <90 mm Hg) and/or low cardiac output (cardiac index <2.2 L/min/m^2) requiring ≥2 intravenous inotropic/pressor drugs, or MCS despite appropriate filling pressures

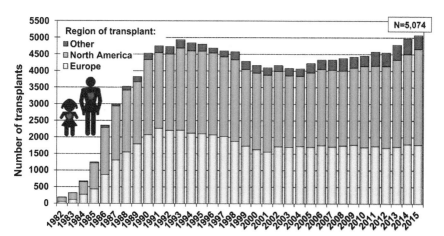

Fig. 3. Number of adult and pediatric heart transplants by year (transplants 1982–2015) and geographic region. (*From* Lund LH, Khush KK, Cherikh WS, et al. The registry of the International Society for Heart and Lung Transplantation: Thirty-fourth Adult Heart Transplantation Report-2017; Focus Theme: Allograft ischemic time. J Heart Lung Transplant 2017;36(10):1039; with permission.)

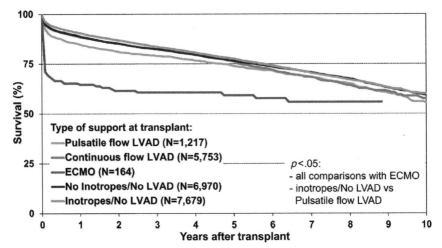

Fig. 4. Kaplan-Meier intermediate-term survival by pretransplant MCS use (adult heart transplants: January 2005 to June 2015). ECMO, extracorporeal membrane oxygenation; LVAD, left ventricular assist device. (*From* Lund LH, Khush KK, Cherikh WS, et al. The registry of the International Society for Heart and Lung Transplantation: Thirty-fourth Adult Heart Transplantation Report-2017; Focus Theme: Allograft ischemic time. J Heart Lung Transplant 2017;36(10):1039; with permission.)

3. Occurrence within 24 hours after HTx
4. Absence of any other obvious cause of graft dysfunction (hyperacute rejection, severe pulmonary hypertension, massive hemorrhage, and technical problems)

Building on this, the International Society for Heart and Lung Transplant (ISHLT) issued a report in 2014 on primary graft dysfunction after HTx.[3] Their classification and definition of severity scale for primary graft dysfunction is presented in **Box 2** and **Table 2**.

Box 1
Traditional cardiac donor selection criteria

Age less than 55 years

No history of chest trauma or cardiac disease

No prolonged hypotension or hypoxemia

Appropriate hemodynamics: mean arterial pressure greater than 60 mm Hg, central venous pressure 8 to 12 mm Hg

Inotropic support less than 10 mcg/kg/min (dopamine or dobutamine)

Normal electrocardiogram

Normal echocardiogram

Normal cardiac angiography (if indicated by donor age and history)

Negative serology (hepatitis B surface antigen, hepatitis C virus, and human immunodeficiency virus)

Adapted from Chiu P, Robbins RC, Ha R. Heart Transplantation. In: Sellke FW, del Nido PJ, Swanson SJ, editors. Sabiston & Spencer surgery of the chest, 9th edition. Philadelphia: Elsevier; 2016; with permission.

Table 1
Criteria used to assess donor lung suitability, defining a "standard lung donor"

Traditional Criteria (Standard Donor)	Extended Criteria (Marginal Donors)
Age ≤55 y	Age >70 y
Clear chest X-ray	Minor diffuse and moderate focal chest radiograph changes acceptable
Pao_2 ≥300 on Fio_2 = 1.0 and positive end-expiratory pressure (PEEP) 5 cm H_2O	Pao_2/Fio_2 <300 mm Hg on PEEP 5 cm H_2O
Tobacco history ≤20 pack yr	Tobacco history <40 pack yr
Absence of chest trauma	Chest trauma not relevant if good pulmonary function
No history of primary pulmonary disease or active pulmonary infection	
No evidence of aspiration/sepsis	Aspiration/sepsis acceptable if good, stable/improving pulmonary function
Absence of pulmonary secretions at bronchoscopy	Purulent secretions not relevant if good, stable/improving pulmonary function
No evidence for human immunodeficiency virus, hepatitis B, hepatitis C, or any other relevant viral disease	
No history or evidence of malignant disease	
ABO compatibility	
Sputum Gram stains: absence of organisms	

From Van Raemdonck D, Coosemans W, Klepetko W, et al. Alternatives to lung donor shortage. Eur Respir Mon 2004;29:89–112. Reproduced with permission of the © ERS 2019.

PGF is the leading cause of early mortality in HTx, accounting for more than 35% of deaths within 30 days postoperatively.[4] Using the PGF criteria from 2011, a study by the same group looked at the incidence of PGF in a multicenter cohort of 857 heart transplants.[5] The incidence of PGF was 22% with a corresponding early mortality of 53%, compared with 7% in patients without PGF (P = .001).

CLINICAL RELEVANCE OF PRIMARY GRAFT DYSFUNCTION IN LUNG TRANSPLANTATION

PGD after lung transplantation describes a clinical syndrome of varying degrees of hypoxemia together with presence of diffuse alveolar infiltrates on chest radiography. In

Box 2
Classification of graft dysfunction after heart transplantation

1. Primary graft dysfunction (PGD):
   a. PGD in left ventricle (PGD-LV): includes left and biventricular dysfunction
   b. PGD in right ventricle (PGD-RV): Includes right ventricular function alone

2. Secondary graft dysfunction: occurs when there is a discernible cause for graft dysfunction (eg, hyperacute rejection, pulmonary hypertension, known surgical complication)

From Kobshigawa J, Zuckermann A, Macdonald P, et al. Report from a consensus conference on primary graft dysfunction after cardiac transplantation. J Heart Lung Transplant 2014;33(4):337; with permission.

Table 2
Definition of severity scale for primary graft dysfunction after heart transplantation

1. PGD in left ventricle (PGD-LV)	*Mild PGD-LV*: one of the following criteria must be met:	LVEF <40% by echocardiography, *or* hemodynamics with RAP >15 mm Hg, PCWP >20 mm Hg, CI <2.0 L/min/m^2 (lasting more than 1 h) requiring low-dose inotropes
	Moderate PGD-LV: must meet one criteria from I and another criteria from II	I. One criterion from the following: • Left ventricular ejection fraction <40%, *or* • Hemodynamic compromise with RAP >15 mm Hg, PCWP >20 mm Hg, CI <2.0 L/min/m^2, hypotension with MAP <70 mm Hg (lasting more than 1 h) II. One criterion from the following: i. High-dose inotropes ii. Newly placed IAPB (regardless of inotropes)
	Severe PGD-LV	Dependence on left or biventricular mechanical support including ECMO, LVAD, BiVAD, or percutaneous LVAD. Excludes requirement for IABP
2. PGD in right ventricle (PGD-RV)	Diagnosis requires either both i and ii, or iii alone:	i. Hemodynamics with RAP >15 mm Hg, PCWP <15 mm Hg, CI <2.0 L/min/m^2 ii. TPG <15 mm Hg and/or pulmonary artery systolic pressure <50 mm Hg, *or* iii. Need for RVAD

Abbreviations: BiVAD, biventricular assist device; CI, cardiac index; ECMO, extracorporeal membrane oxygenation; IABP, intra-aortic balloon pump; LVAD, left ventricular assist device; LVEF, left ventricular ejection fraction; PCWP, pulmonary capillary wedge pressure; RAP, right atrial pressure; RVAD, right ventricular assist device; TPG, transpulmonary pressure gradient.

Adapted from Kobshigawa J, Zuckermann A, Macdonald P, et al. Report from a consensus conference on primary graft dysfunction after cardiac transplantation. J Heart Lung Transplant 2014;33(4):337; with permission.

2005 the first ISHLT Working Group on PGD proposed a standardized definition and grading system[6] (**Table 3**), and a validation of these definitions was performed in 2016.[7] They described that PGD grade 3 was associated with higher mortality in the acute phase after lung transplantation (PGD grade 3 72 hours post transplant was associated with 30-day mortality relative risk of 6.95 compared with no PGD), and that all grades of PGD were associated with greater risk of bronchiolitis obliterans syndrome development in survivors. The literature supports incidences of PGD of ~30% early after transplant and a 15% to 20% incidence of PGD grade 3 at 48 to 72 hours. The time course of PGD progression and resolution has an effect on patient survival outcomes, with patients experiencing severe, persistent PGD having the greatest mortality risk.[8]

Table 3		
Grades of primary graft dysfunction after lung transplantation		
Grade	Pao_2/Fio_2 Ratio	Radiographic Infiltrates Consistent with Pulmonary Edema
0	>300	Absent
1	>300	Present
2	200–300	Present
3	<200	Present

Adapted from Christie JD, Carby M, Bag R, et al. Report of the ISHLT working group on primary lung graft dysfunction part II: Definition. A consensus statement of the International Society for Heart and Lung Transplantation. J Heart Lung Transplant 2005;24(10):1458; with permission.

It is unequivocal that PGD in heart and lung allografts is an important factor in causing early mortality and morbidity and is also strongly associated with late-onset morbidity.[9] The goal of optimizing heart and lung donor allografts must then be to attenuate or treat the underlying causes of PGD. To achieve this, the mechanisms and timing of injury to heart and lung allografts must be identified.

RISK FACTORS FOR PRIMARY GRAFT DYSFUNCTION IN HEART AND LUNG ALLOGRAFTS

Although specific causes and associations have been linked to an increased risk of developing PGD after heart and lung transplant, similarities between the two exist in that a "multihit" model spanning the entire transplantation process may be envisaged. This multihit model may be seen as a heterogeneous, dynamic accumulation of different injuries incurred at different stages in the transplant process, involving:

- Donor comorbidity/social history
- Management of the donor patient
- The donation procedure
- Procurement and preservation of the donor organ
- Organ reperfusion in the recipient
- Recipient comorbidity
- Factors in the transplant procedure and postoperative phase

A large number of studies have highlighted the association of recipient-related risk factors with the development of PGD in lung transplantation. In a systemic review, the incidence of PGD was shown to be highest in patients with a pretransplant diagnosis of sarcoidosis (50%) or idiopathic pulmonary arterial hypertension (30.3%).[10] One study showed an increased risk of PGD of 30% for every 10 mm Hg increase in mean pretransplant pulmonary artery pressure.[11] Another study found that a combination of increased body mass index, moderate to severe pulmonary arterial hypertension, and a pretransplant diagnosis other than chronic obstructive pulmonary disease or cystic fibrosis could identify recipients at higher risk of PGD at 48 to 72 hours.[12]

With respect to donor-related post–lung transplant PGD risk factors, meta-analysis showed that donor cigarette smoking increased PGD risk mainly for "high-risk" recipients[12] while other probable risk factors include an undersized donor relative to the recipient.[8] Another systematic review showed that there was no association of the type of donation procedure, either donation after cardiac death (DCD) or donation after brain death (DBD) with PGD risk.[13]

Operative risk factors for PGD are previous pleurodesis in the recipient,[14] use of cardiopulmonary bypass during the procedure, large-volume intraoperative blood product transfusion, and a higher inspired oxygen fraction (Fio$_2$) at the time of donor lung reperfusion.[11]

There are numerous recurring donor-, intraoperative-, and recipient-related factors seen in the literature that may be linked to the development of PGD in heart allografts. Major recipient-related factors are linked to increasing age, presence of pulmonary arterial hypertension, and worse pretransplant clinical condition (including dependence on intravenous inotropic support, MCS, and mechanical ventilation).[3] The only validated scoring system for the prediction of PGD after HTx is the RADIAL score, which identified 6 factors with similar weight (risk ratio ~2), with 4 recipient-related factors (right atrial pressure >10 mm Hg, Age >60 years, diabetes, inotropic support dependence), 1 related to the donor (age >30 years), and 1 to the procedure (allograft ischemia time >240 minutes).[2] The presence of each of these factors adds 1 point to the total score. The score was validated in a large multicenter cohort showing 3 groups with low (0–1 points), medium (2 points), and high (≥3 points) risk for PGD with an actual incidence in each group of 12%, 19%, and 28%,[6] respectively.

CAUSES OF INJURY IN THE DONOR AND DURING THE DONATION PROCEDURE
Donation after Brain Death

In a donation procedure following DBD, organs are perfused and ventilated with oxygenated blood up until the moment of procurement. Despite this, DBD donor organs may suffer significant injury from numerous insults, including iatrogenic insults (eg, excessive fluid resuscitation or suboptimal ventilation) and injury incurred secondary to processes inherent in brain death. Brain death is associated with a series of events including intense release of myocardial norepinephrine, resulting in massive mitochondrial calcium overload.[15,16] This in turn may activate myocardial apoptosis or necrosis. Furthermore, a catecholamine storm also causes the activation of multiple proinflammatory mediators,[17] leading to numerous sequelae, including injury to lung epithelium and disruption of the capillary-alveolar membrane causing ("neurogenic") lung edema and acute lung injury.

Donation after Determination of Cardiac Death

Uniform agreement on DCD donor candidacy includes ventilator-dependent individuals with nonrecoverable or irreversible neurologic injury not meeting brain death criteria. Such DCD donors, awaiting cardiac death in a controlled (typically intensive care unit [ICU]) setting, are denoted as "Maastricht category III" donors (with categories I, II, IV, and V being in "uncontrolled" settings[18]). After the withdrawal of life-sustaining therapy (WLST) in these donors, functional warm ischemia time (WIT) starts when the hemodynamic status reaches critical levels for satisfactory organ perfusion, denoted by a systolic pressure of ≤50 mm Hg. After the cessation of circulation (cardiopulmonary arrest), a locally determined "no-touch" time interval, typically 5 minutes, will ensue after which verification of death is performed, and the donation procedure may begin. The end of the WIT is denoted by the start of the cold preservation flush in the donor organ. DCD donor organs inevitably suffer hypoxia and hypoperfusion during progression to circulatory arrest and the "no-touch" period of warm, pulseless ischemia. Despite this, and because lungs may be able to better tolerate warm ischemia owing to low metabolic needs and localized storage of oxygen trapped in alveoli, evidence shows that lung allografts show acceptable outcomes after DCD procedures. The 2015 ISHLT DCD Registry Report compared DCD and matched DBD lung transplants and observed a comparable 5-year survival in both groups.[19]

TARGETS FOR OPTIMIZATION OF HEART AND LUNG ALLOGRAFTS IN THE DONOR

Management of both DBD and DCD donors to optimize cardiac and pulmonary function and to limit organ injury in the donor milieu requires hemodynamic, neuroendocrine, and organ-specific approaches. **Table 4** outlines the standard therapies available to optimize allograft function in the donor.[20]

In 2009, a multicenter randomized controlled trial comparing a lung protective ventilation (LPV) strategy with conventional ventilation strategies in DBD donors showed that an LPV strategy improved the preharvest Pao_2/Fio_2 ratio in comparison with conventional ventilation practices.[21,22] The recommended ventilation strategy for donors (**Table 5**)[23] suggests that appropriate LPV plays an important role in attenuating lung injury and optimizing donor lungs.

CAUSES OF INJURY DURING ALLOGRAFT PRESERVATION: STATIC COLD STORAGE

Traditionally, heart and lung allografts are preserved after the initiation of hypothermic (and in the case of heart allografts, cardioplegic) arrest of cell function by static cold storage. This involves the rapid flushing and cooling of the organ with an adapted crystalloid-based fluid, which optimally confers the following protection of the organ:

- Minimizes hypothermia-induced cell injury
- Buffers intracellular acidosis

Table 4	
Standard approach to donor management, and optimizing heart and lung allografts	
Hemodynamics	
Hypovolemic shock	i. Crystalloid repletion to achieve euvolemia ii. Consider albumin 5% for fluid resuscitation iii. Avoid hydroxyethyl starch fluid resuscitation
Vasodilatory shock	i. Goal central venous pressure 6–8 mm Hg ii. Goal mean arterial pressure >60 mm Hg iii. Vasopressin 0.01–0.04 IU/min to maintain hemodynamic goals iv. Consider the administration of inotropes to support LV systolic and diastolic function with excessive fluid requirements
Cardiac shock	i. Consider placement of pulmonary artery catheter to tailor therapy ii. Inotropes to optimize central venous pressure, mean arterial pressure, and mixed oxygen saturation
Hormonal	
Diabetes insipidus (BDB donor)	i. Vasopressin 0.01–0.04 IU/min, consider higher doses with caution ii. Desmopressin if persistent ongoing diabetes insipidus with sodium >145–150 mmol/L
Adrenal insufficiency	Intravenous methylprednisolone 15 mg/kg
Thyroid deficiency	Consider intravenous T3 (4 μg bolus then 3 μg/h) or T4 (20 μg bolus then 10 μg/h) in unstable donor despite hemodynamic optimization
Hyperglycemia	Consider standard ICU management protocol

Adapted from Courtwright A, Cantu E. Evaluation and management of the potential lung donor. Clin Chest Med 2017;38(4):755; with permission.

Table 5
The recommended lung-protective ventilation strategy in potential lung donors

Objective	Parameters Adjusted
Prevention of alveolar overdistention	Tidal volume 6–8 mL/kg IBW, plateau pressure <30 cm H_2O
Maintain alveolar recruitment	Adequate PEEP 8–10 cm H_2O
Prevention of oxygen toxicity	Lowest Fio_2 (≤ 0.5) to keep Spo_2 92%–95%

Abbreviations: IBW, ideal body weight; PEEP, positive end-expiratory pressure; Spo_2, oxygen saturation by pulse oximetry.
Adapted from Mascia L, Pasero D, Slutsky AS, et al. Effect of a lung protective strategy for organ donors on eligibility and availability of lungs for transplantation: a randomized controlled trial. JAMA 2010;304(23):2620–7.

- Prevents expansion of the extracellular space by optimizing oncotic pressure
- Prevents injury from oxygen free radicals
- Prevents reperfusion damage caused by depletion of ATP stores

Static cold storage limits the storage time to a maximum of 4 to 6 hours in heart allografts and approximately 6 to 10 hours in lung allografts. In an ISHLT registry report examining the relationship between outcome of HTx and ischemia time of the allograft,[4] an allograft ischemia time of less than 4 hours was associated with considerably higher survival than an allograft ischemia time of ≥ 4 hours.[4,24] Heart allografts exposed to longer periods of cold ischemia have been shown to confer worse survival in the years post transplant when compared with hearts subjected to shorter cold storage times (**Fig. 5**).

Lung allografts can survive better for longer in cold storage owing to the presence of small stores of oxygen trapped in the alveoli when lungs are preserved in a

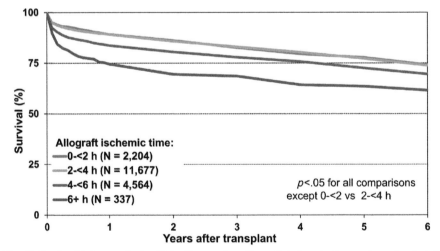

Fig. 5. Kaplan-Meier survival within 6 years by allograft ischemic time categories (adult heart transplants; January 2009 to June 2015). (*From* Lund LH, Khush KK, Cherikh WS, et al. The registry of the International Society for Heart and Lung Transplantation: Thirty-fourth Adult Heart Transplantation Report-2017; Focus Theme: Allograft ischemic time. J Heart Lung Transplant 2017;36(10):1044; with permission.)

semi-inflated state. However, longer ischemia times are associated with poorer 30-day survival post transplant[1] (**Fig. 6**).

This time limit of effectiveness of cold storage geographically confines the donor pool available to a specific recipient, and is also a serious clinical problem if surgical preparation in the recipient is complex and reperfusion of the allograft is delayed. Examples of this are redo sternotomies in heart transplant recipients (eg, explantation of MCS) or pneumonectomy following pleurodesis in lung transplantation.

It is therefore necessary to develop ways of extending the time allografts can be safely preserved. However, other questions also drive the development of alternative methods of allograft preservation:

- Are there ways of functionally assessing allografts in an ex vivo setting?
- Are there techniques available to better preserve and treat allografts to attenuate injury and improve function following implantation?

ALTERNATIVES TO COLD STORAGE ORGAN PRESERVATION
Preservation of Heart Allografts

The feasible alternatives to static cold storage confer differing potential advantages. First, continuous or repetitive cold perfusion of heart allografts during preservation allows one to extend the preservation time. In an experimental porcine model, donor hearts preserved for 24 hours were transplanted and showed acceptable function.[25]

The second alternative is to preserve heart allografts in a functioning, warm state.[26] A platform for ex vivo heart perfusion (EVHP) has been developed and is in clinical use (Organ Care System [OCS]; Transmedics, **Fig. 7**). This facilitated a prospective, randomized, noninferiority trial (PROCEED II trial)[27] comparing standard cold cardioplegic storage of human donor hearts with beating-heart allografts perfused and preserved ex vivo at normothermia with the OCS. In the standard group, the cold ischemia

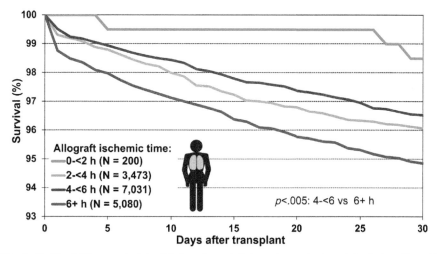

Fig. 6. Kaplan-Meier survival to 30 days for adult lung transplant recipients by allograft ischemic time (transplants: 2009 to June 2015). Log-rank test statistic with adjustments for multiple comparisons using the Scheffe method. (*From* Chambers DC, Yusen RD, Cherikh WS, et al. The registry of the International Society for Heart and Lung Transplantation: Thirty-fourth Adult Lung And Heart-Lung Transplantation Report-2017; Focus Theme: Allograft ischemic time. J Heart Lung Transplant 2017;36(10):1052; with permission.)

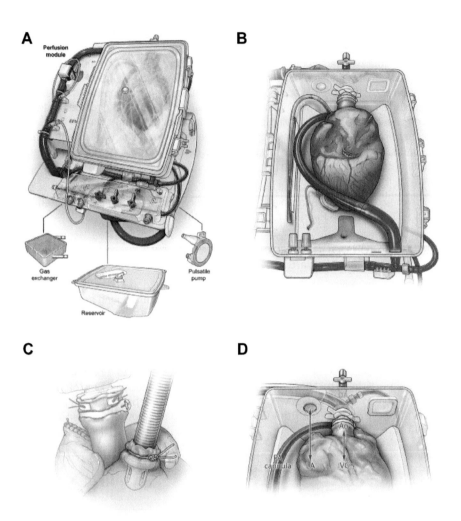

Fig. 7. Ex vivo heart perfusion (EVHP). EVHP is a platform providing the opportunity to perfuse, optimize, preserve in beating-heart state, and assess donor hearts. The only platform currently in clinical use is the Organ Care System, a portable system designed to be taken to the donor hospital and used directly after procurement of the donor heart. (*A*) Depiction of components. (*B*) Placement of donor heart within perfusion module. (*C*) Positioning of pulmonary artery cannula. (*D*) Ascending aortic cannula. (*From* Chan JL, Kobashigawa JA, Reich HJ, et al. Intermediate outcomes with ex-vivo allograft perfusion for heart transplantation. J Heart Lung Transplant 2017;36(3):259; with permission; and *Courtesy of* TransMedics, Andover, MA.)

time was 195 minutes and the 30-day patient and graft survival rate was 97% (n = 61). In the OCS group, the cold ischemia time was 113 minutes with a 30-day patient and graft survival of 94% (n = 63) (P = .45). Rates of cardiac-related adverse events, incidence of severe rejection, and length of ICU stay did not differ significantly between the groups.

The opportunity to limit the cold storage time and to biochemically functionally assess donor hearts on the OCS has emboldened the use of "extended criteria" heart allografts in HTx. A single-center experience described the use of EVHP in high-risk heart transplant procedures,[28] defining high risk as either donor-related factors (estimated ischemic time >4 hours, left ventricular ejection fraction [LVEF] <50%, left ventricular hypertrophy, donor cardiac arrest, alcohol/drug abuse, and coronary artery disease) or recipient factors (MCS, elevated pulmonary vascular resistance, or both). Thirty hearts were preserved with the OCS, of which 26 were transplanted. Only one death was observed within the first year, with the remaining 25 patients demonstrating a well-preserved biventricular allograft function (LVEF of 66.3% ± 5.6%, mean longitudinal right ventricular systolic function of 13.6 ± 3.1 mm). This result demonstrates the role EVHP can play in optimizing outcome in "high-risk" heart transplant procedures, possibly by attenuating injury in "extended criteria" allografts, and allows investigators to explore the possibility of using heart allografts from DCD donors.

Traditionally, heart allografts from DCD donors have been considered unsuitable for transplantation because of the warm ischemia to which the allografts are exposed. The period between the withdrawal of life support and organ harvesting subjects the heart allografts to multiple injuries, including hypoxia, hypoperfusion, and ventricular distension. One study investigated the role of EVHP in DCD HTx in a porcine model looking at DCD hearts exposed to 30 minutes of warm ischemia, which were then preserved with either 4 hours of EVHP or 4 hours of standard cold storage.[29] Five of 6 hearts in the EVHP group displayed favorable lactate profiles during EVHP and were successfully weaned off cardiopulmonary bypass. All hearts transplanted from the cold storage group demonstrated acute severe PGD and could not be weaned. This beneficial role of EVHP in DCD heart allografts is thought to be linked to the restoration of perfusion enabling the return of aerobic cell metabolism and replenishment of cellular nutrients. This prevents ongoing ischemic injury and the reperfusion injury that follows.

In a study in humans comparing the outcome after HTx from DCD and DBD donors,[30] EVHP was used for normothermic preservation, transport, and biochemical assessment in all DCD hearts. DCD heart retrieval used one of two differing techniques: normothermic regional perfusion (NRP) or direct procurement and perfusion (DPP). NRP describes a technique whereby perfusion is restored to the arrested heart while still in situ (with exclusion of the cerebral circulation). This approach enables post–warm-ischemia functional assessment of the heart in the donor by pulmonary artery catheter measurements and transesophageal echocardiography. This technique, however, is limited in numerous countries by ethical objection to the restoration of circulation in a deceased donor. The alternative to NRP is DPP, whereby the heart is removed directly after flush with a cold cardioplegia solution and installed and reperfused on EVHP. In DPP, functional assessment of the DCD heart is not possible and, therefore, levels of biomarkers in the EVHP perfusate are used to reflect allograft viability. The study was a single-center observational matched cohort study to compare patients who received transplants of DCD donor hearts with matched recipients who received transplants of DBD donor hearts. Twenty-eight DCD heart transplants were performed with almost equal numbers of DCD hearts procured by either NRP or DPP. Survival at 90 days (DCD 92%, DBD 96%, $P = 1.0$), hospital length of stay, allograft function, and 1-year survival (DCD 86%, DBD 88%, $P = .98$) were comparable between groups. The retrieval method (NRP vs DPP) was not associated with a difference in outcome. Early cardiac output was, however, better in the DCD group (2.5 vs 2.0 L/min/m^2, $P = .04$), possibly explained by the avoidance of myocardial injury caused by the catecholamine storm during brain death in DBD donors and/or a possible effect of ischemic preconditioning after WLST in DCD donors.

Developments and Controversies in Ex Vivo Heart Perfusion

At present, clinical assessment of the allograft during EVHP relies on sampling lactate levels from the aortic root and pulmonary artery cannulas, using lactate trends as a surrogate for myocardial viability. Other biomarkers of myocardial injury, such a troponin, are of limited use[31] given their elevation caused by nonspecific stresses during donation procedures. Currently there are no modalities to functionally assess heart allografts on EVHP, primarily as it is not possible to fully load and challenge a heart allograft on the OCS platform. Alternative platforms aiming to preserve heart allografts in a beating state while assessing function using pressure-volume loops generated under clinical loading conditions are being investigated.

Myocardial edema has been identified as an issue associated with prolonged preservation of heart allografts on EVHP, although it is uncertain whether the weight gain of the allograft translates to adverse outcomes.[31] To attenuate myocardial edema, alternatives to the current perfusion solution and technique are being explored, aiming to optimize the oncotic pressures of the perfusion fluid and attempting to improve diastolic coronary perfusion while limiting excessive aortic root pressures.[32]

ALTERNATIVES TO COLD STORAGE ORGAN PRESERVATION
Preservation of Lung Allografts

Cold storage is an acceptable method of preserving donor lungs provided that minimal injury has been incurred in the donor and that the ischemia times are not excessively long. There are, however, techniques offering alternatives to static cold storage, which have come through several noninferiority trials[33,34] and which play vital roles in the use of marginal lung allografts.

The techniques make use of ex vivo lung perfusion (EVLP) technology enabling the perfusion, rewarming, and ventilation of donor lungs in a controlled setting. The first EVLP technique (Lund protocol) was originally designed with the intent of short-term evaluation of DCD lungs ex vivo[35]:

- Lund protocol
  - Open left atrium
  - Perfusate with type-matched red blood cells
  - Performed on a static protocol-specific integrated system (Vivoline, XVIVO).

In 2016 a single-center study compared the short-term and long-term outcomes of recipients transplanted with initially rejected-for-transplant lungs that were then subjected to EVLP using the Lund protocol (n = 27) with recipients of non-EVLP (standard) lungs (n = 145) during the same period. There was no significant difference between short-term and long-term outcomes between the 2 groups.[36]

To achieve stable ex vivo perfusion of lungs for periods of up to 12 hours, the Toronto group developed several lung-protective strategies as additions to the Lund protocol,[37,38] including reducing the flow through the lungs from 100% of the predicted cardiac output to 40% with the aim of reducing the incidence of hydrostatic lung edema:

- Toronto protocol (**Fig. 8**)
  - Acellular perfusate
  - Closed left atrium
  - Performed on a static system encompassing equipment consisting of either individual parts or integrated in one unit (XPS perfusion system, XVIVO)

Furthermore, they preserved the left atrium in a closed state, facilitating maintenance of a positive left atrial pressure of 3 to 5 mm Hg during EVLP. This approach

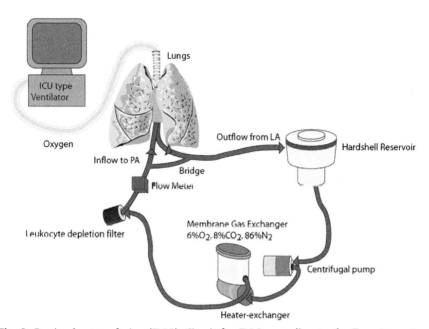

Fig. 8. Ex vivo lung perfusion (EVLP). Circuit for EVLP according to the Toronto protocol. EVLP is performed according to 3 protocols: the Toronto, Lund, and Organ Care System protocols. These protocols describe the perfusion and ventilation strategies of donor lungs (based on the predicted body weight of the donor). All protocols use a technique to deoxygenate the perfusate leaving the left atrium. The function of the donor lungs to oxygenate the perfusate is then possible by comparing the oxygen content of perfusate in the left atrium and pulmonary artery. Indications for EVLP: a poor to worsening Pao_2/Fio_2 ratio in the donor (<300 with a positive end-expiratory pressure of 5 cm H_2O and an Fio_2 of 1.0), a requirement to functionally assess the lungs, and logistics. Contraindications to EVLP: aspiration, bilateral infection, and diffuse traumatic contusion. The goals of the EVLP include functional assessment, improvement of lung function to a stable and sustainable situation, and protection from further injury. Lungs are assessed and accepted according to major criteria, which reflect the ability of the lungs to perform adequate gas exchange and also include assessment of the pulmonary vascular resistance and compliance of the lungs. A plain radiograph may aid in determining the etiology of lung injury. (*Adapted from* Cypel M, Yeung JC, Hirayama S, et al. Technique for prolonged normothermic ex vivo lung perfusion. J Heart Lung Transplant 2008;27(12):1320; with permission.)

was designed to tent open postcapillary venules in the lung and thus prevent their cyclical collapse, which occurs during ventilation. This adaptation was based on studies showing that absence of positive left atrial pressure can lead to unstable alveolar geometry[39] and a reduction in lung compliance.[40] The group published their first major study in 2011,[41] demonstrating that the incidence of PGD in high-risk donor lungs subjected to 4 hours of EVLP was comparable with that of conventional lung allografts (EVLP group n = 20 vs conventional lung group n = 116, incidence PGD III 15% vs 30% in the control group, P = .11). On the background of these positive clinical results, Slama and colleagues[34] investigated whether EVLP would affect or improve outcome when used for "standard" lung allografts. In a single-center trial, 41 standard lungs in a conventional (non-EVLP) group were compared with 39 standard lungs subjected to 4 hours of EVLP before transplantation. Although short-term clinical outcomes did not differ between the groups, the incidence of PGD (grade >1) was lower in the EVLP group at all time points compared with the control group (24 hours: 5.7% vs 19.5%, $P = .10$).

An alternative EVLP technique puts emphasis on reducing the cold ischemia time of lung allografts. A mobile EVLP unit (OCS system, Transmedics) has been developed to be taken to lung procurement procedures:

- OCS protocol
  - Open left atrium
  - Perfusate with type-matched red blood cells
  - Portable equipment designed to be taken to the donor hospital and run during the transport of donor lungs

After cold flush, donor lungs are installed on the EVLP unit, perfused, rewarmed, and ventilated. The lungs are then kept on the EVLP for normothermic perfusion during transport and preservation for up to 5 hours until the lungs are cooled for a short period of cold ischemia to facilitate the surgical implantation procedure. Similar to the study using the Toronto protocol, a multicenter noninferiority, randomized trial[33] (INSPIRE) comparing outcomes of transplant following preservation of standard lungs with either portable EVLP with the OCS (n = 141) or static cold storage (n = 165) demonstrated no clear short-term survival benefit from preservation with the OCS. However, there was a notable decrease in PGD in the EVLP arm of the study, with an incidence of PGD grade 3 within 72 hours post transplant of 17.7% in the OCS group and 29.7% in the static cold storage group ($P = .015$).

Developments and Controversies in Ex Vivo Lung Perfusion

A platform providing access to perfusate, substrate obtained by bronchoalveolar lavage, and lung tissue in the context of normothermic, functional preservation of donor lungs is a hugely welcome research tool in understanding the etiology and pathophysiology of donor lung injury.

Further research strategies of interest include the role of (ultra-)protective ventilation strategies of lungs during EVLP to attenuate lung injury and eventual lung-induced biotrauma. Targeted protective ventilation strategies adapted to the individual lung, including concepts of open lung ventilation and prone ventilation,[42] may lead to increased future use of marginal donor lungs (Video 1).

Still to be performed is a direct comparison of the EVLP protocols and platforms, and whether indeed certain platforms confer a clinically relevant optimization of allograft function in the context of specific injuries.

PERIOPERATIVE MANAGEMENT OF LUNG ALLOGRAFTS

Studies have shown that gradual reintroduction of blood flow during the reperfusion phase, over a 10-minute period, can significantly improve graft function.[43] This prevents reperfusion of cold, atelectatic lungs with full normothermic cardiac output, which can lead to epithelial shear stress injury,[44] inflammation, and lung edema.

In accordance with the principles of protective lung ventilation, the ventilation strategy after reperfusion of the lung allograft should maximize the tidal volume to 4 to 6 mL/kg predicted body weight of the donor. This also includes keeping the Fio_2 low during the early reperfusion period (ie, 0.21–0.5).[11]

Novel therapies for the optimization of donor lung function and attenuation of PGD are listed in **Table 6**. One of the most encouraging therapies is the prophylactic use of surfactant in donor lungs. A pilot study in 2017[45] investigated the presence of surfactant proteins in lung allografts and concurrent rate of PGD in the recipient. The results

Table 6
Novel therapies for the optimization of donor lung allograft function and the attenuation of primary graft dysfunction

Therapy	Rationale	Design	Results	References
N-acetylcysteine (intravenous)	Limit generation of reactive oxygen species (ROS)	Porcine model of lung transplant	NAC-treated animals developed less pulmonary edema as measured by EVLW index and less protein and inflammatory cytokines in BAL. NAC therapy to both donor and recipient improved oxygenation, airway pressure, and lung compliance	Inci et al,[48] 2010
Adenosine A2A receptor agonist (intravenous)	Limit ROS-dependent cytokine production by natural killer T cells via modulation of NAPDH oxidase 2 (NOX2)[54]	Murine hilar clamping model of EVLP and murine EVLP	limits IRI-mediated lung injury, less neutrophil inflammation, cytokine production, and pulmonary edema formation	Sharma et al,[49] 2016
Diannexin (recombinant homodimer of annexin V) via pulmonary flush and intravenous to the recipient at time of reperfusion	Inhibition of apoptosis	Rat model of lung transplantation	Reduced peak airway pressure, limited EVLW, attenuated proinflammatory cytokine production, suppressed apoptosis	Hashimoto et al,[50] 2016
α1-antitrypsin (A1AT) intravenous direct before ischemia	Inhibition of apoptosis	Rat IRI model,[51] pig model of lung transplantation[52]	Reduced pulmonary edema formation, reduced lung injury scores, improved Pao_2/Fio_2 ratios and lung compliance	Gao et al,[51] 2014; Iskender et al,[52] 2016

(continued on next page)

Table 6
(continued)

Therapy	Rationale	Design	Results	References
Soluble RAGE ligand (sRAGE)/RAGE knockout	Inhibiting receptor for advanced glycation end products (RAGE), a critical mediator of acute lung injury	Mouse model of IRI using hilar clamping	Less pulmonary edema and less histologic evidence of lung injury	Sternberg et al,[53] 2008
Aspirin and intrabronchial DNase I treatment	Reducing neutrophil extracellular trap formation, extracellular deposits of chromatin extruded by activated neutrophils, which sequester inflammatory mediators	Murine PGD model, BAL from human lung transplant recipients	Limited lung injury within 8 h of reperfusion, improved lung permeability, improved oxygenation	Sayah et al,[54] 2015
Mesenchymal stem (stromal) cells engineered to deliver IL-10	Using the anti-inflammatory and immunosuppressive effects of IL-10 (inhibiting cytokine synthesis, downgrades the expression of helper T cells)	Rat model of IRI	Improved oxygenation, reduced pulmonary edema, reduced apoptosis, and reduced T cell infiltration after hilar clamping	Manning et al,[55] 2010
Plasmin administration in the EVLP perfusate	Induces fibrinolysis, destroying (micro)thrombi in the donor lungs	Rat EVLP model	Improved pulmonary vascular res stance, improved lung compliance, and reduced pulmonary edema formation	Motoyama et al,[56] 2013
Prone ventilation	Protective lung ventilation strategy aimed at reducing or attenuating lung injury	Porcine EVLP model	Improved Pao_2/Fio_2 ratios, reduced extravascular lung water, lowered interleukin-1β levels	Niikawa et al,[42] 2019

Abbreviations: BAL, bronchoalveolar lavage; EVLW, extravascular lung water; IRI, ischemia-reperfusion injury; NAC, *N*-acetylcysteine.

showed that low levels of surfactant protein gene expression in the lung donor before preservation and implantation was linked to the development of PGD grade 3. Other studies showed that donor lungs exposed to endogenous surfactant before retrieval had significantly higher pulmonary function 1 month after transplantation, but that the benefit disappeared by the end of the first post-transplant year.[46] There remains, however, a lack of prospective, randomized studies regarding the use of surfactant in lung allografts and its role in the prevention or treatment of PGD.

PERIOPERATIVE MANAGEMENT OF HEART ALLOGRAFTS

If the factors linked to the development of PGD have been taken into account and, where possible, attenuated, the perioperative management of heart transplant recipients remains mainly supportive, ensuring adequate oxygen delivery to, and perfusion of, the heart allograft combined with optimizing and supporting other organ systems. In the case of the development of PGD, supportive treatment involves a combination of inotropes and pulmonary vasodilators.[47] If there is no response to escalating medical treatment, early initiation of short-term MCS is warranted.[3]

SUMMARY

Injuries sustained by donor heart and lung allografts during the transplantation process are multiple and cumulative. Optimization of allograft function plays an essential role in the short-term and long-term outcome of the recipient in terms of not only mortality and morbidity but also quality of life. Therapeutic targets to prevent or attenuate injury are to be found in the donor, during the preservation process, intraoperatively during transplantation, and in the postoperative management of the recipient. The newest and most promising methods of optimizing donor heart and lung allografts are to be found in alternative preservation strategies, which enable concomitant functional assessment of donor organs and also provide a modality to initiate therapies to treat injured allografts or prevent injury during reperfusion in the recipient.

SUPPLEMENTARY DATA

Supplementary data related to this article can be found online at https://doi.org/10.1016/j.anclin.2019.08.010.

REFERENCES

1. Chambers C, Yusen RD, Cherikh WS, et al. The registry of the ISHLT report—2017. J Heart Lung Transplant 2017;36(10):1047–59.
2. Segovia J, Cosío MD, Barceló JM, et al. RADIAL: a novel primary graft failure risk score in heart transplantation. J Heart Lung Transplant 2011;30(6):644–51.
3. Kobshigawa J, Zuckerman A, Macdonald P, et al. Report from a consensus conference on PGD after cardiac transplantation. J Heart Lung Transplant 2014; 33(4):327–40.
4. Lund LH, Khush KK, Cherikh WS, et al. The registry of the ISHLT report—2017. J Heart Lung Transplant 2017;36(10):1037–46.
5. Cosío MD, Gomez Bueno M, Almenar L, et al. Primary graft failure after heart transplantation. J Heart Lung Transplant 2013;32(12):1187–95.
6. Christie JD, Carby M, Bag R, et al. Report of the ISHLT working group on primary lung graft dysfunction part II: definition. J Heart Lung Transplant 2005;24(10): 1454–9.

7. Snell GI, Yusen RD, Weill D, et al. Report of the ISHLT working group on primary lung graft dysfunction, part I. J Heart Lung Transplant 2017;36(10):1097–103.

8. Diamond JM, Arcasoy S, Kennedy CC, et al. Report of the ISHLT working group on primary lung graft dysfunction, part II: epidemiology. J Heart Lung Transplant 2017;36(10):1104–13.

9. Whitson BA, Prekker ME, Herrington CS, et al. PGD and long-term pulmonary function after lung transplantation. J Heart Lung Transplant 2007;26:1004–11.

10. Liu Y, Lui Y, Su L, et al. Recipient-related clinical risk factors for PGD after lung transplantation. PLoS One 2014;9(3):e92773.

11. Diamond JM, Lee JC, Kawut SM, et al, Lung Transplant Outcomes Group. Clinical risk factors for PGD after lung transplantation. Am J Respir Crit Care Med 2013; 187(5):527–34.

12. Shah RJ, Diamond JM, Cantu E, et al. Objective estimates improve risk stratification for PGD after lung transplantation. Am J Transplant 2015;15:2188–96.

13. Krutsingcr D, Rccd RM, Blcvins A, ct al. Lung transplantation from donation after cardiac death. J Heart Lung Transplant 2015;34(5):675–84.

14. Shigemura N, Bhama J, Gries CJ, et al. Lung transplantation in patients with prior cardiothoracic surgical procedures. Am J Transplant 2012;12:1249–55.

15. Steen S, Sjöberg T, Liao Q, et al. Pharmacological normalization of circulation after acute brain death. Acta Anaesthesiol Scand 2012;56:1006–12.

16. Bezovic G, Steen S, Sjöberg T, et al. Circulation stabilizing therapy and pulmonary high-resolution CT in a porcine brain death model. Acta Anaesthesiol Scand 2015;60:93–102.

17. Atkinson C, FLoerchinger B, Qiao F, et al. Donor brain death exacerbates complement-dependent ischemia/reperfusion injury in transplanted hearts. Circulation 2013;127:1290–9.

18. Kootstra G, Daemen JH, Oomen AP. Categories of non-heart-beating donors. Transplant Proc 1995;27(5):2893–4.

19. Cypel M, Levvey BJ, van Raemdonck D, et al. ISHLT DCD registry report. J Heart Lung Transplant 2015;74:1278–82.

20. Courtwright A, Cantu E. Evaluation and management of the potential lung donor. Clin Chest Med 2017;38:751–9.

21. Mascia L, Pasero D, Slutsky AS, et al. Effect of a lung protective strategy for organ donors on eligibility and availability of lungs for transplantation. JAMA 2010; 304(23):2620–7.

22. Bansal R, Esan A, Hess D, et al. Mechanical ventilatory support in potential lung donor patients. Chest 2014;146(1):220–7.

23. Belzer FO, Southard JH. Principles of solid organ preservation by cold storage. Transplantation 1988;45:673–6.

24. Budrikis A, Bolys R, Liao Q, et al. Function of adult pig hearts after 2 and 12 hours of cold cardioplegic preservation. Ann Thorac Surg 1998;66:73–8.

25. Steen S, Paskevicius A, Liao Q, et al. Safe orthotopic transplantation of hearts harvested 24 hours after brain death and preserved for 24 hours. Scand Cardiovasc J 2016;50(3):193–200.

26. Hassanein WH, Zellos L, Tyrrell TA, et al. Continuous perfusion of donor hearts in the beating state extends preservation time and improves recovery of function. J Thorac Cardiovasc Surg 1998;116:821–30.

27. Ardehali A, Esmailian F, Deng M, et al. Ex-vivo perfusion of donor hearts for human heart transplantation (PROCEED II). Lancet 2015;385:2577–84.

28. Garcia Sáez D, Bartlomiej Z, Sabashnikov A, et al. Evaluation of the OCS in heart transplantation with an adverse donor/recipient profile. Ann Thorac Surg 2014;98: 2099–106.
29. Iyer A, Gao L, Doyle A, et al. Normothermic *ex vivo* perfusion provides superior organ preservation and enables viability assessment of hearts from DCD donors. Am J Transplant 2015;15:371–80.
30. Messer S, Page A, Axell R, et al. Outcome after heart transplantation from DCD donors. J Heart Lung Transplant 2017;36(12):1311–8.
31. Collins MJ, Moainie SL, Griffith BP, et al. Preserving and evaluating hearts with ex vivo machine perfusion. Eur J Cardiothorac Surg 2008;34:318–25.
32. Beuth J, Falter F, Pinto Ribeiro RV. New strategies to expand and optimize heart donor pool.ex vivo heart perfusion and donation after circulatory death: a review of current research and future trends. Anesth Analg 2019;128(3):406–13.
33. Warnecke G, Van Raemdonck D, Smith MA, et al. Normothermic ex-vivo preservation with portable OCS Lung device for bilateral lung transplantation (INSPIRE). Lancet Respir Med 2018;6:357–67.
34. Slama A, Schillab L, Barta M, et al. Standard donor lung procurement with normothermic EVLP. J Heart Lung Transplant 2017;36(7):744–53.
35. Steen S, Liao Q, Wierup PN, et al. Transplantation of lungs from non-heart-beating donors after functional assessment ex vivo. Ann Thorac Surg 2003;76:244–52.
36. Wallinder A, Riise GC, Ricksten SE, et al. Transplantation after EVLP. J Heart Lung Transplant 2016;35:1303–10.
37. Cypel M, Yeung JC, Hirayama S, et al. Technique for prolonged normothermic EVLP. J Heart Lung Transplant 2008;27:1319–25.
38. Cypel M, Keshavjee S. Extracorporeal lung perfusion (EVLP). Curr Opin Organ Transplant 2016;21:329–35.
39. Petak F, Habre W, Hantos Z, et al. Effect of pulmonary vascular pressures and flow on airway and parenchymal mechanics in isolated rat lungs. J Appl Physiol (1985) 2002;92:169–78.
40. Broccard AF, Vannay C, Feihl F, et al. Impact of low pulmonary vascular pressure on ventilator-induced lung injury. Crit Care Med 2002;30:2183–90.
41. Cypel M, Teung J, Liu M, et al. Normothermic EVLP in clinical lung transplantation. N Engl J Med 2011;364:1431–40.
42. Niikawa H, Okamoto T, Ayyat KA, et al. The protective effect of prone position on ischemia-reperfusion injury and lung function in an ex vivo porcine lung model. J Heart Lung Transplant 2019;157:425–33.
43. Bhabra MS, Hopkinson DN, Shaw TE, et al. Critical importance of the first 10 minutes of lung graft reperfusion after hypothermic storage. Ann Thorac Surg 1996; 61:1631–5.
44. Pierre AF, DeCampos KN, Liu M, et al. Rapid reperfusion causes stress failure in ischemic rat lungs. J Thorac Cardiovasc Surg 1998;116:932–42.
45. Belhaj A, Boven C, Dewachter L, et al. Influence of donor lung surfactant-A and -B protein expression on the development of PGD after lung transplantation. Ann Transplant 2017;22:361–9.
46. Strüber M, Fischer S, Niedermeyer J, et al. Effects of exogenous surfactant instillation in clinical lung transplantation. J Thorac Cardiovasc Surg 2007;133: 1620–5.
47. Rabin J, Kaczorowski DJ. Perioperative management of the cardiac transplant recipient. Crit Care Clin 2019;35:45–60.

48. Inci I, Eme B, Jungraithmayr W, et al. Prevention of PGD in lung transplantation by N-acetylcysteine after prolonged cold ischemia. J Heart Lung Transplant 2010; 29(11):1293–301.
49. Sharma AK, LaPar DJ, Stone ML, et al. NOX2 activation of natural killer T cells is blocked by the adenosine A2A receptor to inhibit lung ischemia-reperfusion injury. Am J Respir Crit Care Med 2016;193(9):988–99.
50. Hashimoto K, Kim H, Oishi H, et al. Annexin V homodimer protects against ischemia-induced acute lung injury in lung transplantation. J Thorac Cardiovasc Surg 2016;151(3):861–9.
51. Gao W, Zhao J, Kim H, et al. alpha1-antitrypsin inhibits ischemia reperfusion-induced lung injury by reducing inflammatory response and cell death. J Heart Lung Transplant 2014;33(3):309–15.
52. Iskender I, Sakamoto J, Nakajima D, et al. Human alpha1-antitrypsin improves early post-transplant lung function. J Heart Lung Transplant 2016;35(7):913–21.
53. Sternberg DI, Gowda R, Mehra D, et al. Blockade of receptor for advanced gly-cation end product attenuates pulmonary reperfusion injury in mice. J Thorac Cardiovasc Surg 2008;136(6):1576–85.
54. Sayah DM, Mallavia B, Liu F, et al. Neutrophil extracellular traps are pathogenic in PGD after lung transplantation. Am J Respir Crit Care Med 2015;191(4):455–63.
55. Manning E, Pham S, Li S, et al. Interleukin-10 delivery via mesenchymal stem cells. Hum Gene Ther 2010;21(6):713–27.
56. Motoyama H, Chen F, Oshumi A, et al. Protective effect of plasmin in marginal donor lungs in an EVLP model. J Heart Lung Transplant 2013;32(5):505–10.

Ethical Considerations for Mechanical Support

Darryl Abrams, MD[a,*], J. Randall Curtis, MD, MPH[b], Kenneth M. Prager, MD[c],
A. Reshad Garan, MD[d], Jonathan Hastie, MD[e], Daniel Brodie, MD[a]

KEYWORDS

- Extracorporeal life support • ECMO • Ethics • Bridge to nowhere
- Withdrawal of life support

KEY POINTS

- Extracorporeal life support can support circulation and gas exchange in patients with severe cardiopulmonary failure.
- Extracorporeal life support in respiratory failure can be a bridge to recovery or a bridge to transplantation; in cardiac failure, it can be a bridge to recovery, a ventricular assist device, or transplantation.
- A "bridge to nowhere" refers to the situation in which patients dependent on extracorporeal life support can neither recover nor undergo transplantation.
- Where it is serving only as a bridge to nowhere, removing the device against the express wishes of a sentient patient violates autonomy and, although opinions vary, some consider doing so to be unethical.
- Extracorporeal life support has made determination of circulatory or neurologic death more challenging and calls attention to issues of potentially inappropriate care and medical futility.

INTRODUCTION

Extracorporeal life support (ECLS) refers to the use of mechanical devices designed to maintain gas exchange and circulation even in severe forms of respiratory and cardiac

Disclosure Statement: D. Brodie reports fees to his university from ALung Technologies, personal fees from Baxter, and anticipated fees from BREETHE, outside the submitted work. All other authors have no conflicts of interest to report.
[a] Division of Pulmonary, Allergy, and Critical Care, Columbia University College of Physicians and Surgeons, 622 West 168th Street, PH 8E, 101, New York, NY 10032, USA; [b] Division of Pulmonary and Critical Care Medicine, Harborview Medical Center, University of Washington, 325 Ninth Avenue, Box 359762, Seattle, WA 98104, USA; [c] Division of Pulmonary, Allergy, and Critical Care, Columbia University College of Physicians and Surgeons, 161 Ft. Washington Avenue, Room 307, New York, NY 10032, USA; [d] Division of Cardiology, Columbia University College of Physicians and Surgeons, 177 Ft. Washington Avenue, 5th Floor, Room 5-435, New York, NY 10032, USA; [e] Department of Anesthesiology, Columbia University College of Physicians and Surgeons, 622 West 168th Street, PH 5-505, New York, NY 10032, USA
* Corresponding author.
E-mail address: da2256@cumc.columbia.edu

Anesthesiology Clin 37 (2019) 661–673
https://doi.org/10.1016/j.anclin.2019.08.001
1932-2275/19/© 2019 Elsevier Inc. All rights reserved.
anesthesiology.theclinics.com

failure. With technological improvements, there has been increasing adoption of ECLS in the management of patients for whom conventional management strategies alone are inadequate or suboptimal.[1,2] For example, in severe cases of the acute respiratory distress syndrome in which invasive mechanical ventilation may be unable to maintain adequate gas exchange, or can do so only at the expense of exacerbating lung injury, ECLS can correct hypoxemia and hypoventilation, facilitate more protective ventilator settings, and may improve mortality.[3,4] In severe, refractory cardiogenic shock, ECLS and ventricular assist devices (VADs) both have the ability to maintain systemic circulation and end-organ perfusion beyond what can be accomplished with medical management alone.[5]

The indications, contraindications, and optimal patient populations remain a source of debate in the medical community, especially when considering the resource-intensive nature of the technology and the severity of illness of the patient population. Patients who would normally not be able to survive with severe, refractory respiratory failure or cardiogenic shock often are able to be sustained with ECLS for prolonged periods of time, and have even recovered. However, despite the great potential for efficacy of ECLS in patients with cardiopulmonary failure, there remains uncertainty in predicting who will benefit and in determining how long patients should be supported when prognosis remains uncertain. One particularly vexing dilemma is what to do when a patient cannot recover or undergo transplantation, but is unable to survive without extracorporeal support. For these reasons, specific ethically challenging situations may arise with the use of ECLS—particularly in the context of initiation, management, and withdrawal of life-sustaining therapy—when compared with other technologies and procedures in medicine.[6] When considering the use of ECLS in patients with cardiopulmonary failure, it is important to anticipate and mitigate these scenarios, whenever possible.[6]

ETHICAL DILEMMAS IN EXTRACORPOREAL LIFE SUPPORT FOR RESPIRATORY FAILURE

ECLS is a temporary form of support for patients with respiratory failure, with 2 broad categories of indications. When ECLS is instituted for acute, potentially reversible, respiratory failure (eg, acute respiratory distress syndrome), where the ultimate goal is native lung recovery, it is referred to as a bridge to recovery (BTR). Alternatively, when the patient has advanced, irreversible lung disease, ECLS may be used as a bridge to transplantation (BTT). Because there is no long-term form of ECLS (ie, destination device) for respiratory failure, patients supported by ECLS are necessarily confined to an intensive care unit (ICU). When patients have become dependent on ECLS for respiratory support, but no longer have the opportunity for recovery or transplantation, ECLS may be thought of as a "bridge to nowhere."[6] Because such scenarios can be particularly difficult to manage, especially when a patient is awake, alert, and wishes to continue receiving extracorporeal support, many of the decisions regarding ECLS initiation and management revolve around attempting to avoid this potential bridge to nowhere. The occurrence of these scenarios can be minimized with careful patient selection and preparation, but these scenarios are inevitable owing to unforeseen events and imperfect decision making.

ECLS in respiratory failure can be either a BTR or a BTT.

When a patient is dependent on ECLS but can neither recover nor undergo transplantation, the situation may be referred to as a "bridge to nowhere."

Patient Selection and Initiation

The decision to initiate ECLS must take into consideration an assessment of benefits and risks, resource use, and specific patient factors. Because of the invasive nature of ECLS, one should select patients in whom the benefit is likely to outweigh the potential risks, as should be the case for other forms of life-sustaining therapy (eg, invasive mechanical ventilation, renal replacement therapy).[7] Unlike the ventilator or dialysis, which have become routine interventions in most intensive care settings, ECLS typically involves a significantly greater resource burden. This impact is measured both in staffing needs and equipment costs. Additional risks relate to the need for large cannulae and systemic anticoagulation, which is typically used with current technology. With a substantial cost of therapy, should the threshold for initiation of ECLS be higher than that of other critical care interventions? Even if one believes that it should—and it is not clear that it should—ECLS has the potential to become significantly more cost effective in the future, meaning that any decisions regarding resource allocation and initiation thresholds would need to be revisited. Economic analyses may help to clarify the current cost of ECLS,[8–10] although they must be made in the context of the health systems in which they are performed.

ECLS is an invasive and very resource-intensive supportive therapy for severe cardiopulmonary failure.

Whether a high cost–benefit ratio should factor into the decision to initiate ECLS remains controversial.

This then raises the question: to whom should ECLS be offered? ECLS outcomes depend significantly on the etiology of respiratory failure, among other patient characteristics. The primary indications for ECLS in acute respiratory failure are extreme impairments of either gas exchange or respiratory system compliance, where the risk of death without ECLS is likely to be greater than the risks of ECLS.[3,8,11] Several prediction models have been proposed that may help to guide patient selection and optimize outcomes for ECLS as a BTR.[12–17] Older age, extrapulmonary organ failures, immunocompromised status, and prolonged duration of mechanical ventilation have been shown to portend a worse prognosis in acute respiratory failure supported with ECLS, and must be considered before initiating ECLS.[13,14,18,19] In the extreme, patients who are moribund or otherwise have very poor prognoses, such as advanced, untreatable malignancy, should not be offered ECLS because it will not change the overall outcome and will only prolong suffering (and likely cause harm).

In cases of BTT, in which extracorporeal support is used to maintain both gas exchange and physical conditioning, the first consideration must be whether the patient is a lung transplant candidate. Because of the lack of destination device therapy, the only absolute contraindication to ECLS for respiratory failure are cases of advanced, irreversible lung disease in which transplantation will not be considered, because this will produce a bridge to nowhere.[20] Even when a patient is eligible for transplantation, certain patient characteristics (eg, septic shock, multiorgan dysfunction, severe arterial occlusive disease, heparin-induced thrombocytopenia, prior prolonged mechanical ventilation, advanced age, and obesity) have been associated with worse outcomes for ECLS as BTT and should be carefully assessed by clinicians contemplating ECLS in this setting.[21,22] Likewise, factors associated with longer transplant wait times, such as short stature or certain blood types,[23] should be considered when offering ECLS, as longer duration of ECLS use may expose the patient to an increased cumulative risk of ECLS complications that may compromise transplant candidacy. Although these factors should not necessarily preclude the use of ECLS, it is important for health care professionals to recognize the possibility that a patient could start as a BTT but later becomes a bridge to nowhere if the patient is subsequently delisted for transplantation owing to either ECLS or non-ECLS complications. Ultimately, similar to patient selection for lung transplantation candidacy itself, the decision to offer ECLS as a BTT should follow a multidisciplinary discussion that weighs both the likelihood of transplantation and the potential ECLS-related complications that may lead to transplant ineligibility.

The decision to initiate ECLS in acute or chronic respiratory failure should take into consideration both the prognosis without ECLS and the likelihood that ECLS will achieve the desired outcome.

An absolute contraindication to ECLS is end-stage respiratory failure when lung transplantation will not be considered.

Chronic obstructive pulmonary disease (COPD) has emerged as a potential indication for ECLS as BTR, and this application has increased potential to lead to ethical dilemmas. COPD benefits primarily from extracorporeal carbon dioxide removal ($ECCO_2R$), a form of ECLS focused on removing carbon dioxide. $ECCO_2R$ is already accepted as an indication for BTT when COPD is in its end stages,[22] but $ECCO_2R$ may be used as a BTR during acute exacerbations as well.[24,25]

Conceptually, $ECCO_2R$ may facilitate the minimization or avoidance of invasive mechanical ventilation during exacerbations of COPD, thereby improving outcomes by reducing ventilator-associated complications.[26] Whether $ECCO_2R$ is superior to conventional ventilation in acute exacerbations of COPD is the subject of ongoing investigation.[27] However, this population is older, already has underlying lung disease, and is likely to have other comorbidities that will limit survival. By introducing a technology with the potential to replace the ventilator while maintaining patient wakefulness, but not necessarily ensuring recovery of lung function and an ability to be liberated from extracorporeal support, $ECCO_2R$ may lead to a greater number of bridges to nowhere.[28] As ECLS is applied with a greater range of indications, it is important to carefully evaluate patients' candidacy for support and discuss all potential outcomes before initiation, including the possible need to withdraw life-sustaining therapy if the desired goal cannot be achieved.

In its current form, ECLS falls within the standard of care of management of certain forms of severe respiratory failure,[29] but is not currently required to achieve the standard of care given the controversies surrounding the existing data,[3,30,31] along with variability of outcomes based on both patient comorbidities and center experience.[32–34] If the technology and the data supporting ECLS improve to the point that ECLS becomes the standard of care, it may become important to discuss the use of ECLS as part of advance care planning, and patients may even be asked their "ECLS status" (ie, do not ECLS).[6,28] As ECLS technology advances and becomes more widespread, it is important both to establish appropriate indications and contraindications for its use and to allow for continued physician judgment in its application, rather than to consider the use of ECLS to become the default.

***

The use of ECCO$_2$R as BTR for acute exacerbations of COPD has the potential to minimize ventilator-associated complications and improve outcomes compared with conventional management.

Its use for this indication also has the potential to create bridges to nowhere because of the uncertainty of recovery in this patient population with preexisting lung disease.

***

Maintenance, Escalation, and Withdrawal of Extracorporeal Life Support in Respiratory Failure

Once a patient has been initiated on ECLS as a BTR or BTT, management strategies are typically similar to those for other critically ill patients, with escalation of support (eg, vasopressors, renal replacement therapy) as clinically indicated, so long as there remains a prospect of achieving the desired outcome (ie, recovery or transplantation). Likewise, the use of cardiopulmonary resuscitation (CPR) during cardiac arrest should be guided in much the same way, namely, by an informed decision by the patient or surrogate decision makers who weigh the prospect of meaningful recovery against potential harm. If the likelihood of either recovery or transplantation is deemed to be unachievable, it may be reasonable to consider withdrawal of life-sustaining therapy, including ECLS. For the unconscious patient, withdrawal of ECLS does not differ from other life-sustaining therapies. The involved health care professionals should meet with the surrogate and communicate as accurately as possible the prognosis and medical options. The medical team ensures the surrogate's understanding, and a decision is reached together with the patient's best interests in mind.

What makes ECLS potentially more challenging than other life-sustaining therapies, such as invasive mechanical ventilation or continuous hemodialysis, is when a patient with capacity to make a decision does not wish to undergo withdrawal of ECLS. Although such a scenario may similarly be encountered with the ventilator or dialysis, those interventions have equivalent forms that may be continued outside the ICU setting, and patients can be transferred to other locations. In contrast, ECLS currently requires ongoing management in the ICU. Although withholding and withdrawing are considered ethical equivalents, in practice these 2 concepts have important differences for clinicians, patients, and family members. These actions may be particularly complicated for the awake patient with capacity. Withholding ECLS from a patient who has no options for recovery or transplantation is a prudent and medically justifiable decision. It is generally accepted that patient autonomy cannot dictate the use of costly medical or surgical interventions that might offer only minimal prolongation of life in an ICU setting. In contrast, some would consider withdrawing ECLS from an awake and competent patient against their expressed wishes to be cruel and unethical.[6] Once there has been a commitment to initiate ECLS, some suggest that the doctor–patient relationship evolves into a stronger ethical bond, which makes these decisions even more complicated. Much as one would not withdraw the ventilator from a dying patient who objects to its removal, it seems unethical to withdraw life support from an objecting patient for whom ECLS is a bridge to nowhere, despite the greater human and technological resources consumed by ECLS. Beyond the principle of patient autonomy, withdrawal against the wishes of an objecting patient would certainly lead to emotional distress of the patient, caregivers, and family. In such circumstances in which the patient opposes withdrawal, a reframing of the goals of care may be appropriate, with a focus instead on optimization of patient comfort and a consideration of the limitations in the escalation of life support, including CPR. When the patient has no capacity, the issues surrounding withdrawal of ECLS over the objections of surrogate decision makers are similar to withdrawal of life-sustaining therapy in ICU patients not receiving ECLS.[35] To facilitate end-of-life decision making, whenever feasible, patients and surrogates should be informed of all possible outcomes at the time of ECLS initiation. This discussion should include the potential for this modality becoming a bridge to nowhere, to prepare patients and surrogates for circumstances in which withdrawal of life support may be medically and ethically appropriate.[6] In addition, consultation with palliative care or ethics specialists is especially important in supporting these patients and their families.

Despite the high resource burden of continuing ECLS in a situation where it is serving only as a bridge to nowhere, removing the device against the express wishes of an awake patient with capacity would violate autonomy and, although opinions vary, some would consider doing so to be unethical.

Anticipation of and discussions regarding the possibility of bridge to nowhere may help to prepare patients and surrogates for decisions about the withdrawal of life support.

ETHICAL DILEMMAS IN EXTRACORPOREAL LIFE SUPPORT FOR CARDIAC FAILURE
Patient Selection and Initiation

ECLS presents similar challenges when used in cardiac failure as it does in respiratory failure; a range of indications with widely variable prognoses, a high degree of complexity, and substantial use of resources. However, unlike ECLS for respiratory failure, which is limited to BTR and BTT, ECLS for cardiac failure may be used as a bridge to destination therapy in the form of a long-term (ie, "durable" or dischargeable) VAD.[5] Both because of the broader range of potential bridging options and because of uncertainty regarding prognosis in many cases of severe cardiac failure, ECLS is often used as a bridge to decision. Patients may be supported until it can be determined whether cardiac function will recover, and, if not, whether the patient is a candidate for long-term VAD or heart transplantation. Despite more bridging options, survival is generally lower in these patients compared with those with respiratory failure.[2] Furthermore, the acceptable duration of support is often much shorter than for respiratory ECLS, typically on the order of days as compared with weeks to months, owing in large part to the complications (eg, embolic events or vascular injury) that can develop during cardiac ECLS that limit recovery or eligibility for VAD or heart transplantation. Each of these factors make careful patient selection a priority, which is all the more difficult because of the emergent nature of ECLS initiation in most cases of cardiac failure, when there may be limited information about a patient's comorbidities or prognosis at the time the decision regarding ECLS needs to be made. To aid in the appropriate selection of patients who are most likely to benefit from ECLS, prognostic scores have been developed.[36] However, because of the acceptance of relatively low success rates for cardiac ECLS, these scoring systems may be more appropriately used to exclude ECLS candidates with the highest expected mortality.

> ECLS in cardiac failure can be used as a BTR, transplantation, destination device (long-term VAD), or decision when the prognosis is uncertain.
>
> Decision making for the initiation of ECLS in cardiac failure, as compared with respiratory failure, should account for lower survival rates, the shorter acceptable duration of support, and the more frequent need to make initiation decisions emergently, with limited information on patients' comorbidities and prognosis.

Extracorporeal CPR (ECPR), which refers to the implementation of ECLS during cardiac arrest, is an indication for ECLS that exemplifies the need for rapid decision making with limited patient information. The clinician must decide within minutes whether to implement this therapy, and often without the availability of important test results. As a consequence of the underlying disease state and the uncertainty of prognosis, neurologically intact survival rates with ECPR are much lower than survival rates with ECLS for cardiogenic shock owing to other etiologies (eg, fulminant myocarditis, acute myocardial infarction).[37–41] For this reason, well-defined inclusion and exclusion criteria consisting of clinical characteristics known to impact outcomes in cardiac arrest should be delineated and adhered to within hospitals with ECPR capabilities.[5] Clinical factors may include duration of arrest and high-quality CPR, patient age, comorbid conditions, concomitant organ failures, and neurologic injury. A systematic approach such as this one may help to both optimize outcomes and facilitate rapid decision making. In the absence of guidelines, ECPR could easily become an expected intervention during cardiac arrest, leading to its widespread use in patients unlikely to benefit and necessitating advanced directives surrounding ECPR (ie, do not ECLS).[28]

> Hospitals offering ECPR for cardiac arrest should have clearly delineated inclusion and exclusion criteria to facilitate rapid decision making, optimize outcomes, and avoid the inappropriate or excessive use of ECPR.

Withdrawal of Life Support and Determination of Death

Many of the considerations previously discussed in the withdrawal of ECLS for respiratory failure apply to ECLS for cardiac failure (eg, bridge to nowhere, withdrawal of life support in a sentient patient, discussions of expectations with patient and family when goals cannot be achieved). However, there are unique aspects to cardiac ECLS given its direct contribution to circulation. Patients receiving ECLS for cardiac failure may be receiving enough circulatory support that death does not result from cardiac arrest, making the concept of "code status" (ie, do not resuscitate orders) irrelevant.[6] In other cases, ECLS may only be providing partial support, such that cardiac arrest would in fact lead to death in the absence of additional resuscitative efforts. Because of the uncertainty of whether death will ensue from cardiac arrest during cardiac ECLS, code status should be discussed in all cases, regardless of the amount of circulatory support provided, and readdressed throughout the clinical course, as appropriate.

> ECLS, when used for cardiac failure, may provide enough circulatory support to maintain adequate end-organ perfusion in the absence of native cardiac function, calling into question the role of CPR during cardiac arrest in certain patients.
>
> Because there may still be a role for CPR depending on the amount of extracorporeal support provided, it is important to determine code status (eg, do not resuscitate status) in all cases of ECLS for cardiac and respiratory failure.

With the development of increasingly sophisticated technology, ECLS has the ability to support circulation and end-organ perfusion well beyond what can be done with medical therapy alone. Traditionally, death has been defined by irreversible cessation of either circulatory or neurologic function, but the usual assessments of heart rhythm and pulsatility are less useful when ECLS continues to provide circulation even in the absence of native cardiac function. In the extreme, when there is cessation of cardiac function with no chance for recovery, VAD, or heart transplantation, what would have once be called circulatory death is transformed by ECLS into a new state of existence, because technology can potentially provide this support for prolonged periods of time, even with no cardiac function.[42] Even declaration of death by neurologic criteria (commonly referred to as "brain death") has become more complicated with extracorporeal support, because certain traditional tests to determine irreversibility (ie, apnea test) are confounded by extracorporeal gas exchange. Ancillary tests to declare death by neurologic criteria may be required.[43]

These scenarios, in which ongoing physiologic functions preclude traditional determinations of cardiac death, may raise questions about the physician's obligation to continue extracorporeal support in what may be viewed as potentially inappropriate care or even medical futility[35]—not necessarily physiologic futility given the potential to preserve end-organ function, but rather futility in supporting the life of a person as a whole. Prolongation of such support, when it is unable to meet the goals set forth at its initiation, runs the risk of compromising a patient's dignity and may run counter to the ethical or moral views of clinicians, although it is important to acknowledge that such circumstances are not unique to ECLS and may be encountered with other forms of life-sustaining therapy.

ECLS has made declaration of death, by either circulatory or neurologic criteria, more difficult because of its ability to maintain circulation and gas exchange in the absence of native cardiac or brain function.

This ability to maintain physiologic functions for prolonged periods of time when there is no prospect of meaningful recovery may represent a form of potentially inappropriate care or medical futility. This can compromise the ethical and moral obligations of clinicians to provide care that benefits patients.

Whether or not there are legal avenues to pursue withdrawal of ECLS against the wishes of surrogates (in the United States, individual state law may vary),[44,45] health care professionals should engage in shared decision making. Shared decision making includes a discussion of the prognosis and options with the surrogates, followed by a consensus decision regarding end-of-life care that will be most consistent with the patient's wishes. In these situations, using an approach of "informed assent" may provide an opportunity for an informed patient or surrogate to allow the clinicians to make a decision that they agree with but are not emotionally or psychologically equipped to make themselves.[46] If a consensus cannot be achieved on withdrawal of ECLS, an appropriate next step would be a discussion of withholding escalation of treatment. Given the extraordinary amount of resource use involved in ECLS, a societal consensus may eventually develop, outlining the circumstances in which physicians may unilaterally withdraw ECLS when the original goals of its implementation cannot be achieved. Just as conventional CPR can be stopped when the physician's professional judgment is that it cannot succeed, could ECPR be similarly stopped if, for example, the patient cannot regain native cardiac function despite ongoing resuscitative efforts? Over what timeframe does ECPR evolve into sustained organ replacement therapy and no longer qualify as CPR? Although there are no guidelines or precedents to support unilateral withdrawal of extracorporeal support in these scenarios, in an ethical analysis it seems that there would be some circumstances in which CPR and ECPR are conceptually the same, and either could be withdrawn with a similar rationale.

Physicians can unilaterally discontinue CPR when it has no meaningful chance of achieving its goal of restoring circulation. Should physicians have the same authority with ECPR?

ROLE OF PALLIATIVE CARE, ETHICS CONSULTATION, AND SPIRITUAL CARE

In light of the myriad ethical dilemmas and difficult end-of-life situations created by ECLS, there may be an increasing role for palliative care, ethics consultations, and spiritual care.[47,48] Palliative care involvement through automatic consultation has been described in the pediatric literature,[48] although consultation on cases with little medical complexity or prognostic uncertainty may not be the preferred use of palliative care resources. Palliative care may have a role in shortening the ICU and hospital length of stay for adults receiving short-term mechanical circulatory support, although the optimal timing of consultation has yet to be determined.[49] Palliative care specialists who work closely with ICU teams are also well-positioned to address distress on the part of nurses and therapists during the care of these patients. Ethics consultations may be useful to reconcile disagreements between health care providers, patients, and surrogates regarding discontinuation of ECLS, although such circumstances may be similar to other forms of life-sustaining therapy and do not necessarily reflect unique dilemmas with ECLS.[50] Although much of the discussion has revolved around dilemmas encountered by physicians and surrogate decision makers, one should not underestimate the emotional and spiritual distress a patient may encounter as a bridge to nowhere. Increasingly, spiritual care is being recognized as an important aspect of patient care.[51,52] Consultation with hospital chaplains and incorporation of a novel spiritual care card for mechanically ventilated patients have been associated with significantly reduced stress and anxiety in the ICU.[53] Such interventions may likewise have a favorable impact for some patients supported with ECLS.

Overall, given the technological complexity, potential for a bridge to nowhere, and the ethically challenging dilemmas that may arise from such advanced forms of life support, an early multidisciplinary team approach should be used for patients managed with ECLS, including palliative care, ethics, and spiritual care, as appropriate.

There is an evolving role for palliative care, ethics consultation, and spiritual care in the management of patients supported with ECLS. Which patients are most likely to benefit from these services, and to what degree they will benefit, remains to be determined.

SUMMARY

ECLS is a sophisticated technology that offers the ability to support patients who would otherwise die from severe, refractory organ failures. With these potential benefits come significant limitations in what ECLS can accomplish. Ultimately, many ethical issues encountered with ECLS are analogous to those encountered with other forms of life-sustaining therapy, though there are some key differences. Whenever possible, physicians should recognize its limitations and plan for these potentially difficult situations.

REFERENCES

1. Karagiannidis C, Brodie D, Strassmann S, et al. Extracorporeal membrane oxygenation: evolving epidemiology and mortality. Intensive Care Med 2016;42: 889–96.
2. Thiagarajan RR, Barbaro RP, Rycus PT, et al. Extracorporeal life support organization registry international report 2016. ASAIO J 2017;63:60–7.
3. Combes A, Hajage D, Capellier G, et al. Extracorporeal membrane oxygenation for severe acute respiratory distress syndrome. N Engl J Med 2018;378:1965–75.
4. Goligher EC, Tomlinson G, Hajage D, et al. Extracorporeal membrane oxygenation for severe acute respiratory distress syndrome and posterior probability of mortality benefit in a post hoc Bayesian analysis of a randomized clinical trial. JAMA 2018;320:2251–9.
5. Abrams D, Garan AR, Abdelbary A, et al. Position paper for the organization of ECMO programs for cardiac failure in adults. Intensive Care Med 2018;44: 717–29.
6. Abrams DC, Prager K, Blinderman CD, et al. Ethical dilemmas encountered with the use of extracorporeal membrane oxygenation in adults. Chest 2014;145: 876–82.
7. Abrams DC, Prager K, Blinderman CD, et al. The appropriate use of increasingly sophisticated life-sustaining technology. Virtual Mentor 2013;15:1050–5.
8. Peek GJ, Mugford M, Tiruvoipati R, et al. Efficacy and economic assessment of conventional ventilatory support versus extracorporeal membrane oxygenation for severe adult respiratory failure (CESAR): a multicentre randomised controlled trial. Lancet 2009;374:1351–63.
9. Oude Lansink-Hartgring A, Dos Reis Miranda D, Donker DW, et al. Cost-effectiveness in extracorporeal life support in critically ill adults in the Netherlands. BMC Health Serv Res 2018;18:172.
10. Harvey MJ, Gaies MG, Prosser LA. U.S. and international in-hospital costs of extracorporeal membrane oxygenation: a systematic review. Appl Health Econ Health Policy 2015;13:341–57.
11. Brodie D, Bacchetta M. Extracorporeal membrane oxygenation for ARDS in adults. N Engl J Med 2011;365:1905–14.
12. Pappalardo F, Pieri M, Greco T, et al. Predicting mortality risk in patients undergoing venovenous ECMO for ARDS due to influenza A (H1N1) pneumonia: the ECMOnet score. Intensive Care Med 2013;39:275–81.
13. Schmidt M, Zogheib E, Roze H, et al. The PRESERVE mortality risk score and analysis of long-term outcomes after extracorporeal membrane oxygenation for severe acute respiratory distress syndrome. Intensive Care Med 2013;39: 1704–13.
14. Schmidt M, Bailey M, Sheldrake J, et al. Predicting survival after extracorporeal membrane oxygenation for severe acute respiratory failure. The Respiratory Extracorporeal Membrane Oxygenation Survival Prediction (RESP) score. Am J Respir Crit Care Med 2014;189:1374–82.
15. Roch A, Hraiech S, Masson E, et al. Outcome of acute respiratory distress syndrome patients treated with extracorporeal membrane oxygenation and brought to a referral center. Intensive Care Med 2014;40:74–83.

16. Enger T, Philipp A, Videm V, et al. Prediction of mortality in adult patients with severe acute lung failure receiving veno-venous extracorporeal membrane oxygenation: a prospective observational study. Crit Care 2014;18:R67.
17. Cheng YT, Wu MY, Chang YS, et al. Developing a simple preinterventional score to predict hospital mortality in adult venovenous extracorporeal membrane oxygenation: a pilot study. Medicine 2016;95:e4380.
18. Schmidt M, Schellongowski P, Patroniti N, et al. Six-month outcome of immunocompromised severe ARDS patients rescued by ECMO. An international multicenter retrospective study. Am J Respir Crit Care Med 2018. [Epub ahead of print].
19. Rozencwajg S, Pilcher D, Combes A, et al. Outcomes and survival prediction models for severe adult acute respiratory distress syndrome treated with extracorporeal membrane oxygenation. Crit Care 2016;20:392.
20. Abrams D, Brodie D. Extracorporeal circulatory approaches to treat acute respiratory distress syndrome. Clin Chest Med 2014;35:765–79.
21. Weill D, Benden C, Corris PA, et al. A consensus document for the selection of lung transplant candidates: 2014–an update from the Pulmonary Transplantation Council of the International Society for Heart and Lung Transplantation. J Heart Lung Transplant 2015;34:1–15.
22. Abrams D, Brodie D, Arcasoy SM. Extracorporeal life support in lung transplantation. Clin Chest Med 2017;38:655–66.
23. Sell JL, Bacchetta M, Goldfarb SB, et al. Short stature and access to lung transplantation in the United States. A cohort study. Am J Respir Crit Care Med 2016;193:681–8.
24. Abrams DC, Brenner K, Burkart KM, et al. Pilot study of extracorporeal carbon dioxide removal to facilitate extubation and ambulation in exacerbations of chronic obstructive pulmonary disease. Ann Am Thorac Soc 2013;10:307–14.
25. Del Sorbo L, Pisani L, Filippini C, et al. Extracorporeal CO2 removal in hypercapnic patients at risk of noninvasive ventilation failure: a matched cohort study with historical control. Crit Care Med 2014;43(1):120–7.
26. Abrams D, Brodie D. Emerging indications for extracorporeal membrane oxygenation in adults with respiratory failure. Ann Am Thorac Soc 2013;10:371–7.
27. Alung Technologies. Extracorporeal CO2 removal with the hemolung RAS for mechanical ventilation avoidance during acute exacerbation of COPD (VENT-AVOID). Bethesda (MD): National Library of Medicine (US); 2000. NLM Identifier: NCT03255057. Available at: ClinicalTrials.gov http://clinicaltrials.gov/ct2/show/NCT03255057. Accessed January 20, 2019.
28. Brodie D, Curtis JR, Vincent JL, et al. Treatment limitations in the era of ECMO. Lancet Respir Med 2017;5:769–70.
29. Abrams D, Ferguson ND, Brochard L, et al. ECMO for ARDS: from salvage to standard of care? Lancet Respir Med 2019;7(2):108–10.
30. Harrington D, Drazen JM. Learning from a trial stopped by a data and safety monitoring board. N Engl J Med 2018;378:2031–2.
31. Hardin CC, Hibbert K. ECMO for severe ARDS. N Engl J Med 2018;378:2032–4.
32. Combes A, Brodie D, Bartlett R, et al. Position paper for the organization of extracorporeal membrane oxygenation programs for acute respiratory failure in adult patients. Am J Respir Crit Care Med 2014;190:488–96.
33. Barbaro RP, Odetola FO, Kidwell KM, et al. Association of hospital-level volume of extracorporeal membrane oxygenation cases and mortality. Analysis of the extracorporeal life support organization registry. Am J Respir Crit Care Med 2015;191:894–901.

34. Hayes D Jr, Tobias JD, Tumin D. Center volume and extracorporeal membrane oxygenation support at lung transplantation in the lung allocation score era. Am J Respir Crit Care Med 2016;194:317–26.

35. Bosslet GT, Pope TM, Rubenfeld GD, et al. An official ATS/AACN/ACCP/ESICM/SCCM policy statement: responding to requests for potentially inappropriate treatments in intensive care units. Am J Respir Crit Care Med 2015;191: 1318–30.

36. Schmidt M, Burrell A, Roberts L, et al. Predicting survival after ECMO for refractory cardiogenic shock: the survival after veno-arterial-ECMO (SAVE)-score. Eur Heart J 2015;36:2246–56.

37. Chen YS, Lin JW, Yu HY, et al. Cardiopulmonary resuscitation with assisted extracorporeal life-support versus conventional cardiopulmonary resuscitation in adults with in-hospital cardiac arrest: an observational study and propensity analysis. Lancet 2008;372:554–61.

38. Shin TG, Jo IJ, Sim MS, et al. Two-year survival and neurological outcome of in-hospital cardiac arrest patients rescued by extracorporeal cardiopulmonary resuscitation. Int J Cardiol 2013;168(4):3424–30.

39. Bougouin W, Aissaoui N, Combes A, et al. Post-cardiac arrest shock treated with veno-arterial extracorporeal membrane oxygenation: an observational study and propensity-score analysis. Resuscitation 2017;110:126–32.

40. Garan AR, Eckhardt C, Takeda K, et al. Predictors of survival and ability to wean from short-term mechanical circulatory support device following acute myocardial infarction complicated by cardiogenic shock. Eur Heart J Acute Cardiovasc Care 2017. https://doi.org/10.1177/2048872617740834.

41. Mirabel M, Luyt CE, Leprince P, et al. Outcomes, long-term quality of life, and psychologic assessment of fulminant myocarditis patients rescued by mechanical circulatory support. Crit Care Med 2011;39:1029–35.

42. Mulaikal TA, Nakagawa S, Prager KM. Extracorporeal membrane oxygenation bridge to no recovery. Circulation 2019;139:428–30.

43. Goswami S, Evans A, Das B, et al. Determination of brain death by apnea test adapted to extracorporeal cardiopulmonary resuscitation. J Cardiothorac Vasc Anesth 2013;27:312–4.

44. Chapter 166 of the Texas Health & Safety Code. Available at: https://statutes. capitol.texas.gov/Docs/HS/htm/HS.166.htm. Accessed January 22, 2019.

45. Halevy A, Brody BA. A multi-institution collaborative policy on medical futility. JAMA 1996;276:571–4.

46. Curtis JR, Burt RA. Point: the ethics of unilateral "do not resuscitate" orders: the role of "informed assent". Chest 2007;132:748–51 [discussion: 755–6].

47. Bein T, Brodie D. Understanding ethical decisions for patients on extracorporeal life support. Intensive Care Med 2017;43:1510–1.

48. Doorenbos AZ, Starks H, Bourget E, et al. Examining palliative care team involvement in automatic consultations for children on extracorporeal life support in the pediatric intensive care unit. J Palliat Med 2013;16:492–5.

49. Nakagawa S, Garan AR, Takeda K, et al. Palliative care consultation in cardiogenic shock requiring short-term mechanical circulatory support: a retrospective cohort study. J Palliat Med 2019;22(4):432–6.

50. Courtwright AM, Robinson EM, Feins K, et al. Ethics committee consultation and extracorporeal membrane oxygenation. Ann Am Thorac Soc 2016;13:1553–8.

51. Hodge DR. A template for spiritual assessment: a review of the JCAHO requirements and guidelines for implementation. Soc Work 2006;51:317–26.

52. Ferrell B, Connor SR, Cordes A, et al. The national agenda for quality palliative care: the National Consensus Project and the National Quality Forum. J Pain Symptom Manage 2007;33:737–44.
53. Berning JN, Poor AD, Buckley SM, et al. A novel picture guide to improve spiritual care and reduce anxiety in mechanically ventilated adults in the intensive care unit. Ann Am Thorac Soc 2016;13:1333–42.

Assessing Right Ventricular Function in the Perioperative Setting, Part I

Echo-Based Measurements

Michael Vandenheuvel, MD[a], Stefaan Bouchez, MD[a],
Patrick Wouters, MD, PhD[a], Eckhard Mauermann, MD, MSc[a,b],*

KEYWORDS

- Right ventricular function and failure • Perioperative assessment
- Echocardiography • Critically ill patients

KEY POINTS

- Perioperative right ventricular failure is an important entity and assessment of function is important for prognosis and management.
- Specific interventricular anatomic and physiologic aspects emphasize the need for right ventricle–specific assessment.
- Echocardiography is an important tool in the assessment of perioperative right ventricular function, but approaches from transthoracic echocardiography cannot be applied uncritically. Novel technologies may have pitfalls of their own.

INTRODUCTION

Heart disease was not only the leading cause of death for the year 2016 in the United States,[1] it also leads to an impressive surgical burden, with some 400,000 annual coronary artery bypass (CABG) grafting operations alone in the United States.[1] Even in noncardiac surgery, cardiac complications are the leading cause of mortality.[2,3]

In the last decade there has been increasing interest in the neglected and/or misunderstood right ventricle.[4–7] Specifically for right ventricular failure (RVF), in-hospital mortality in general is 5% to 17%,[4] and up to 40% in select high-risk populations.[8]

Similarly, in the perioperative setting, RVF also significantly contributes to cardiac morbidity and mortality in both noncardiothoracic[9] and cardiothoracic surgery.[10–12]

Disclosure: The authors have no conflicts of interest.
[a] Department of Anesthesiology and Perioperative Medicine, Ghent University Hospital, C. Heymanslaan 10, Ghent 9000, Belgium; [b] Department for Anesthesia, Surgical Intensive Care, Prehospital Emergency Medicine and Pain Therapy, Basel University Hospital, Spitalstrasse 21, Basel 4031, Switzerland
* Corresponding author.
E-mail address: Eckhard.Mauermann@usb.ch

Several studies have underlined the right ventricle's prognostic value in cardiac surgery for a wide range of procedures, including coronary artery disease,[12] valve surgery,[13,14] congenital/reconstructive surgery,[15–18] ventricular assist device placement/heart transplant,[19,20] and a variety of other disease states altering cardiac function.[21–23] Particularly in the dynamic perioperative setting, accurate and precise assessment of right ventricular performance may be of great importance.[4,5,24–26]

This article focuses on the perioperative evaluation of right ventricular (RV) performance by echocardiography and by catheter-based methods.

Pathophysiologic Considerations

A causal and pathophysiologic understanding of RVF helps to understand diagnostic and management options. Although no universal definition of RVF is accepted, it can be defined as a combination of hypotension, increased right atrial (RA) pressures (>15 mm Hg) and absence of pulmonary edema.[27] Others prefer a more functional approach, defining RVF as the inability of the RV to provide adequate blood flow without excessive use of the Frank-Starling mechanism.[28]

The primary function of the RV is to facilitate blood flow through the lungs and provide the left ventricle with adequate preload, which usually occurs in a low-pressure system.[29] In order to achieve this, the right ventricle is anatomically and physiologically designed as a volume pump, easily expanding to accommodate varying volumes and keeping central venous pressures low. Although early studies from the 1950s seemed to indicate that cauterization of the RV free wall resulted in only modest changes in cardiac output and central venous pressure,[30,31] it has become evident that, particularly in the perioperative setting, the right ventricle and its reaction with the pulmonary vasculature can be of critical importance,[29] especially in the dynamic perioperative setting (eg, the influence of positive pressure ventilation, anesthesia, blood loss, extracorporeal circulation).[32,33] Although, in principle, RV function can be compromised by pressure overload, volume overload, and/or decreased contractility,[34] increased afterload has the greatest relevance.[6,35,36]

There are several mechanisms through which this RVF may be explained.[28,34,37] The homeometric adaptation (Anrep phenomenon) of the RV fails rapidly in critically ill patients. The expected increase in RV contractility in response to a further acute RV afterload augmentation is blunted, predominately because of systemic hypotension and inflammation (both associated with pulmonary hypertension [PHT]). As a result, the RV–pulmonary artery coupling ratio (Ees/Ea) diminishes (i.e., uncoupling occurs), and the RV needs heterometric adaptation (Frank-Starling mechanism), to preserve output. This adaptation aggravates tricuspid regurgitation and can cause a leftward interventricular septum shift, aggravating the negative spiral with ever-diminishing left ventricular (LV) output and RV perfusion pressures.[28] Aside from this, PHT can also be associated with severe LV diastolic dysfunction and/or mitral disease, all of which may explain the observed increased mortality.[6,28]

THE ROLE OF ECHOCARDIOGRAPHY

Perioperative RV function can be assessed clinically, by echocardiography, and by catheter-based measurements. Echocardiography is of great utility in patient management[38,39] and is recommended routinely during cardiac surgery.[40–42] Although qualitative assessment of RV function may be made by experienced echocardiographers,[43,44] it may be arbitrary.[5] Furthermore, the addition of quantitative measurements improves discrimination.[44,45] However, quantifying global RV performance by echocardiography is difficult on account of the ventricle's shape, position, and sequential pistonlike contraction.[5,24,25,37,46,47]

Current guidelines on RV function[5] and chamber quantification exist,[46,48] but these are generally transthoracic echocardiogram (TTE) focused, whereas the transesophageal echocardiography (TEE) guidelines[40,42] largely avoid the right ventricle. Several RV indices are recommended for TTE[5,46]:

1. Tricuspid annular plane systolic excursion (TAPSE; aka tricuspid annular motion)
2. Tricuspid annular velocity (S′)
3. Fractional area change (FAC)
4. Myocardial performance index (MPI, also called Right Ventricular Index of Myocardial Performance or Tei index), and, increasingly:
5. Myocardial deformation imaging (global and free wall strain and strain rate)[18]

For each of these indices, this article:

i. Describes the index with its strengths and weaknesses
ii. Identifies possible means of overcoming limitations (**Table 1**)
iii. Compares these measures in TEE and TTE (**Table 2**)

Tricuspid Annular Displacement: Tricuspid Annular Plane Systolic Excursion

TAPSE is a measure of longitudinal displacement of the lateral tricuspid annulus to the apex during systole. Although a regional measure, it correlates with global RV systolic function[5,26,36,49–53] and clinical outcomes.[36,54] It is easily measured, generally by M mode, giving it excellent temporal resolution, but making it highly susceptible to misalignment. Although the clinician may move the transthoracic probe to optimize alignment, the position of the transesophageal probe is largely limited by the patient's anatomy, leading to significant and systematic underestimation.

Clinicians have long realized that measurements of TAPSE in TEE are not interchangeable with those made by cardiologists before induction. TAPSE measured by M mode in the midesophageal 4-chamber view (ME4C) significantly and substantially underestimates TAPSE measured in the apical 4-chamber view (AP4C) under identical loading conditions. Clearly, clinicians should not be measuring TAPSE by M mode in the ME4C.

Possible solutions for overcoming the issue of misalignment are:

1. To use M mode in alternative views with superior alignment
2. To use an alternative technology

Regarding the alternative TEE views with superior alignment, several such views exist for visualizing the right ventricle.[25,42] In particular, the transgastric RV inflow view (TGRVi) and a modified deep transgastric (dTG) view focusing on the right ventricle seem promising. Flo Forner and colleagues[55] examined 30 patients after induction first by TTE and then by TEE. Echo views were attainable in all 30 patients. However, TAPSE by M mode in the dTG view also systematically underestimated the TAPSE by M mode in the AP4C.[55] Korshin and colleagues[56] performed a similar study in 47 patients and found both the dTG and the TGRVi to underestimate TAPSE by M mode. In addition, the dTG and TGRVi views were only obtainable in some 50% of patents. Our preliminary data examining a randomized order of postinduction TTE and TEE views with both image acquisition and analysis by 2 independent echocardiographers also confirm these results.[57] Possible reasons for continued underestimation of TAPSE by M mode in alternative views may include persistent misalignment, misalignment out of plane (eg, in the sagittal plane; anteflexion/retroflexion in the

Table 1
Overview of studies directly comparing measurements of right ventricular function in transthoracic and transesophageal echocardiography

Author (Year)	Design	Conventional Technology and View	Alternative Technology and View
TAPSE			
		Vs TAPSE by M mode in TTE, AP4C	Vs TAPSE by M mode in TTE, AP4C
Flo Forner et al,[55] 2017	• N = 30 of 30 • TTE and TEE postinduction • Nonrandomized	M mode in dTG: Pearson r = 0.92 Agreement: mean bias −1.5 mm (95% LoA −5.7 to 2.8; shorter in TEE) Intrauser ICC 0.93 (0.85–0.97) Interuser ICC 0.93 (0.70–0.98)	Anatomic M mode in ME4C: Pearsor r = 0.94 Agreement: mean bias −0.5 mm (95% LoA −3.9 to 3.0 mm; shorter in TEE) Intrauser ICC 0.93 (0.83–0.97) Interuser ICC 0.86 (0.44–0.96) Anatomic M mode in dTG: Pearson r = 0.97 Agreement: mean bias −0.4 mm (95% LoA −2.8 to 2.0 mm; shorter in TEE); Intrauser ICC 0.94 (0.78–0.97) Interuser ICC 0.95 (0.78–0.99) 2D (ES image and ED image) in ME4C: Pearson r = 0.93 Agreement: mean bias −1.5 mm (95% LoA −5.4 to 2.5 mm; shorter in TEE) Intrauser ICC 0.86 (0.44–0.95) Interuser ICC 0.87 (0.49–0.97)
Korshin et al,[56] 2018	• N = 44 of 47 • TTE and TEE postinduction • Nonrandomized	M mode in dTG (n = 23): Pearson r = 0.87 Agreement: mean bias −1.2 mm (−8 to 6 mm) M mode in TGRVi: (n = 23) Pearson r = 0.69 Agreement: mean bias −3.2 mm (95% LoA −11 to 5 mm)	Anatomic M mode in dTG (n = 8): Pearson r = 0.96 Agreement: mean bias −0.6 mm (95% LoA 3–4 mm) Anatomic M mode in TGRVi (n = 8): Pearson r = 0.96 Agreement: mean bias −0.3 mm (95% LoA 2–4 mm) 2D (ES image and ED image) in ME4C (n = 44): Pearson r = 0.96 Agreement: mean bias 0.0 mm (95% LoA 8–9 mm)

Shen et al,[65] 2018	• N = 60 of 72 • TTE preinduction (<3 mo): TEE postinduction	NA	Speckle tracking in ME4C: Linear regression: TEE = 0.82TTE + 5.6 Pearson r = 0.87 Agreement: TTE M-mode mean bias 2.4 mm (95% LoA −2.7 to 7.5) Interuser variability ICC = 0.99 Intrauser variability ICC = 0.92
Markin et al,[66] 2017	• N = 84 of 100 • TTE and TEE postinduction • Nonrandomized	M mode in ME4C: Linear regression: TEE = 0.64TTE + b; Pearson r = 0.45 TTE a mean 6.5 mm larger	Speckle tracking in ME4C: TAPSE by M-mode mean 0.6 mm larger Linear regression: TEE = 0.95TTE + b Pearson r = 0.62
Dhawan et al,[64] 2019	• N = 125 of 125 • TTE and TEE postinduction • Nonrandomized	NA	2D (apical-lateral distance in ES and ED images) in ME4C: Pearson r = 0.797 Agreement: mean bias 0.6 mm (95% LoA −3.3 to 4.6 mm)
Skinner et al,[63] 2017	• N = 40 of 43 • TTE and TEE awake/sedated with spontaneous ventilation • Analysis in left lateral decubitus position • Nonrandomized	NA	2D (marking lateral annulus in ES and ED images) in ME4C: 20.5 ± 5.9 mm vs 20.5 ± 5.8 mm (AP4C), P = .9 $R^2 = 0.93$ Agreement: mean bias 0.0 mm (95% LoA −3.2 to 3.1 mm)
Our preliminary data[57]	• N = 24 of 25 • TTE and TEE postinduction • Randomized order	M mode in ME4C: 13.1 ± 3.8 mm vs 17.3 ± 4.0 mm (AP4C) P<.001 M mode in dTG: 14.5 ± 4.7 mm vs 17.3 ± 4.0 mm (AP4C) P<.001 M mode in TGRVi: 12.3 ± 4.0 mm vs 17.3 ± 4.0 mm (AP4C) P<.001	Speckle tracking in ME4C: 16.9 ± 5.4 mm vs 17.3 ± 4.0 mm (AP4C), P = .736 Linear regression: TEE = 0.81TTE + b Pearson r = 0.59 Agreement: TTE M-mode mean bias 0.2 mm (95% LoA −9.1 to 8.6) Interuser variability ICC = 0.56 Intrauser variability ICC = 0.70

(continued on next page)

Table 1
(continued)

Author (Year)	Design	Conventional Technology and View	Alternative Technology and View
Velocity			
		Vs S′ in TTE, AP4C	Vs S′ in TTE, AP4C
Tousignant et al,[67] 2008	• N = 23 of 24 • TTE and TEE postinduction • Nonrandomized	S′ in ME4C 5.9 cm/s ± 1.8 S′ in AP4C 9.0 cm/s ± 2.0	NA
Michaux et al,[71] 2009	• N = 50 • TTE preinduction • TEE postinduction	TDI in ME4C: 7.0 ± 1.4 cm/s vs 14.8 ± 2.7 cm/s (AP4C); P<.001	NA
Our preliminary data[72]	• N = 24 of 25 • TTE and TEE postinduction • Randomized order	TDI in ME4C: 6.9 ± 2.0 cm/s vs 9.1 ± 2.1 cm/s (AP4C); P<.001 TDI in dTG: 6.8 ± 1.7 cm/s vs 9.1 ± 2.1 cm/s; P<.001 TDI in TGRVi: S′ 6.1 ± 1.3 cm/s vs 9.1 ± 2.1 cm/s; P<.001	Speckle tracking in ME4C: Linear regression: TEE = 0.87TTE + 0.60 Pearson r = 0.78 Agreement: TTE M-mode mean bias −0.6 cm/s (95% LoA −3.5 to 2.4) Interuser variability ICC = 0.73 Intrauser variability ICC = 0.78
FAC			
Skinner et al,[63] 2017	• N = 40 of 43 • TTE and TEE awake/sedated with spontaneous ventilation • Analysis in left lateral decubitus position • Nonrandomized	2D (ES image and ED image) in ME4C: 39.4 ± 13.2% vs 37.3 ± 12.5% (AP4C); P = .3	NA
RV MPI			
Michaux et al,[70] 2010	• N = 20 • TTE preinduction • TEE postinduction	PW in ME4C and UEAASax: 0.15 (95% CI 0.09–0.19) vs 0.30 (95% CI 0.23–0.38) in AP4C; P>.001	NA

Michaux et al,[71] 2009	• N = 50 • TTE preinduction • TEE postinduction	PW in ME4C and UEAASax: 0.17 ± 0.12 vs 0.32 ± 0.11 in AP4C	NA
Deformation			
Kurt et al,[94] 2012	• N = 34 of 34 • TTE and TEE postinduction • Nonrandomized	RV strain (6-segment model): TTE −22.2% ± 2.9%, TEE −23.0% ± 3.0%; $P<.21$ Agreement: 0.8 (−6.1 to 7.7) ICC intraobserver variability: 0.94 (0.87–0.97) RV strain rate (6-segment model) TTE −1.37 ± 0.35 TEE −1.49 ± 0.36/s, $P = .21$ Agreement: 0.21 (−0.52 to 0.77) ICC intraobserver variability 0.95 (0.88–0.98)	NA
Tousignant et al,[95] 2010	• N = 21 of 23 • TTE and TEE postinduction • Nonrandomized	RV strain (6-segment model) Only obtained in 73% of TEE and 38% of TTE; 8 patients with both RV strain TEE −20.33 ± 9.71 vs TTE −20.01 ± 3.2 RV strain (lateral segments only) Lateral apical TEE −23.3 ± 7.0 vs TTE −20.6 ± 10.6 Lateral mid-TEE −29.8 ± 5.2 vs TEE −22.5 ± 7.7 Lateral basal −31.5 ± 8.1 vs TEE −22.8 ± 13.2	NA

Abbreviations: 2D, two-dimensional; AP4C, apical 4-chamber view; CI, confidence interval; dTG, deep transgastric; ED, enddiastolic; ES, endsystolic; ICC, intraclass correlation coefficient; LoA, limit of agreement; ME4C, midesophageal 4-chamber view; NA, not available; PW, pulsed wave doppler; TDI, tissue Doppler imaging; TGRVi, transgastric RV inflow view; UEAASax, upper esophageal aortic arch short axis.

Table 2
Practical considerations for performing measurements of right ventricular function

Measurement	Established Technology	Alternative Technology	Suggested Views	Benefit	Important Limitations	Normal Values (TTE[a])	Abnormal Cutoffs (TTE[a])
TAPSE	M mode	—	Not suggested (TGRVi or dTG)	• Simple, quick, reproducible • Not dependent on high-quality 2D images • Good temporal resolution • Available on all machines	• Angle dependent • Visualized portion of annulus not strictly lateral (alterative views) • Assume motion of base representative of whole RV (cave: after pericardiectomy) • Load dependent	24 ± 3.5 mm	<17 mm
—	—	Anatomic M mode	ME4C	• Largely angle independent	• Not available on all machines	NA	NA
—	—	2D (apical-lateral distance)	ME4C	• Largely angle independent • Analysis from any previous 2D loop	• Requires several manual steps • Foreshortening leads to overestimation	NA	NA
—	—	2D (marking lateral annulus)	ME4C	• Largely angle independent • Analysis from any previous 2D loop	• Requires several manual steps	NA	NA
—	—	STE	ME4C	• Largely angle independent • Analysis from any previous 2D loop • Automated with option of manual correction	• Not available on all machines • Vendor variation/ unknown tracking algorithms	NA	NA

S′	TDI	—	Not suggested (TGRVi or dTG)	• Simple, quick, reproducible • Not dependent on high-quality 2D images • Good temporal resolution • Available on all machines • Less load dependent than TAPSE	• Angle dependent • Visualized portion of annulus not strictly lateral (alternative views) • Assume motion of base representative of whole RV (cave: after pericardiectomy)	14.1 ± 2.3 cm/s	<9.5 cm/s
	STE	ME4C	—	• Largely angle independent • Analysis from any previous 2D loop • Systolic and diastolic values	• Not available on all machines • Vendor variation/unknown tracking algorithms • Off-line, not commercially available • Framerate sensitive	NA	NA
Strain/strain rate	TDI	ME4C	—	• Suboptimal 2D images can be used	• Angle dependent	NA	NA
	STE	—	—	• Largely angle independent • Assesses regional and global function	• Temporal resolution (especially for strain rate) • Most software optimized for LV and TTE • Vendor variation, black box of tracking algorithms	−29 ± 4.5	>−20%

(continued on next page)

Table 2
(continued)

Measurement	Established Technology	Alternative Technology	Suggested Views	Benefit	Important Limitations	TTE[a]	
						Normal Values	Abnormal Cutoffs
FAC	2D	—	ME4C	• Largely angle independent • Reflects longitudinal and radial contraction	• Tracing of trabeculated endocardia boarder • Higher variability/lower reproducibility • Foreshortening may overestimate • Neglects RV outflow tract contraction	49% ± 7%	<35%
MPI	PW	—	ME4C or ME RVOT, UE AA SAX, or TG pulmonic value view	• Feasible in many patients • Independent of geometry • Less affected by heart rate • Incorporates systolic and diastolic aspects	• Varies with pressure and volume status • Unreliable with differing R-R intervals (eg, atrial fibrillation) • Load dependent • Unreliable when RA pressure increased	0.26 ± 0.09	>0.43
—	TDI	—	TGRVi	—	—	0.38 ± 0.08	>0.54

Abbreviations: ME RVOT, Mid esophageal right ventricular inflow outflow; STE, speckle-tracking echocardiography; TG, Transgastric; UE AA SAX, Upper esophageal aortic arch short axis.

[a] Values as recommended by current TTE guidelines: Badano and colleagues (2018)[48] and Lang and colleagues (2015).[46]

ME4C), and visualization of a less mobile part of the tricuspid annulus (eg, the inferior portion).[58,59] In summary, TAPSE by M mode in TEE, regardless of the view, also underestimates TTE measurements.

Regarding alternative technologies, the use of a less angle-dependent technology may be promising. Three possible options, all based on two-dimensional (2D) loops, have been examined.

The first possible approach is to measure TAPSE by anatomic M mode, which examines 2D pixel samples along a freely positioned cursor line,[60] and has been shown to increase accuracy.[61] Both Flo Forner and colleagues[55] and Korshin and colleagues[56] examined this option,[55,56] and found not only more accurate but also unbiased TAPSE measurements when using anatomic M mode compare with conventional M mode in the ME4C, dTG, and TGRVi. Although interesting and promising, only 38 patients were examined in total. Importantly, anatomic M mode is not available on all echo machines.

A second approach is to simply use the end-diastolic and end-systolic 2D frames, either measuring the distance from the tricuspid annulus to the apex in both frames[62] or marking the position of the tricuspid annulus in both frames.[63,64] However, this requires the user to select the appropriate frames and also place annular and apical points, potentially leading to the observed slight systematic underestimation[55] and greater variability than with anatomic M mode.[55,56]

A third approach is use speckle tracking–based software, which tracks speckles in an area of interest at the lateral tricuspid annulus and at the apex, yielding a displacement-time curve over the cardiac cycle. Shen and colleagues[65] compared postinduction speckle tracking–based TAPSE in the ME4C with TAPSE by M mode in the AP4C of examinations taken in the 3 months before surgery in 60 of 72 eligible patients. They found both measurements to correlate, with longer measurements in the AP4C. Markin and colleagues[66] also examined TAPSE by M mode and speckle tracking in both the ME4C and AP4C views, both during anesthesia, in 84 of 112 patients. They found TAPSE by speckle tracking in the AP4C to correlate with TAPSE by M mode in the ME4C. The investigators explicitly state that reproducibility may be a crux of this method because, of the 100 available 2D loops acquired by an experienced echocardiographer, only 84 could be analyzed by the novice. Our data in a similar trial analyzing 24 of 25 patients with randomized views and image acquisition and analysis by 2 echocardiographers confirm correlation and show TAPSE by speckle tracking to be an unbiased but imprecise surrogate for the reference standard TAPSE.[57] Taken together, these data in nearly 200 patients seem promising and unbiased, but there is uncertainty about precision and reliability.

Furthermore, in any of these postprocessing options, the frame rate of 2D loops may also be an important factor, potentially limiting their use in tachycardic right ventricles.

Tricuspid Annular Systolic Velocity: S'

Tricuspid annular systolic velocity measures the speed of displacement and has many similarities to TAPSE. The rationale for longitudinal regional measurements as a surrogate for global function are the same and S' has been shown to correlate with measures of global RV function[5,26,50,52] and correlate with outcomes.[5,26] Potential advantages compared with TAPSE include a lesser degree of dependence on loading conditions[5,46] and the possibility of also assessing diastolic velocities. Nonetheless, S' has not been studied extensively in TEE, potentially on account of its extreme angle dependence by its usual determination by tissue Doppler. Again similar to TAPSE, potential means of overcoming the problem of misalignment are alternative TEE views and alternative technologies.

Regarding alternative views, Tousignant and colleagues[67] found S' velocities measured by tissue Doppler imaging (TDI) in the TGRVi to underestimate those measured in the AP4C. Similarly, other studies have shown mean tricuspid annular velocity to be systematically lower in the TGRVi than the AP4C.[68,69] Both author groups explained this difference through measurements of the tricuspid annulus at the less mobile inferior site.[69] Michaux and colleagues[70,71] also found significant differences in S' measured in anesthetized and ventilated ME4C with awake TTE. In our previously mentioned diagnostic study, we also measured systematic underestimation in the ME4C, TGRVi, and dTG compared with the AP4C.[57]

Regarding alternative technologies for examining S', only one study could be identified. Recently, the authors were able to show that S' may be derived by differentiating TAPSE by speckle tracking in the ME4C with respect to time.[72] The resultant speckle tracking–based velocities correlated with the TDI gold standard measured in the AP4C. The same limitations for this technology exist as in TAPSE by speckle tracking, although the effect of far-field noise is greater.

Fractional Area Change

Although TAPSE and S' are regional measures of longitudinal performance, FAC is a more global marker of contractility. FAC is defined as the difference between end-diastolic and end-systolic area, divided by end-diastolic area, usually measured in the ME4C for TEE. In TTE it correlates with RV ejection faction (RVEF) as determined by MRI,[73–75] and three-dimensional ejection faction (EF)[74,76] as well as with mortality and morbidity.[13,77,78] In TEE, some data have also shown an association with mortality and morbidity.[79–82]

An advantage to this approach is that it also accounts for the action of the superficial layer of circumferential fibers facilitating inward contraction, which have received increased attention.[26] In cardiac surgery, with the known decrease in longitudinal function following pericardiectomy, this may be particularly useful.[68,83]

Surprisingly, data explicitly comparing FAC in TTE with TEE are scarce. Skinner and colleagues[63] found TTE and TEE measurements of RV FAC not to vary significantly, although this study was performed in spontaneously breathing patients in the left lateral decubitus position.

Myocardial Performance Index (Right Ventricular Index of Myocardial Performance or Tei Index)

The RV MPI is a nongeometric measure of global RV performance accounting for both systolic and diastolic performance. Specifically, the RV MPI is the ratio between the sum of the isovolumetric contraction and relaxation times divided by the ejection time. Measurements may either be made using tissue Doppler at the lateral annulus or using pulsed-wave Doppler at the leaflet tips of both the inflow and outflow tract,[84] but requires exact measurement of times as shown by different definitions according to the method used. The RV MPI has also been shown to be a predictor of adverse events,[84] particularly for PAH.[85] In TEE, preincision RV MPI and RV FAC were independently associated with mortality and morbidity after valvular heart surgery.[13]

Two studies comparing RV MPI by pulsed-wave Doppler in TTE and TEE could be found. Michaux and colleagues[70] found that although the MPI could be measured in all 20 patients undergoing CABG surgery, those measured by TEE and under anesthesia were significantly lower than those measured in the same patients by TTE on the previous day. However, variability was 4-fold higher in TEE measurements, prompting the investigators to conclude that the RV MPI may be a questionable indicator of global RV function in anesthetized and ventilated patients.[70] Similarly, data from the same group in 50 patients undergoing CABG surgery confirmed significantly lower values of the MPI in anesthetized TEE compared with awake TTE.[71]

Deformation Imaging: Global and Free Wall Strain/Strain Rate

Deformation imaging refers to changes in myocardial shape over time and can be complex. Deformations may occur in 3 dimensions (longitudinal, circumferential, or radial strain) may be relative to the original length (Lagrangian strain) or the length at the immediately previous time (natural or Eulerian strain), and may be examined at the end of systole or as a peak value. Furthermore, deformation may also be expressed as velocities (ie, strain rate). However, for the right ventricle, Lagrangian longitudinal strain is generally reported either for the (lateral) free wall only or for both the free wall and septum. RV strain in TTE has been shown to correlate with RVEF measured by cardiac MRI (CMRI),[73,86] and outcomes.[87,88] Current guidelines explicitly for RV strain exist[48] but fail to mention TEE. Studies examining RV strain in TEE and outcomes have shown mixed results at best[79,89,90] and problems with acceptable image acquisition.[91]

Originally, strain was assessed by TDI, but the need for high frame rates, strong angle dependence, and nondifferentiation between the 3 dimensions has severely limited its use, particularly in TEE.[92] In contrast, speckle tracking–based myocardial deformation is a largely angle-independent technology.[46,93] Major limitations include frame rate, the number of available speckles in the (nonhypertrophied) right ventricle, different software with unknown algorithms generally developed for the left ventricle in TTE, and the composition of the acquired 2D image.

Kurt and colleagues[94] found global strain between AP4C and ME4C to show good agreement for the right ventricle when examining both the septum and RV free wall together. Similarly, Tousignant and colleagues[95] found global RV longitudinal strain to be comparable between ME4C and AP4C. However, in the same study, examining only the RV free wall showed a relevant systematic overestimation in ME4C in the basal, mid, and apical segments. Although several reasons could explain why this could be a problem in the right ventricle, higher values of strain have also been shown for the left ventricle when comparing TTE and TEE, albeit to a lesser degree (mean bias, 3.4 ± 4.9).[96]

Despite its appeal, several reasons should caution clinicians from uncritically applying speckle tracking–based strain to the right ventricle in TEE. First, the right ventricle in the ME4C is a long, thin-walled lateral structure in the far field, which means that (1) a wide sector is needed (increases in sector width lead to less robust tracking)[97] of substantial depth, both of which decrease temporal resolution, to (2) track a thin-walled structure with a limited number of speckles (fewer trackable speckles yield poorer tracking),[96] moving laterally (poorer resolution than longitudinal motion) in the noisy far field of TEE probes (higher frequencies yield poorer far-field resolution.) In addition, acoustic shadows from valvular structures, catheters, and so forth may decrease the quality of (apical) tracking. Taken together, these factors significantly increase noise, in part challenging the notion that speckle tracking is a fully angle-independent technology.[93] To make matters worse, tracking algorithms of speckle-tracking software show significant intervendor variability[98] and are generally optimized for the left ventricle in TTE. A recent study examining the same TEE images by commonly available dedicated LV software and dedicated off-line RV software concluded that the two softwares cannot be used interchangeably, although both were sensitive measures for identifying RV dysfunction.[99]

Putting It All Together for Clinical Use

Clearly there is no simple solution. An ideal measurement of RV function would be easy and quick to perform, precise, accurate, and reproducible, and would correlate with gold standard measurements and clinical outcomes.

For TTE, a meta-analysis of 17 studies and 1280 patients compared TAPSE and FAC with MRI as the gold standard.[100] FAC correlated better than TAPSE with CMRI-based EF (0.56 vs 0.40; P = .018). Other TTE studies have underscored the utility of the most commonly used measures of RV function.[101,102] Increasingly, RV strain and strain rate are also being recommended for TTE and may be preferable to conventional measures.[48,102]

This article shows that data examining comparability between TTE and TEE measurements of RV function are scarce and largely unconvincing. The most data are available for TAPSE (see **Table 1**), which may be unfortunate because longitudinal function is known to decrease with pericardiectomy, whereas global function is not as affected.[26,68,83,103] However, independent of the issue of transferability from TTE and TEE, there is evidence for an association between RV FAC, RV MPI, and TAPSE[54] measured by TEE with adverse outcomes.

In summary, clinicians should utilize multiple quantitative measures with their respective benefits and drawbacks to visual assessment when assessing RV function. Each measurement alone only describes an aspect of RV function, adeptly described by the tale of the elephant being examined by blind men, each describing a different part of the elephant.[47] In addition, our clinical assessment should also consider forward stroke volume, valve disorders, regional dysfunction, contractile pattern, as well as the clinical context, particularly in the dynamic perioperative setting.[26]

REFERENCES

1. Xu J, Murphy SL, Kochanek KD, et al. National vital statistics reports volume 67, number 5 July 26, 2018, deaths: final data for 2016. vol. 67. 2018. Available at: https://www.cdc.gov/. Accessed January 30, 2019.

2. Devereaux PJ, Xavier D, Pogue J, et al. Characteristics and short-term prognosis of perioperative myocardial infarction in patients undergoing noncardiac surgery. Ann Intern Med 2011;154(8):523.

3. Lee TH, Marcantonio ER, Mangione CM, et al. Derivation and prospective validation of a simple index for prediction of cardiac risk of major noncardiac surgery. Circulation 1999;100(10):1043–9. Available at: http://www.ncbi.nlm.nih.gov/pubmed/10477528. Accessed January 31, 2019.

4. Harjola V-P, Mebazaa A, Čelutkienė J, et al. Contemporary management of acute right ventricular failure: a statement from the Heart Failure Association and the Working Group on Pulmonary Circulation and Right Ventricular Function of the European Society of Cardiology. Eur J Heart Fail 2016;18(3):226–41.

5. Rudski LG, Lai WW, Afilalo J, et al. Guidelines for the echocardiographic assessment of the right heart in adults: a report from the American Society of Echocardiography. J Am Soc Echocardiogr 2010;23(7):685–713.

6. Haddad F, Couture P, Tousignant C, et al. The right ventricle in cardiac surgery, a perioperative perspective: i. anatomy, physiology, and assessment. Anesth Analg 2009;108(2):407–21.

7. Haddad F, Doyle R, Murphy DJ, et al. Right ventricular function in cardiovascular disease, part II: pathophysiology, clinical importance, and management of right ventricular failure. Circulation 2008;117(13):1717–31.

8. Campo A, Mathai SC, Le Pavec J, et al. Outcomes of hospitalisation for right heart failure in pulmonary arterial hypertension. Eur Respir J 2011;38(2):359–67.

9. Jasudavisius A, Arellano R, Martin J, et al. A systematic review of transthoracic and transesophageal echocardiography in non-cardiac surgery: implications for point-of-care ultrasound education in the operating room. Can J Anaesth 2016; 63(4):480–7.

10. Bartels K, Karhausen J, Sullivan BL, et al. Update on perioperative right heart assessment using transesophageal echocardiography. Semin Cardiothorac Vasc Anesth 2014;18(4):341–51.

11. Grønlykke L, Ravn HB, Gustafsson F, et al. Right ventricular dysfunction after cardiac surgery – diagnostic options. Scand Cardiovasc J 2017;51(2):114–21.

12. Maslow AD, Regan MM, Panzica P, et al. Precardiopulmonary bypass right ventricular function is associated with poor outcome after coronary artery bypass grafting in patients with severe left ventricular systolic dysfunction. Anesth Analg 2002;95(6):1507–18. Available at: http://www.ncbi.nlm.nih.gov/pubmed/12456409. Accessed January 30, 2019.

13. Haddad F, Denault AY, Couture P, et al. Right ventricular myocardial performance index predicts perioperative mortality or circulatory failure in high-risk valvular surgery. J Am Soc Echocardiogr 2007;20(9):1065–72.

14. Ito S, Pislaru SV, Soo WM, et al. Impact of right ventricular size and function on survival following transcatheter aortic valve replacement. Int J Cardiol 2016;221: 269–74.

15. Couperus LE, Delgado V, Palmen M, et al. Right ventricular dysfunction affects survival after surgical left ventricular restoration. J Thorac Cardiovasc Surg 2017;153(4):845–52.

16. Gatzoulis MA, Clark AL, Cullen S, et al. Right ventricular diastolic function 15 to 35 years after repair of tetralogy of Fallot. Restrictive physiology predicts superior exercise performance. Circulation 1995;91(6):1775–81. Available at: http://www.ncbi.nlm.nih.gov/pubmed/7882487. Accessed January 31, 2019.

17. Therrien J, Provost Y, Merchant N, et al. Optimal timing for pulmonary valve replacement in adults after tetralogy of Fallot repair. Am J Cardiol 2005;95(6): 779–82.

18. Ohye RG, Schranz D, D'Udekem Y. Current therapy for hypoplastic left heart syndrome and related single ventricle lesions. Circulation 2016;134(17): 1265–79.

19. Neyer J, Arsanjani R, Moriguchi J, et al. Echocardiographic parameters associated with right ventricular failure after left ventricular assist device: a review. J Heart Lung Transplant 2016;35(3):283–93.

20. Ravis E, Theron A, Mancini J, et al. Severe right ventricular dysfunction is an independent predictor of pre- and post-transplant mortality among candidates for heart transplantation. Arch Cardiovasc Dis 2017;110(3):139–48.

21. Beckmann E, Ismail I, Cebotari S, et al. Right-sided heart failure and extracorporeal life support in patients undergoing pericardiectomy for constrictive pericarditis: a risk factor analysis for adverse outcome. Thorac Cardiovasc Surg 2017;65(8):662–70.

22. Bodez D, Ternacle J, Guellich A, et al. Prognostic value of right ventricular systolic function in cardiac amyloidosis. Amyloid 2016;23(3):158–67.

23. Cannon JE, Su L, Kiely DG, et al. Dynamic risk stratification of patient long-term outcome after pulmonary endarterectomy: results from the United Kingdom National Cohort. Circulation 2016;133(18):1761–71.

24. Kossaify A. Echocardiographic assessment of the right ventricle, from the conventional approach to speckle tracking and three-dimensional imaging, and insights into the "Right Way" to explore the forgotten chamber. Clin Med Insights Cardiol 2015;9:65–75.

25. Kasper J, Bolliger D, Skarvan K, et al. Additional cross-sectional transesophageal echocardiography views improve perioperative right heart assessment. Anesthesiology 2012;117(4):726–34.

26. Portnoy SG, Rudski LG. Echocardiographic evaluation of the right ventricle: a 2014 perspective. Curr Cardiol Rep 2015;17(4):21.

27. Kinch J, Ryan T. Right ventricular infraction. N Engl J Med 1994;330(17):1211–7.

28. Vieillard-Baron A, Naeije R, Haddad F, et al. Diagnostic workup, etiologies and management of acute right ventricle failure: A state-of-the-art paper. Intensive Care Med 2018;44(6):774–90.

29. Pinsky MR. The right ventricle: interaction with the pulmonary circulation. Crit Care 2016;20(1):266.

30. Starr I, Jeffers WA, Meade RH. The absence of conspicuous increments of venous pressure after severe damage to the right ventricle of the dog, with a discussion of the relation between clinical congestive failure and heart disease. Am Heart J 1943;26(3):291–301.

31. Kagan A. Dynamic Responses of the Right Ventricle following Extensive Damage by Cauterization. Circulation 1952;5(6):816–23.

32. Freiermuth D, Skarvan K, Filipovic M, et al. Volatile anaesthetics and positive pressure ventilation reduce left atrial performance: a transthoracic echocardiographic study in young healthy adults. Br J Anaesth 2014;112(6):1032–41.

33. Skarvan K, Lambert A, Filipovic M, et al. Reference values for left ventricular function in subjects under general anaesthesia and controlled ventilation assessed by two-dimensional transoesophageal echocardiography. Eur J Anaesthesiol 2001;18(11):713–22. Available at: http://www.ncbi.nlm.nih.gov/pubmed/11580777. Accessed January 31, 2019.

34. Vandenheuvel M a, Bouchez S, Wouters PF, et al. A pathophysiological approach towards right ventricular function and failure. Eur J Anaesthesiol 2013;30(7):386–94.

35. Brooks H, Kirk ES, Vokonas PS, et al. Performance of the right ventricle under stress: relation to right coronary flow. J Clin Invest 1971;50(10):2176–83.

36. Kaul TK, Fields BL. Postoperative acute refractory right ventricular failure: incidence, pathogenesis, management and prognosis. Cardiovasc Surg 2000;8(1):1–9. Available at: http://www.ncbi.nlm.nih.gov/pubmed/10661697. Accessed January 30, 2019.

37. Haddad F, Hunt S a, Rosenthal DN, et al. Right ventricular function in cardiovascular disease, part I: Anatomy, physiology, aging, and functional assessment of the right ventricle. Circulation 2008;117(11):1436–48.

38. Galal W, Hoeks SE, Flu WJ, et al. Relation between preoperative and intraoperative new wall motion abnormalities in vascular surgery patients: a transesophageal echocardiographic study. Anesthesiology 2010;112(3):557–66.

39. Kolev N, Brase R, Swanevelder J, et al. The influence of transoesophageal echocardiography on intra-operative decision making. A European multicentre study. European Perioperative TOE Research Group. Anaesthesia 1998;53(8):767–73. Available at: http://www.ncbi.nlm.nih.gov/pubmed/9797521. Accessed January 15, 2019.

40. American Society of Anesthesiologists and Society of Cardiovascular Anesthesiologists Task Force on Transesophageal Echocardiography. Practice

guidelines for perioperative transesophageal echocardiography. An updated report by the American Society of Anesthesiologists and the Society of Cardiovascular Anesthesiologists Task Force on Transesophageal Echocardiography. Anesthesiology 2010;112(5):1084–96.

41. Flachskampf FA, Wouters PF, Edvardsen T, et al. Recommendations for transoesophageal echocardiography: EACVI update 2014. Eur Heart J Cardiovasc Imaging 2014;15(4):353–65.

42. Hahn RT, Abraham T, Adams MS, et al. Guidelines for performing a comprehensive transesophageal echocardiographic examination: recommendations from the American Society of Echocardiography and the Society of Cardiovascular Anesthesiologists. J Am Soc Echocardiogr 2013;26(9):921–64.

43. Magunia H, Schmid E, Hilberath JN, et al. 2D echocardiographic evaluation of right ventricular function correlates with 3D volumetric models in cardiac surgery patients. J Cardiothorac Vasc Anesth 2017;31(2):595–601.

44. Orde S, Slama M, Yastrebov K, et al, College of Intensive Care Medicine of Australia and New Zealand [CICM] Ultrasound Special Interest Group [USIG]. Subjective right ventricle assessment by echo qualified intensive care specialists: assessing agreement with objective measures. Crit Care 2019;23(1):70.

45. Ling LF, Obuchowski NA, Rodriguez L, et al. Accuracy and interobserver concordance of echocardiographic assessment of right ventricular size and systolic function: a quality control exercise. J Am Soc Echocardiogr 2012; 25(7):709–13.

46. Lang RM, Badano LP, Mor-Avi V, et al. Recommendations for cardiac chamber quantification by echocardiography in adults: an update from the American Society of Echocardiography and the European Association of Cardiovascular Imaging. Eur Heart J Cardiovasc Imaging 2015;16(3):233–71.

47. Rudski LG, Afilalo J. The blind men of Indostan and the elephant in the echo lab. J Am Soc Echocardiogr 2012;25(7):714–7.

48. Badano LP, Kolias TJ, Muraru D, et al. Standardization of left atrial, right ventricular, and right atrial deformation imaging using two-dimensional speckle tracking echocardiography: a consensus document of the EACVI/ASE/Industry Task Force to standardize deformation imaging. Eur Heart J Cardiovasc Imaging 2018;19(6):591–600.

49. Miller D, Farah MG, Liner A, et al. The relation between quantitative right ventricular ejection fraction and indices of tricuspid annular motion and myocardial performance. J Am Soc Echocardiogr 2004;17(5):443–7.

50. Tamborini G, Marsan NA, Gripari P, et al. Reference values for right ventricular volumes and ejection fraction with real-time three-dimensional echocardiography: evaluation in a large series of normal subjects. J Am Soc Echocardiogr 2010;23(2):109–15.

51. Kaul S, Tei C, Hopkins JM, et al. Assessment of right ventricular function using two-dimensional echocardiography. Am Heart J 1984;107(3):526–31. Available at: http://www.ncbi.nlm.nih.gov/pubmed/6695697. Accessed January 31, 2019.

52. Sato T, Tsujino I, Ohira H, et al. Validation study on the accuracy of echocardiographic measurements of right ventricular systolic function in pulmonary hypertension. J Am Soc Echocardiogr 2012;25(3):280–6.

53. Sato T, Tsujino I, Oyama-Manabe N, et al. Simple prediction of right ventricular ejection fraction using tricuspid annular plane systolic excursion in pulmonary hypertension. Int J Cardiovasc Imaging 2013;29(8):1799–805.

54. Schmid E, Hilberath JN, Blumenstock G, et al. Tricuspid annular plane systolic excursion (TAPSE) predicts poor outcome in patients undergoing acute

pulmonary embolectomy. Heart Lung Vessel 2015;7(2):151–8. Available at: http://www.ncbi.nlm.nih.gov/pubmed/26157741. Accessed March 13, 2019.

55. Flo Forner A, Hasheminejad E, Sabate S, et al. Agreement of tricuspid annular systolic excursion measurement between transthoracic and transesophageal echocardiography in the perioperative setting. Int J Cardiovasc Imaging 2017;33(9):1385–94.

56. Korshin A, Grønlykke L, Nilsson JC, et al. The feasibility of tricuspid annular plane systolic excursion performed by transesophageal echocardiography throughout heart surgery and its interchangeability with transthoracic echocardiography. Int J Cardiovasc Imaging 2018;34(7):1017–28.

57. Mauermann E, Vandenheuvel M, Francois K, et al. Differences in right ventricular displacement, velocity, and myocardial deformation by transesophageal vs. transthoracic echocardiography. SCA Phoenix; 2018.

58. Hammarström E, Wranne B, Pinto FJ, et al. Tricuspid annular motion. J Am Soc Echocardiogr 1991;4(2):131–9. Available at: http://www.ncbi.nlm.nih.gov/pubmed/2036225. Accessed January 31, 2019.

59. Atsumi A, Ishizu T, Kameda Y, et al. Application of 3-dimensional speckle tracking imaging to the assessment of right ventricular regional deformation. Circ J 2013;77.

60. Mele D, Pedini I, Alboni P, et al. Anatomic M-mode: a new technique for quantitative assessment of left ventricular size and function. Am J Cardiol 1998; 81(12):82G–5G.

61. Yumi Hayashi S, Lind BI, Seeberger A, et al. Analysis of mitral annulus motion measurements derived from M-mode, Anatomic M-mode, tissue doppler displacement, and 2-dimensional strain imaging. J Am Soc Echocardiogr 2006;19(9):1092–101.

62. Morita Y, Nomoto K, Fischer GW. Modified tricuspid annular plane systolic excursion using transesophageal echocardiography for assessment of right ventricular function. J Cardiothorac Vasc Anesth 2016;30(1):122–6.

63. Skinner H, Kamaruddin H, Mathew T. Tricuspid annular plane systolic excursion: comparing transthoracic to transesophageal echocardiography. J Cardiothorac Vasc Anesth 2017;31(2):590–4.

64. Dhawan I, Makhija N, Choudhury M, et al. Modified tricuspid annular plane systolic excursion for assessment of right ventricular systolic function. J Cardiovasc Imaging 2019;27(1):24–33.

65. Shen T, Picard MH, Hua L, et al. Assessment of tricuspid annular motion by speckle tracking in anesthetized patients using transesophageal echocardiography. Anesth Analg 2018;126(1):62–7.

66. Markin NW, Chamsi-Pasha M, Luo J, et al. Transesophageal speckle-tracking echocardiography improves right ventricular systolic function assessment in the perioperative setting. J Am Soc Echocardiogr 2017;30(2):180–8.

67. Tousignant CP, Bowry R, Levesque S, et al. Regional differences in color tissue Doppler-derived measures of longitudinal right ventricular function using transesophageal and transthoracic echocardiography. J Cardiothorac Vasc Anesth 2008;22(3):400–5.

68. David J-S, Tousignant CP, Bowry R. Tricuspid annular velocity in patients undergoing cardiac operation using transesophageal echocardiography. J Am Soc Echocardiogr 2006;19(3):329–34.

69. Nikitin NP, Witte KK, Thackray SD, et al. Longitudinal ventricular function: normal values of atrioventricular annular and myocardial velocities measured with

quantitative two-dimensional color doppler tissue imaging. J Am Soc Echocardiogr 2003;16(9):906–21.

70. Michaux I, Seeberger M, Schuman R, et al. Feasibility of measuring myocardial performance index of the right ventricle in anesthetized patients. J Cardiothorac Vasc Anesth 2010;24(2):270–4.

71. Michaux I, Filipovic M, Seeberger M, et al. Are normal echocardiographic values obtained by transthoracic echocardiography in awake patients suitable for evaluation of cardiac function in anesthetized and mechanically ventilated patients? Anesth Analg 2009;109(5):1701 [author reply: 1702–3].

72. Mauermann E, Vandenheuvel M, François K, et al. A novel speckle-tracking based method for quantifying tricuspid annular velocities in TEE. J Cardiothorac Vasc Anesth 2019;33(10):2636–44.

73. Focardi M, Cameli M, Carbone SF, et al. Traditional and innovative echocardiographic parameters for the analysis of right ventricular performance in comparison with cardiac magnetic resonance. Eur Heart J Cardiovasc Imaging 2015; 16(1):47–52.

74. Gopal AS, Chukwu EO, Iwuchukwu CJ, et al. Normal values of right ventricular size and function by real-time 3-dimensional echocardiography: comparison with cardiac magnetic resonance imaging. J Am Soc Echocardiogr 2007; 20(5):445–55.

75. Horton KD, Meece RW, Hill JC. Assessment of the right ventricle by echocardiography: a primer for cardiac sonographers. J Am Soc Echocardiogr 2009; 22(7):776–92 [quiz: 861–2].

76. Imada T, Kamibayashi T, Ota C, et al. Intraoperative right ventricular fractional area change is a good indicator of right ventricular contractility: a retrospective comparison using two- and three-dimensional echocardiography. J Cardiothorac Vasc Anesth 2015;29(4):831–5.

77. Zornoff LAM, Skali H, Pfeffer MA, et al. Right ventricular dysfunction and risk of heart failure and mortality after myocardial infarction. J Am Coll Cardiol 2002; 39(9):1450–5. Available at: http://www.ncbi.nlm.nih.gov/pubmed/11985906. Accessed January 30, 2019.

78. Anavekar NS, Skali H, Bourgoun M, et al. Usefulness of right ventricular fractional area change to predict death, heart failure, and stroke following myocardial infarction (from the VALIANT ECHO Study). Am J Cardiol 2008;101(5): 607–12.

79. Silverton NA, Patel R, Zimmerman J, et al. Intraoperative transesophageal echocardiography and right ventricular failure after left ventricular assist device implantation. J Cardiothorac Vasc Anesth 2018;32(5):2096–103.

80. Younan D, Pigott DC, Gibson CB, et al. Right ventricular fractional area of change is predictive of ventilator support days in trauma and burn patients. Am J Surg 2018;216(1):37–41.

81. Kim J, Di Franco A, Seoane T, et al. Right ventricular dysfunction impairs effort tolerance independent of left ventricular function among patients undergoing exercise stress myocardial perfusion imaging. Circ Cardiovasc Imaging 2016; 9(11). https://doi.org/10.1161/CIRCIMAGING.116.005115.

82. Muresian H. The clinical anatomy of the right ventricle. Clin Anat 2016;29(3): 380–98.

83. Maus TM. TAPSE: a red herring after cardiac surgery. J Cardiothorac Vasc Anesth 2018;32(2):779–81.

84. Tei C, Ling LH, Hodge DO, et al. New index of combined systolic and diastolic myocardial performance: a simple and reproducible measure of cardiac

function–a study in normals and dilated cardiomyopathy. J Cardiol 1995;26(6): 357–66. Available at: http://www.ncbi.nlm.nih.gov/pubmed/8558414. Accessed March 13, 2019.

85. Tei C, Dujardin KS, Hodge DO, et al. Doppler echocardiographic index for assessment of global right ventricular function. J Am Soc Echocardiogr 1996; 9(6):838–47. Available at: http://www.ncbi.nlm.nih.gov/pubmed/8943444. Accessed March 13, 2019.

86. Lu KJ, Chen JXC, Profitis K, et al. Right ventricular global longitudinal strain is an independent predictor of right ventricular function: a multimodality study of cardiac magnetic resonance imaging, real time three-dimensional echocardiography and speckle tracking echocardiography. Echocardiography 2015;32(6): 966–74.

87. Park SJ, Park J-H, Lee HS, et al. Impaired RV global longitudinal strain is associated with poor long-term clinical outcomes in patients with acute inferior STEMI. JACC Cardiovasc Imaging 2015;8(2):161–9.

88. Rajagopal S, Forsha DE, Risum N, et al. Comprehensive assessment of right ventricular function in patients with pulmonary hypertension with global longitudinal peak systolic strain derived from multiple right ventricular views. J Am Soc Echocardiogr 2014;27(6):657–65.e3.

89. Beck DR, Foley L, Rowe JR, et al. Right ventricular longitudinal strain in left ventricular assist device surgery-a retrospective cohort study. J Cardiothorac Vasc Anesth 2017;31(6):2096–102.

90. Ting P-C, Chou A-H, Liao C-C, et al. Comparison of right ventricular measurements by perioperative transesophageal echocardiography as a predictor of hemodynamic instability following cardiac surgery. J Chin Med Assoc 2017; 80(12):774–81.

91. Duncan AE, Sarwar S, Kateby Kashy B, et al. Early left and right ventricular response to aortic valve replacement. Anesth Analg 2017;124(2):406–18.

92. Silverton N, Meineri M. Speckle tracking strain of the right ventricle: an emerging tool for intraoperative echocardiography. Anesth Analg 2017;125(5):1475–8.

93. Forsha D, Risum N, Rajagopal S, et al. The influence of angle of insonation and target depth on speckle-tracking strain. J Am Soc Echocardiogr 2015;28(5): 580–6.

94. Kurt M, Tanboga IH, Isik T, et al. Comparison of transthoracic and transesophageal 2-dimensional speckle tracking echocardiography. J Cardiothorac Vasc Anesth 2012;26(1):26–31.

95. Tousignant C, Desmet M, Bowry R, et al. Speckle tracking for the intraoperative assessment of right ventricular function: a feasibility study. J Cardiothorac Vasc Anesth 2010;24(2):275–9.

96. Marcucci CE, Samad Z, Rivera J, et al. A comparative evaluation of transesophageal and transthoracic echocardiography for measurement of left ventricular systolic strain using speckle tracking. J Cardiothorac Vasc Anesth 2012;26(1): 17–25.

97. Teske AJ, De Boeck BWL, Melman PG, et al. Echocardiographic quantification of myocardial function using tissue deformation imaging, a guide to image acquisition and analysis using tissue Doppler and speckle tracking. Cardiovasc Ultrasound 2007;5(1):27.

98. Mirea O, Pagourelias ED, Duchenne J, et al. Variability and reproducibility of segmental longitudinal strain measurement. JACC Cardiovasc Imaging 2018; 11(1):15–24.

99. Silverton NA, Lee JP, Morrissey CK, et al. A comparison of left- and right-sided strain software for the assessment of intraoperative right ventricular function. J Cardiothorac Vasc Anesth 2018. https://doi.org/10.1053/j.jvca.2018.10.038.

100. Lee JZ, Low S-W, Pasha AK, et al. Comparison of tricuspid annular plane systolic excursion with fractional area change for the evaluation of right ventricular systolic function: a meta-analysis. Open Heart 2018;5(1):e000667.

101. Hamilton-Craig CR, Stedman K, Maxwell R, et al. Accuracy of quantitative echocardiographic measures of right ventricular function as compared to cardiovascular magnetic resonance. Int J Cardiol Heart Vasc 2016;12:38–44.

102. Longobardo L, Suma V, Jain R, et al. Role of two-dimensional speckle-tracking echocardiography strain in the assessment of right ventricular systolic function and comparison with conventional parameters. J Am Soc Echocardiogr 2017; 30(10):937–46.e6.

103. Sullivan TP, Moore JE, Klein AA, et al. Evaluation of the clinical utility of transesophageal echocardiography and invasive monitoring to assess right ventricular function during and after pulmonary endarterectomy. J Cardiothorac Vasc Anesth 2018;32(2):771–8.

Assessing Right Ventricular Function in the Perioperative Setting,
Part II: What About Catheters?

Michael Vandenheuvel, MD[a], Stefaan Bouchez, MD[a],
Patrick Wouters, MD, PhD[a], Eckhard Mauermann, MD, MSc[a,b],*

KEYWORDS

- Right ventricular function and failure • Perioperative assessment
- Right ventricular pressure • Three-dimensional echocardiography
- Pressure-volume loops • Critically ill patients

KEY POINTS

- Perioperative right ventricular failure is an important entity, and assessment of function is critical for prognosis and management.
- Specific interventricular anatomic and physiologic aspects emphasize the need for right ventricular–specific assessment.
- In specific perioperative settings, tailored additional right ventricular monitoring can be of great use to the perioperative physician. This includes pressure-based and flow-based measurements.
- A combination of pressure-based and 3-dimensional echocardiography technologies may be clinically promising.

INTRODUCTION

As reviewed in the Michael Vandenheuvel and colleagues' article, "Assessing Right Ventricular Function in the Perioperative Setting, Part I – Echo-Based Measurements," in this issue, 2-dimensional (2-D) echocardiography can provide valuable insights into the right ventricular (RV) function. It is considered standard monitoring in the cardiac surgery perioperative setting.[1–3] In selected perioperative settings, however, RV

Disclosure Statement: All authors state to have no conflicts of interest.
[a] Department of Anesthesiology and Perioperative Medicine, Ghent University Hospital, C. Heymanslaan 10, Ghent 9000, Belgium; [b] Department for Anesthesia, Surgical Intensive Care, Prehospital Emergency Medicine and Pain Therapy, Basel University Hospital, Spitalstrasse 21, Basel 4031, Switzerland
* Corresponding author.
E-mail address: Eckhard.Mauermann@usb.ch

Anesthesiology Clin 37 (2019) 697–712
https://doi.org/10.1016/j.anclin.2019.08.004
1932-2275/19/© 2019 Elsevier Inc. All rights reserved.
anesthesiology.theclinics.com

failure (RVF) is known to be more prevalent,[4–6] which may warrant a more extensive monitoring strategy. This can be provided by RV catheterization, adding pressure-based and/or flow-based information. This may also allow a more functional approach, not solely dependent on visualized anatomy.

Categories of perioperative patients that may need additional RV monitoring include patients with pulmonary hypertension (PHT),[7–10] preexisting RVF, and multiple types of congenital heart disease.[11–17] Similarly, patients undergoing pulmonary endarterectomy,[18,19] left ventricular assist device implantation, and heart and/or lung transplantation[20–25] are well known to be at risk for severe RVF, all having an impact on perioperative morbidity and mortality.

Catheter-based assessment also has the advantage of providing global, functional, and continuous operator-independent information, which can be a major advantage in the intensive care setting. Additional settings in which nonechocardiographic assessment of RV function may be of interest include contraindications for transesophageal echocardiography (TEE) probe placement (eg, esophageal pathology) or during off-pump coronary artery bypass, where imaging can be obstructed during critical operative phases.[26,27] All of these settings warrant a detailed review of the available additional (non–2-D echocardiographic) monitoring modalities that can be deployed in the perioperative setting.

CATHETER-BASED METHODS

Catheter-based modalities for the evaluation of RV function provide invasive hemodynamic measurements,[28] usually by simple measures (eg, pulmonary artery catheter [PAC], also known as Swan-Ganz catheter).[29] More sensitive, sophisticated conductance catheters or alternatives to create pressure-volume (PV) loops of the RV are also an option traditionally used in the experimental setting.[30] These are discussed in the following paragraphs. Combining different approaches may allow a more complete evaluation of the RV is emphasized.

Pressure-Based Assessment

Since the clinical introduction of the PAC in 1970, there has been much debate about its usefulness in different perioperative settings. Earlier studies showed increased harm, whereas the PAC-Man (Assessment of the clinical effectiveness of pulmonary artery catheters in management of patients in intensive care) trial subsequently suggested it can be used safely (showing no change in in-hospital mortality).[31] Although studies have never demonstrated an alteration in mortality from the use of PACs,[32] it is possible that in selected (compromised) patients it may be of use. It must be taken into account, however, that severe complications can result from its insertion and use (eg, arrhythmia, pulmonary artery [PA] rupture, and pulmonary embolus).[33]

Broadly speaking, the technology is used to assess right-sided pressures (right atrial, RV, PA, and pulmonary capillary wedge pressures) as well as evaluate cardiac output and sample true mixed venous blood. It also can be used to pace the (right) heart and measure central temperature. Additionally, careful analysis of the pressure waveforms can yield additional information of RV performance. In allowing an early and adequate recognition of the negative spiral of RVF (described in Michael Vandenheuvel and colleagues' article, "Assessing Right Ventricular Function in the Perioperative Setting, Part I – Echo-Based Measurements," in this issue), the use of PACs may be beneficial in select patients, especially those at risk for acute RVF (eg, a history of significant PHT or after left ventricular assist device insertion) or patients not responding to conventional treatment may benefit.

Pressure Measurement Evaluation

The availability of continuous right-sided pressure measurements can be of use in multiple perioperative settings. It readily demonstrates PHT, because a resting mean PA pressure above 25 mm Hg is proposed as a cutoff for PHT by the World Health Organization.[34] It also can assess pulmonary vascular resistance (where a threshold of 250 dyn·s·cm^{-5} commonly is used) when combined with cardiac output measurements. Especially useful in the dynamic perioperative setting, a PAC can help diagnose acute RV dysfunction in a real-time manner. When the RA pressure is higher than the PA occlusion pressure, severe isolated RVF is documented. In biventricular failure, both RA and LA pressures are elevated. A PAC also can be supportive in differentiating shock types and in the diagnosis of tamponade and can help monitor fluid status.[33]

When interpreting right-sided pressures, some caveats need to be kept in mind. First, it cannot be stressed enough that PA pressures should always be compared with the simultaneously measured systemic pressures, because both are coupled.[35] Second, raised intrathoracic or intra-abdominal pressures rise RA pressures even when no RV dysfunction is present.[36] Third, a decompensating patient with known PA hypertension shows pseudonormalization of PA pressures. In this patient, however, the RA pressures are elevated, and the systemic pressures are diminished. This further underlines the importance of evaluating the mean PA pressures as a ratio to mean systemic pressures.[36,37]

Pressure Waveform Evaluation

RA pressure waveforms can reveal a host of abnormalities. A selection of these is discussed, because they are most frequently encountered in the perioperative setting. Of particular interest is an elevated v-wave, or fused c-wave and v-wave. The normal v-wave, generated during venous return, is superimposed by a retrograde influx of blood during systolic ventricular contraction, suggesting an incompetent tricuspid valve. In cardiac tamponade, venous blood flow is obstructed toward the RA. The elevated venous pressures result in prominent a-waves and v-waves, which makes the x-descent look steep, and the short diastolic window results in a very short y-descent. Elevated a-waves (cannon a-waves) typically are encountered when the right atrium contracts against a closed tricuspid valve, as occurs in junctional rhythms.[38]

Careful analysis of the RV and PA pressure waveforms can yield additional information on RV function and ischemia,[39–41] especially in the acute setting. Simultaneous display of both PA and RV pressures allows online assessment,[37,41,42] especially when plotted on top of each other (**Fig. 1**):[41]

- During diastole, the high compliance of the normal RV results in a horizontal slope (see **Fig. 1**A). This slope tilts upward in the setting of RV diastolic dysfunction (see **Fig. 1**B), culminating in the square root sign. The RV pressures align in parallel with the diastolic PA pressures (see **Fig. 1**).
- In RV systolic failure, the systolic upstroke is slowed, reflecting a diminished dP/dt (see **Fig. 1**).
- RV outflow tract obstruction (RVOTO) is also readily diagnosed using this strategy, where the difference in peak systolic PA and peak RV pressures is larger than 6 mm Hg.

Dynamic RVOTO may be present in up to 4% of patients undergoing cardiac surgery (with a gradient above 25 mm Hg). It often results in hemodynamic instability, and in this setting inotropic agents are contraindicated and volume loading and slowing of heart rate beneficial.[37,42]

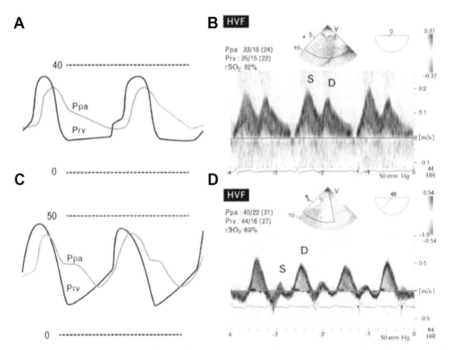

Fig. 1. Simultaneous display of RV and PA pressure waveforms over time allows further evaluation of diastolic and systolic RV function. (*A, B*) Normal waveforms, with a steep systolic and a horizontal diastolic RV pressure trace. (*C, D*) The blunted upward RV systolic slope suggests systolic dysfunction. RV diastolic dysfunction can be recognized by the upward sloping diastolic RV pressure trace. Ppa, pressure in the pulmonary artery; Prv, pressure in the right ventricle. (*From* Denault AY, Haddad F, Jacobsohn E, et al. Perioperative right ventricular dysfunction. Curr Opin Anaesthesiol 2013;26(1):74.2; with permission.)

Flow-Based Assessment

PACs allow the estimation of right-sided cardiac output. The thermodilution methodology consists of injecting cold fluid proximal to the tip, where the temperature change is recorded. Using a time-concentration curve (Stewart-Hamilton), cardiac output can be quantified. Modifying the original PAC with a thermistor, continuous cardiac output measurement is possible. Small quantities of heat are generated in the proximal thermistor in order to stabilize catheter tip temperatures. The energy requirement correlates with the cardiac output. In both methods, respiratory effects on PA blood flow are considerable—it is suggested to measure during expiration. Even after averaging 3 measurements, variability of up to 15% is a known concern. Additionally, tricuspid insufficiency results in an underestimation of cardiac output.[31] Nonetheless, continuous assessment of mixed venous saturation and cardiac output is of interest to clinicians and may help guide therapeutic measures and their effects.

Supportive Monitoring

As discussed previously, venous congestion associated with RVF can result in decreased flow in several important organs. This can be readily shown using brain near-infrared spectroscopy, where a drop in tissue oxygenation index and (if available) a rise in deoxygenated hemoglobin can be appreciated. This should prompt therapeutic action.[33] The systemic venous congestion that occurs because of RVF affects multiple organs, exemplified in a raised liver panel or renal dysfunction.

Three-Dimensional Echocardiography

3-D echocardiography has become an important complementary imaging modality to 2-D echocardiography, as emphasized in current guidelines.[43,44] Overall, however, although 3-D transthoracic echocardiography (TTE) and TEE have made imaging of the RV feasible[44–47] and promising,[28,30,44,48,49] it remains underutilized.[1,44,48]

Real-time 3-D imaging enables the visualization of moving structures within a defined depth or volume. Traditionally, 3-D TEE has been used to examine valves and facilitate communication with the surgeon.[44] Dynamic visualization with the surrounding structures also improves visualization of cardiac structures, defects, and devices and may be used for preplanning procedures and intraprocedural guidance.[44,50–53]

An additional major benefit of 3-D echocardiography—and the focus in this article—is for assessing global volumes and ejection fraction (EF). Despite minor differences, alternatives for estimating volumes by 2-D echocardiography for the other 3 cardiac chambers exist.[48,54,55] For the RV, however, only 3-D can accurately quantify volumes and EF. This has been examined in large cohort studies for normal RV volumes.[56,57]

Because ultrasound imaging inherently involves a trade-off of spatiotemporal resolution, 3-D imaging of a large structure in the far-field is subject to poor temporal resolution. This may be overcome by (1) decreases in spatial resolution or (2) the use of electrocardiographic gating for slice-wise construction of the entire ventricle from multiple regular beats in apnea. These techniques allow for a sufficient temporal resolution for creating an accurate volume-time relationship.

3-D echocardiography-derived RV volume measurements correlate well with cardiac MRI volume measurements[58–73] across a wide range of pathologic conditions in adults,[58,68–73] children,[66,67] and animals.[64,65] Furthermore, this correlation also seems to hold in single-beat 3-D acquisitions.[74,75] Additionally, right ventricular 3-D echocardiography volumes have been shown to correlate better than 2-D measurements,[47,71] despite moderate systematic underestimation of volumes, again in both humans[68,76,77] and animals.[64,65] Finally, several studies have shown excellent intraobserver and interobserver variability.[58,59,64] Evidence from 3-D TEE suggests that reproducible information regarding RV size and function also exist in the dynamic perioperative setting of cardiac surgery.[78] Unlike with systolic function, qualitative estimation of 3-D volumes by expert echocardiographers is inaccurate compared with 3-D.[79]

Increasingly, 3-D volumes may be used as the basis of other measurements, such as RV free-wall tricuspid annular plane systolic excursion (TAPSE) or strain analyses. 3-D volumes of the entire ventricle eliminate the problem of identifying the optimal 2-D slice for analysis (eg, the true lateral annulus for TAPSE measurements). As such, 3-D imaging may yield more accurate measures of displacement, velocities, and deformation at the clearly identified lateral annulus or free wall, which requires and is dependent on postprocessing software.

PRESSURE-VOLUME LOOPS: A PLACE FOR THREE-DIMENSIONAL ECHOCARDIOGRAPHY?

In the experimental setting, ventricular PV loops are recognized as the gold standard for ventricular assessment. Plotting the instantaneous intraventricular pressure and volume allows a PV loop to be created for a heartbeat. Multiple loop-derived indices are available to quantify ventricular function as well as loading conditions and ventriculo-arterial interaction. The slope of the end-systolic PV relationship (end-systolic elastance [Ees]), which is classically derived from multiple PV loops acquired during fast and controlled preload reduction, has been shown to be relatively loading independent (**Fig. 2**).[80–83] The preload recruitable stroke work, which is calculated by plotting the ventricular stroke work (quantified by the area of the loop) to the end-diastolic volume, is a second robust measure of ventricular contractile state.[84,85]

The arterial elastance (Ea), or the ratio of end-systolic pressure over stroke volume, seems a reliable index for afterload.[86,87] By combining Ees and Ea as a ratio, ventricular-arterial coupling can be assessed.[88] Ventricular-arterial coupling describes the relationship of a source of energy (eg, the ventricle) and the load attached to it (eg, the arterial system).[89] In essence, this relationship is a measure of hemodynamic and metabolic efficiency with uncoupling signaling a reduction in ejection efficiency[90] and poorer outcomes.[91]

Thus, PV loops offer a great deal of information generally not available to the clinician. In the dynamic perioperative setting of patients undergoing cardiac surgery, the information afforded by visualizing the main determinants of cardiac performance (preload, afterload, and inotropy) as well as relative interactions (eg, ventriculo-arterial coupling) may be of great benefit.[92]

Originally described in 1895 by Otto Frank,[49] conductance catheters are the gold standard in the experimental setting to construct PV loops.[93] These catheters generate a low-voltage electric field, between multiple electrodes. This allows an accurate estimation of the surrounding ventricular blood volumes. After calibration, instantaneous ventricular volumes are generated, which can be combined with simultaneously measured micromanometer pressures. The impractical nature, inherent invasiveness, and high costs, however, associated with conductance catheter use precludes routine clinical use in the perioperative setting.[45,94–96] Increasingly, clinical studies have begun to illustrate the benefit of left-sided PV loops in heart failure,[97–101] resynchronization,[102–106] and left-sided surgical procedures.[107–109] Interest in right-sided PV loops is increasing[30,110,111] and conductance catheters can be used in the RV.[112–116]

From a clinical perspective, echocardiography and the PAC still remain the gold standard for RV function assessment in the perioperative period.[117] Some groups,

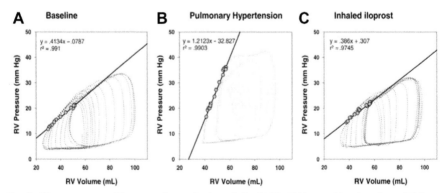

Fig. 2. Measurement of inotropy by occlusion of the IVC in PV loops: Ees rises from (*A*) baseline to the (*B*) PHT state. (*C*) Effects of a pulmonary vasodilator also can be appreciated. RV, right ventricle. (*From* Rex S, Missant C, Claus P, et al. Effects of inhaled iloprost on right ventricular contractility, right ventriculo-vascular coupling and ventricular interdependence: a randomized placebo-controlled trial in an experimental model of acute pulmonary hypertension. Crit Care 2008;12(5):R113; with permission.)

including the authors',[118] are investigating the combined use of RV 3-D TEE volumetry with continuous RV pressure measurements. In 2004, Uebing and colleagues[119] constructed RV PV loops combining angiographic volumes with instantaneous RV pressures in 56 postoperative tetralogy of Fallot patients. They were able to quantify RV load. Also in 2005, Kuehne and colleagues[120] combined MRI-derived volumes

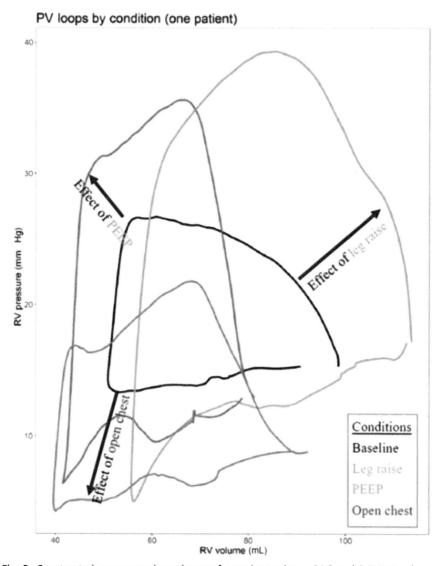

Fig. 3. Constructed pressure-volume loops of a patient using a PAC and 3-D TEE volumes. Acquisitions were made in steady state in 3 conditions: closed chest baseline after passive leg raise and during sustained PEEP (20 mm Hg). The resulting loops reflect expected physiologic changes. PEEP, positive end exspiratory pressure; PV, pressure volume; RV, right ventricle. (*From* Vandenheuvel M, Mauermann E, Bouchez S, et al. Perioperative right ventricular pressure-volume loops based on 3D-echo and pulmonary artery catheter. Eacta Annual Congress 2018:P01.2; with permission.)

Table 1
Results of constructed pressure-volume loops in 16 patients

Pooled Data (16 Patients)	Baseline to Leg Raise (Relative Change [CI] and P Value)		Baseline to Positive End-Expiratory Pressure (Relative Change [CI] and P Value)	
End-diastolic volume	**1.13** [1.08–1.25]	<.001	**0.82** [0.68–0.98]	.033
Stroke volume	**1.19** [1.10–1.28]	.001	**0.71** [0.63–0.83]	<.001
Cardiac output	**1.15** [1.08–1.27]	.001	**0.66** [0.55–0.76]	.001
Stroke work	**1.47** [1.35–1.65]	<.001	0.86 [0.68–1.11]	.376
Arterial elastance	1.04 [0.95–1.15]	.323	**1.94** [1.56–2.29]	<.001

Effects of leg raise and positive end-expiratory pressure are apparent and statistically significant after paired Wilcoxon testing.
Bold text indicates statistical significance.
From Vandenheuvel M, Mauermann E, Bouchez S, et al. Perioperative right ventricular pressure-volume loops based on 3D-echo and pulmonary artery catheter. Eacta Annual Congress 2018:P01.2; with permission.

with a 6F catheter RV pressure, creating PV loops in 6 patients without and 6 patients with PHT. They also used this methodology in 6 swine, showing good levels of agreements by Bland-Altman analysis versus conductance catheter technology. In 2014, Witschey and colleagues[121] were also able to construct left-sided PV loops using semiautomated active contour recognition on MRI and a microtip pressure measurement.

In 2013, Herberg and colleagues[122] used 3-D (TTE or TEE) echocardiography and a miniature pressure wire in a pilot study to determine the feasibility of creating ventricular PV loops in 31 children and adolescents with congenial heart defects undergoing routine catherization procedures. They found that combining these volume-time and pressure-time relationships was possible in all patients, with low intraobserver and interobserver variability ($3.6 \pm 1.3\%$ and $5.6 \pm 1.5\%$, respectively).[122] Data from the authors' group in 16 elective adult coronary artery bypass graft patients suggest the feasibility of a purely clinical approach, using a regular fluid-filled PAC and 3-D TEE, showing physiologically expected effects of leg raise, high sustained positive end-expiratory pressure (PEEP), and chest opening (**Fig. 3**).[118] These changes were significant after paired Wilcoxon testing (**Table 1**). The authors currently are determining the level of distortion of the fluid-filled pressure signal as well as validating against conductance catheter technology.

SUMMARY

Although in the past decade the importance of the RV has been acknowledged, dysfunction remains a considerable source of morbidity and mortality, especially in certain subsets of perioperative patients. Selective, tailored additional monitoring modalities can be deployed in these patients to construct a comprehensive assessment of RV function. Ongoing investigations have underlined the specific advantages and disadvantages of proposed assessment modalities. The authors believe an integrative approach may be beneficial. Directed evaluation of acute and chronic RV function (and consequent tailored management) is facilitated by combining different sources of information. Multiple promising research paths are being investigated by the community in search of ways to allow constructing a more detailed, but easily visualizable, picture of a specific patient's RV function.

REFERENCES

1. Rudski LG, Lai WW, Afilalo J, et al. Guidelines for the echocardiographic assessment of the right heart in adults: a report from the american society of echocardiography. J Am Soc Echocardiogr 2010;23(7):685–713.

2. Hahn RT, Abraham T, Adams MS, et al. Guidelines for performing a comprehensive transesophageal echocardiographic examination: recommendations from the American Society of Echocardiography and the Society of Cardiovascular Anesthesiologists. J Am Soc Echocardiogr 2013;26(9):921–64.

3. American Society of Anesthesiologists and Society of Cardiovascular Anesthesiologists Task Force on Transesophageal Echocardiography. Practice guidelines for perioperative transesophageal echocardiography. An updated report by the American Society of Anesthesiologists and the Society of Cardiovascular Anesthesiologists Task Force on Transesophageal Echocardiography. Anesthesiology 2010;112(5):1084–96.

4. Reichert CLA, Visser CA, van den Brink RBA, et al. Prognostic value of biventricular function in hypotensive patients after cardiac surgery as assessed by transesophageal echocardiography. J Cardiothorac Vasc Anesth 1992;6(4):429–32.

5. Maslow AD, Regan MM, Panzica P, et al. Precardiopulmonary bypass right ventricular function is associated with poor outcome after coronary artery bypass grafting in patients with severe left ventricular systolic dysfunction. Anesth Analg 2002;95(6):1507–18. Available at: http://www.ncbi.nlm.nih.gov/pubmed/12456409. Accessed January 31, 2019.

6. Campo A, Mathai SC, Le Pavec J, et al. Outcomes of hospitalisation for right heart failure in pulmonary arterial hypertension. Eur Respir J 2011;38(2):359–67.

7. Galiè N, Hoeper MM, Humbert M, et al. Guidelines for the diagnosis and treatment of pulmonary hypertension: the Task Force for the Diagnosis and Treatment of Pulmonary Hypertension of the European Society of Cardiology (ESC) and the European Respiratory Society (ERS), endorsed by the Internat. Eur Heart J 2009;30(20):2493–537.

8. Jasudavisius A, Arellano R, Martin J, et al. A systematic review of transthoracic and transesophageal echocardiography in non-cardiac surgery: implications for point-of-care ultrasound education in the operating room. Can J Anaesth 2016;63(4):480–7.

9. Bartels K, Karhausen J, Sullivan BL, et al. Update on perioperative right heart assessment using transesophageal echocardiography. Semin Cardiothorac Vasc Anesth 2014;18(4):341–51.

10. Grønlykke L, Ravn HB, Gustafsson F, et al. Right ventricular dysfunction after cardiac surgery – diagnostic options. Scand Cardiovasc J 2017;51(2):114–21.

11. Cullen S, Shore D, Redington A. Characterization of right ventricular diastolic performance after complete repair of tetralogy of Fallot. Restrictive physiology predicts slow postoperative recovery. Circulation 1995;91(6):1782–9. Available at: http://www.ncbi.nlm.nih.gov/pubmed/7882488. Accessed January 31, 2019.

12. Gatzoulis MA, Clark AL, Cullen S, et al. Right ventricular diastolic function 15 to 35 years after repair of tetralogy of Fallot. Restrictive physiology predicts superior exercise performance. Circulation 1995;91(6):1775–81. Available at: http://www.ncbi.nlm.nih.gov/pubmed/7882487. Accessed January 31, 2019.

13. Webb G, Gatzoulis MA. Atrial Septal Defects in the Adult. Circulation 2006;114(15):1645–53.

14. Filippov AA, Del Nido PJ, Vasilyev NV. Management of systemic right ventricular failure in patients with congenitally corrected transposition of the great arteries. Circulation 2016;134(17):1293–302.
15. Kamata M, Stiver C, Naguib A, et al. A retrospective analysis of the influence of ventricular morphology on the perioperative outcomes after fontan surgery. J Cardiothorac Vasc Anesth 2017;31(1):128–33.
16. Ohye RG, Schranz D, D'Udekem Y. Current therapy for hypoplastic left heart syndrome and related single ventricle lesions. Circulation 2016;134(17): 1265–79.
17. Raj R, Puri GD, Jayant A, et al. Perioperative echocardiography-derived right ventricle function parameters and early outcomes after tetralogy of Fallot repair in mid-childhood: a single-center, prospective observational study. Echocardiography 2016;33(11):1710–7.
18. Banks DA, Pretorius GVD, Kerr KM, et al. Pulmonary endarterectomy. Semin Cardiothorac Vasc Anesth 2014;18(4):331–40.
19. Banks DA, Pretorius GVD, Kerr KM, et al. Pulmonary endarterectomy. Semin Cardiothorac Vasc Anesth 2014;18(4):319–30.
20. Loghmanpour NA, Kormos RL, Kanwar MK, et al. A bayesian model to predict right ventricular failure following left ventricular assist device therapy. JACC Heart Fail 2016;4(9):711–21.
21. Vivo RP, Cordero-Reyes AM, Qamar U, et al. Increased right-to-left ventricle diameter ratio is a strong predictor of right ventricular failure after left ventricular assist device. J Heart Lung Transplant 2013;32(8):792–9.
22. Cameli M, Lisi M, Righini FM, et al. Speckle tracking echocardiography as a new technique to evaluate right ventricular function in patients with left ventricular assist device therapy. J Heart Lung Transplant 2013;32(4):424–30.
23. Houston BA, Kalathiya RJ, Hsu S, et al. Right ventricular afterload sensitivity dramatically increases after left ventricular assist device implantation: a multicenter hemodynamic analysis. J Heart Lung Transplant 2016;35(7):868–76.
24. Neyer J, Arsanjani R, Moriguchi J, et al. Echocardiographic parameters associated with right ventricular failure after left ventricular assist device: a review. J Heart Lung Transplant 2016;35(3):283–93.
25. Ravis E, Theron A, Mancini J, et al. Severe right ventricular dysfunction is an independent predictor of pre- and post-transplant mortality among candidates for heart transplantation. Arch Cardiovasc Dis 2017;110(3):139–48.
26. Kapoor P, Chowdhury U, Mandal B, et al. Trans-esophageal echocardiography in off-pump coronary artery bypass grafting. Ann Card Anaesth 2009;12(2):174.
27. Sung T-Y, Kwon M-Y, Muhammad HB, et al. Placing a saline bag underneath the heart enhances transgastric transesophageal echocardiographic imaging during cardiac displacement for off-pump coronary artery bypass surgery. J Cardiothorac Vasc Anesth 2014;28(1):42–8.
28. Freed BH, Tsang W, Bhave NM, et al. Right ventricular strain in pulmonary arterial hypertension: a 2D echocardiography and cardiac magnetic resonance study. Echocardiography 2015;32(2):257–63.
29. Harjola V-P, Mebazaa A, Čelutkienė J, et al. Contemporary management of acute right ventricular failure: a statement from the Heart Failure Association and the Working Group on Pulmonary Circulation and Right Ventricular Function of the European Society of Cardiology. Eur J Heart Fail 2016;18(3):226–41.
30. McCabe C, White PA, Rana BS, et al. Right ventricle functional assessment: have new techniques supplanted the old faithful conductance catheter? Cardiol Rev 2014;22(5):233–40.

31. Harvey S, Harrison DA, Singer M, et al. Assessment of the clinical effectiveness of pulmonary artery catheters in management of patients in intensive care (PAC-Man): a randomised controlled trial. Lancet 2005;366(9484):472–7.

32. Rajaram SS, Desai NK, Kalra A, et al. Pulmonary artery catheters for adult patients in intensive care. Cochrane Database Syst Rev 2013;(2):CD003408.

33. Vieillard-Baron A, Naeije R, Haddad F, et al. Diagnostic workup, etiologies and management of acute right ventricle failure: a state-of-the-art paper. Intensive Care Med 2018;44(6):774–90.

34. Simonneau G, Gatzoulis MA, Adatia I, et al. Updated clinical classification of pulmonary hypertension. J Am Coll Cardiol 2013;62(25):D34–41.

35. Robitaille A, Denault AY, Couture P, et al. Importance of relative pulmonary hypertension in cardiac surgery: the mean systemic-to-pulmonary artery pressure ratio. J Cardiothorac Vasc Anesth 2006;20(3):331–9.

36. Haddad F, Hunt SA, Rosenthal DN, et al. Right ventricular function in cardiovascular disease, part I: anatomy, physiology, aging, and functional assessment of the right ventricle. Circulation 2008;117(11):1436–48.

37. Denault A, Deschamps A, Tardif J-C, et al. Pulmonary hypertension in cardiac surgery. Curr Cardiol Rev 2010;6(1):1–14.

38. Massaer B, Bouchez S, Poelaer J. Central venous pressure: an old lady in new clothes? Acta Clin Belg 2006;61(5):228–35.

39. Kinch J, Ryan T. Right ventricular infraction. N Engl J Med 1994;330(17):1211–7.

40. Goldstein JA, Barzilai B, Rosamond TL, et al. Determinants of hemodynamic compromise with severe right ventricular infarction. Circulation 1990;82(2):359–68. Available at: http://www.ncbi.nlm.nih.gov/pubmed/2372887. Accessed January 15, 2019.

41. Denault AY, Haddad F, Jacobsohn E, et al. Perioperative right ventricular dysfunction. Curr Opin Anaesthesiol 2013;26(1):71–81.

42. Raymond M, Grønlykke L, Couture EJ, et al. Perioperative right ventricular pressure monitoring in cardiac surgery. J Cardiothorac Vasc Anesth 2018. https://doi.org/10.1053/j.jvca.2018.08.198.

43. Vegas A, Meineri M. Three-dimensional transesophageal echocardiography is a major advance for intraoperative clinical management of patients undergoing cardiac surgery. Anesth Analg 2010;110(6):1548–73.

44. Lang RM, Badano LP, Tsang W, et al. EAE/ASE recommendations for image acquisition and display using three-dimensional echocardiography. Eur Heart J Cardiovasc Imaging 2012;13(1):1–46.

45. Portnoy SG, Rudski LG. Echocardiographic evaluation of the right ventricle: a 2014 perspective. Curr Cardiol Rep 2015;17(4):21.

46. Tamborini G, Brusoni D, Torres Molina JE, et al. Feasibility of a new generation three-dimensional echocardiography for right ventricular volumetric and functional measurements. Am J Cardiol 2008;102(4):499–505.

47. van der Zwaan HB, Geleijnse ML, McGhie JS, et al. Right ventricular quantification in clinical practice: two-dimensional vs. three-dimensional echocardiography compared with cardiac magnetic resonance imaging. Eur J Echocardiogr 2011;12(9):656–64.

48. Lang RM, Badano LP, Mor-Avi V, et al. Recommendations for cardiac chamber quantification by echocardiography in adults: an update from the American Society of Echocardiography and the European Association of Cardiovascular Imaging. Eur Heart J Cardiovasc Imaging 2015;16(3):233–71.

49. Frank O. Zur Dynamik des Herzmuskels. Z Biol 1895;32:370–447.

50. Asch FM, Bieganski SP, Panza JA, et al. Real-time 3-dimensional echocardiography evaluation of intracardiac masses. Echocardiography 2006;23(3):218–24.
51. Müller S, Feuchtner G, Bonatti J, et al. Value of transesophageal 3D echocardiography as an adjunct to conventional 2D imaging in preoperative evaluation of cardiac masses. Echocardiography 2008;25(6):624–31. Available at: http://www.ncbi.nlm.nih.gov/pubmed/18652008. Accessed January 31, 2019.
52. Almomani A, Morsy M, Dimaano M, et al. Incremental value of transthoracic real time three-dimensional echocardiography in assessment of a right ventricular mass. Echocardiography 2013;30(6):E175–8.
53. Surkova E, Muraru D, Aruta P, et al. Current clinical applications of three-dimensional echocardiography: when the technique makes the difference. Curr Cardiol Rep 2016;18(11):109.
54. Badano LP, Miglioranza MH, Mihăilă S, et al. Left atrial volumes and function by three-dimensional echocardiography: reference values, accuracy, reproducibility, and comparison with two-dimensional echocardiographic measurements. Circ Cardiovasc Imaging 2016;9(7). https://doi.org/10.1161/CIRCIMAGING.115.004229.
55. Peluso D, Badano LP, Muraru D, et al. Right atrial size and function assessed with three-dimensional and speckle-tracking echocardiography in 200 healthy volunteers. Eur Heart J Cardiovasc Imaging 2013;14(11):1106–14.
56. Tamborini G, Marsan NA, Gripari P, et al. Reference values for right ventricular volumes and ejection fraction with real-time three-dimensional echocardiography: evaluation in a large series of normal subjects. J Am Soc Echocardiogr 2010;23(2):109–15.
57. Maffessanti F, Muraru D, Esposito R, et al. Age-, body size-, and sex-specific reference values for right ventricular volumes and ejection fraction by three-dimensional echocardiography: a multicenter echocardiographic study in 507 healthy volunteers. Circ Cardiovasc Imaging 2013;6(5):700–10.
58. Kim J, Cohen SB, Atalay MK, et al. Quantitative assessment of right ventricular volumes and ejection fraction in patients with left ventricular systolic dysfunction by real time three-dimensional echocardiography versus cardiac magnetic resonance imaging. Echocardiography 2015;32(5):805–12.
59. Laser KT, Horst J-P, Barth P, et al. Knowledge-based reconstruction of right ventricular volumes using real-time three-dimensional echocardiographic as well as cardiac magnetic resonance images: comparison with a cardiac magnetic resonance standard. J Am Soc Echocardiogr 2014;27(10):1087–97.
60. Morikawa T, Murata M, Okuda S, et al. Quantitative analysis of right ventricular function in patients with pulmonary hypertension using three-dimensional echocardiography and a two-dimensional summation method compared to magnetic resonance imaging. Am J Cardiol 2011;107(3):484–9.
61. Shimada YJ, Shiota M, Siegel RJ, et al. Accuracy of right ventricular volumes and function determined by three-dimensional echocardiography in comparison with magnetic resonance imaging: a meta-analysis study. J Am Soc Echocardiogr 2010;23(9):943–53.
62. Calcutteea A, Chung R, Lindqvist P, et al. Differential right ventricular regional function and the effect of pulmonary hypertension: three-dimensional echo study. Heart 2011;97(12):1004–11.
63. Inaba T, Yao A, Nakao T, et al. Volumetric and functional assessment of ventricles in pulmonary hypertension on 3-dimensional echocardiography. Circ J 2013;77(1):198–206. Available at: http://www.ncbi.nlm.nih.gov/pubmed/23018765. Accessed January 15, 2019.

64. Sieslack AK, Dziallas P, Nolte I, et al. Quantification of right ventricular volume in dogs: a comparative study between three-dimensional echocardiography and computed tomography with the reference method magnetic resonance imaging. BMC Vet Res 2014;10(1):242.
65. Heusch A, Koch JA, Krogmann ON, et al. Volumetric analysis of the right and left ventricle in a porcine heart model: comparison of three-dimensional echocardiography, magnetic resonance imaging and angiocardiography. Eur J Ultrasound 1999;9(3):245–55. Available at: http://www.ncbi.nlm.nih.gov/pubmed/10657599. Accessed January 15, 2019.
66. Laser KT, Karabiyik AA, K€ Orperich H, et al. Validation and reference values for three-dimensional echocardiographic right ventricular volumetry in children: a multicenter study. J Am Soc Echocardiogr 2018;31:1050–63.
67. Lu X, Nadvoretskiy V, Bu L, et al. Accuracy and reproducibility of real-time three-dimensional echocardiography for assessment of right ventricular volumes and ejection fraction in children. J Am Soc Echocardiogr 2008;21(1):84–9.
68. Knight DS, Grasso AE, Quail MA, et al. Accuracy and reproducibility of right ventricular quantification in patients with pressure and volume overload using single-beat three-dimensional echocardiography. J Am Soc Echocardiogr 2015;28(3):363–74.
69. Tadic M, Celic V, Cuspidi C, et al. Right heart mechanics in untreated normotensive patients with prediabetes and type 2 diabetes mellitus: a two- and three-dimensional echocardiographic study. J Am Soc Echocardiogr 2015;28(3):317–27.
70. Leibundgut G, Rohner A, Grize L, et al. Dynamic assessment of right ventricular volumes and function by real-time three-dimensional echocardiography: a comparison study with magnetic resonance imaging in 100 adult patients. J Am Soc Echocardiogr 2010;23(2):116–26.
71. Jenkins C, Chan J, Bricknell K, et al. Reproducibility of right ventricular volumes and ejection fraction using real-time three-dimensional echocardiography: comparison with cardiac MRI. Chest 2007;131(6):1844–51.
72. Fujimoto S, Mizuno R, Nakagawa Y, et al. Estimation of the right ventricular volume and ejection fraction by transthoracic three-dimensional echocardiography. A validation study using magnetic resonance imaging. Int J Card Imaging 1998;14(6):385–90. Available at: http://www.ncbi.nlm.nih.gov/pubmed/10453393. Accessed January 30, 2019.
73. Gopal AS, Chukwu EO, Iwuchukwu CJ, et al. Normal values of right ventricular size and function by real-time 3-dimensional echocardiography: comparison with cardiac magnetic resonance imaging. J Am Soc Echocardiogr 2007;20(5):445–55.
74. Park J-B, Lee S-P, Lee J-H, et al. Quantification of right ventricular volume and function using single-beat three-dimensional echocardiography: a validation study with cardiac magnetic resonance. J Am Soc Echocardiogr 2016;29(5):392–401.
75. Zhang QB, Sun JP, Gao RF, et al. Feasibility of single-beat full-volume capture real-time three-dimensional echocardiography for quantification of right ventricular volume: validation by cardiac magnetic resonance imaging. Int J Cardiol 2013;168(4):3991–5.
76. Crean AM, Maredia N, Ballard G, et al. 3D Echo systematically underestimates right ventricular volumes compared to cardiovascular magnetic resonance in adult congenital heart disease patients with moderate or severe RV dilatation. J Cardiovasc Magn Reson 2011;13(1):78.

77. Sugeng L, Mor-Avi V, Weinert L, et al. Multimodality comparison of quantitative volumetric analysis of the right ventricle. JACC Cardiovasc Imaging 2010; 3(1):10–8.
78. Karhausen J, Dudaryk R, Phillips-Bute B, et al. Three-dimensional transesophageal echocardiography for perioperative right ventricular assessment. Ann Thorac Surg 2012;94(2):468–74.
79. Magunia H, Schmid E, Hilberath JN, et al. 2D echocardiographic evaluation of right ventricular function correlates with 3D volumetric models in cardiac surgery patients. J Cardiothorac Vasc Anesth 2017;31(2):595–601.
80. Dell'Italia LJ, Walsh RA. Application of a time varying elastance model to right ventricular performance in man. Cardiovasc Res 1988;22(12):864–74. Available at: http://www.ncbi.nlm.nih.gov/pubmed/3256426. Accessed January 15, 2019.
81. Brown KA, Ditchey RV. Human right ventricular end-systolic pressure-volume relation defined by maximal elastance. Circulation 1988;78(1):81–91. Available at: http://www.ncbi.nlm.nih.gov/pubmed/3383413. Accessed January 15, 2019.
82. Kass DA, Maughan WL. From "Emax" to pressure-volume relations: a broader view. Circulation 1988;77(6):1203–12. Available at: http://www.ncbi.nlm.nih.gov/pubmed/3286035.
83. Rex S, Missant C, Claus P, et al. Effects of inhaled iloprost on right ventricular contractility, right ventriculo-vascular coupling and ventricular interdependence: a randomized placebo-controlled trial in an experimental model of acute pulmonary hypertension. Crit Care 2008;12(5):R113.
84. Glower DD, Spratt JA, Snow ND, et al. Linearity of the Frank-Starling relationship in the intact heart: the concept of preload recruitable stroke work. Circulation 1985;71(5):994–1009.
85. Pasipoularides AD, Shu M, Shah A, et al. Right ventricular diastolic relaxation in conscious dog models of pressure overload, volume overload, and ischemia. J Thorac Cardiovasc Surg 2002;124(5):964–72.
86. Kelly RP, Ting CT, Yang TM, et al. Effective arterial elastance as index of arterial vascular load in humans. Circulation 1992;86(2):513–21. Available at: http://www.ncbi.nlm.nih.gov/pubmed/1638719.
87. Segers P, Stergiopulos N, Westerhof N. Relation of effective arterial elastance to arterial system properties. Am J Physiol Heart Circ Physiol 2002;282(3): H1041–6.
88. Fourie PR, Coetzee AR, Bolliger CT. Pulmonary artery compliance: its role in right ventricular-arterial coupling. Cardiovasc Res 1992;26(9):839–44. Available at: http://www.ncbi.nlm.nih.gov/pubmed/1451160. Accessed January 15, 2019.
89. Cholley B, Le Gall A. Ventriculo-arterial coupling: the comeback? J Thorac Dis 2016;8(9):2287–9.
90. Pinsky MR. The right ventricle: interaction with the pulmonary circulation. Crit Care 2016;20(1):266.
91. Vanderpool RR, Pinsky MR, Naeije R, et al. RV-pulmonary arterial coupling predicts outcome in patients referred for pulmonary hypertension. Heart 2015; 101(1):37–43.
92. Ryan JJ, Tedford RJ. Diagnosing and treating the failing right heart. Curr Opin Cardiol 2015;30(3):292–300.
93. Baan J, van der Velde ET, de Bruin HG, et al. Continuous measurement of left ventricular volume in animals and humans by conductance catheter. Circulation 1984;70(5):812–23. Available at: http://www.ncbi.nlm.nih.gov/pubmed/6386218. Accessed January 15, 2019.

94. Burkhoff D. Pressure-volume loops in clinical research. J Am Coll Cardiol 2013; 62(13):1173–6.
95. Sagawa K. The end-systolic pressure-volume relation of the ventricle: definition, modifications and clinical use. Circulation 1981;63(6):1223–7. Available at: http://www.ncbi.nlm.nih.gov/pubmed/7014027. Accessed January 15, 2019.
96. Wei AE, Maslov MY, Pezone MJ, et al. Use of pressure-volume conductance catheters in real-time cardiovascular experimentation. Heart Lung Circ 2014; 23(11):1059–69.
97. Penicka M, Bartunek J, Trakalova H, et al. Heart failure with preserved ejection fraction in outpatients with unexplained dyspnea: a pressure-volume loop analysis. J Am Coll Cardiol 2010;55(16):1701–10.
98. Warriner DR, Brown AG, Varma S, et al. Closing the loop: modelling of heart failure progression from health to end-stage using a meta-analysis of left ventricular pressure-volume loops. PLoS One 2014;9(12):e114153.
99. Spevack DM, Karl J, Yedlapati N, et al. Echocardiographic left ventricular end-diastolic pressure volume loop estimate predicts survival in congestive heart failure. J Card Fail 2013;19(4):251–9.
100. He K-L, Burkhoff D, Leng W-X, et al. Comparison of ventricular structure and function in Chinese patients with heart failure and ejection fractions >55% versus 40% to 55% versus. Am J Cardiol 2009;103(6):845–51.
101. Ky B, French B, May Khan A, et al. Ventricular-arterial coupling, remodeling, and prognosis in chronic heart failure. J Am Coll Cardiol 2013;62(13):1165–72.
102. Delnoy PPHM, Ottervanger JP, Vos DHS, et al. Upgrading to biventricular pacing guided by pressure-volume loop analysis during implantation. J Cardiovasc Electrophysiol 2011;22(6):677–83.
103. Eberhardt F, Hanke T, Fitschen J, et al. AV interval optimization using pressure volume loops in dual chamber pacemaker patients with maintained systolic left ventricular function. Clin Res Cardiol 2012;101(8):647–53.
104. Padeletti L, Pieragnoli P, Ricciardi G, et al. Acute hemodynamic effect of left ventricular endocardial pacing in cardiac resynchronization therapy. Circ Arrhythm Electrophysiol 2012;5(3):460–7.
105. Pappone C, Ćalović Ž, Vicedomini G, et al. Multipoint left ventricular pacing in a single coronary sinus branch improves mid-term echocardiographic and clinical response to cardiac resynchronization therapy. J Cardiovasc Electrophysiol 2015;26(1):58–63.
106. Pieragnoli P, Perego GB, Ricciardi G, et al. Cardiac resynchronization therapy acutely improves ventricular-arterial coupling by reducing the arterial load: assessment by pressure-volume loops. Pacing Clin Electrophysiol 2015;38(4): 431–7.
107. Gaemperli O, Biaggi P, Gugelmann R, et al. Real-time left ventricular pressure-volume loops during percutaneous mitral valve repair with the MitraClip system. Circulation 2013;127(9):1018–27.
108. Lavall D, Reil J-C, Segura Schmitz L, et al. Early hemodynamic improvement after percutaneous mitral valve repair evaluated by noninvasive pressure-volume analysis. J Am Soc Echocardiogr 2016;29(9):888–98.
109. Lim DS, Gutgesell HP, Rocchini AP. Left ventricular function by pressure-volume loop analysis before and after percutaneous repair of large atrial septal defects. J Interv Cardiol 2014;27(2):204–11.
110. McCabe C, White PA, Hoole SP, et al. Right ventricular dysfunction in chronic thromboembolic obstruction of the pulmonary artery: a pressure-volume study using the conductance catheter. J Appl Physiol 2014;116(4):355–63.

111. Mueller I, Jansen-Park S-H, Neidlin M, et al. Design of a right ventricular mock circulation loop as a test bench for right ventricular assist devices. Biomed Tech (Berl) 2017;62(2):131–7.
112. Bishop A, White P, Oldershaw P, et al. Clinical application of the conductance catheter technique in the adult human right ventricle. Int J Cardiol 1997;58(3):211–21. Available at: http://www.ncbi.nlm.nih.gov/pubmed/9076547. Accessed January 15, 2019.
113. Tedford RJ, Mudd JO, Girgis RE, et al. Right ventricular dysfunction in systemic sclerosis–associated pulmonary arterial hypertension. Circ Heart Fail 2013;6(5):953–63.
114. Danton MHD, Greil GF, Byrne JG, et al. Right ventricular volume measurement by conductance catheter. Am J Physiol Heart Circ Physiol 2003;285(4):H1774–85.
115. Chaturvedi RR, Kilner PJ, White PA, et al. Increased airway pressure and simulated branch pulmonary artery stenosis increase pulmonary regurgitation after repair of tetralogy of Fallot. Real-time analysis with a conductance catheter technique. Circulation 1997;95(3):643–9. Available at: http://www.ncbi.nlm.nih.gov/pubmed/9024152. Accessed January 15, 2019.
116. Derrick GP, Narang I, White PA, et al. Failure of stroke volume augmentation during exercise and dobutamine stress is unrelated to load-independent indexes of right ventricular performance after the Mustard operation. Circulation 2000;102(19 Suppl 3):III154–9. Available at: http://www.ncbi.nlm.nih.gov/pubmed/11082379. Accessed January 15, 2019.
117. Itagaki S, Hosseinian L, Varghese R. Right ventricular failure after cardiac surgery: management strategies. Semin Thorac Cardiovasc Surg 2012;24(3):188–94.
118. Vandenheuvel M, Mauermann E, Bouchez S, et al. Perioperative right ventricular pressure-volume loops based on 3D-echo and pulmonary artery catheter. In: Eacta Annual Congress; 2018:P01.2. Manchester, September 19-21, 2018.
119. Uebing A, Fischer G, Schmiel F, et al. Angiocardiographic pressure volume loops in the analysis of right ventricular function after repair of tetralogy of Fallot. Int J Cardiovasc Imaging 2005;21(5):469–80.
120. Kuehne T, Yilmaz S, Steendijk P, et al. Magnetic resonance imaging analysis of right ventricular pressure-volume loops: in vivo validation and clinical application in patients with pulmonary hypertension. Circulation 2004;110(14):2010–6.
121. Witschey WRT, Contijoch F, McGarvey JR, et al. Real-time magnetic resonance imaging technique for determining left ventricle pressure-volume loops. Ann Thorac Surg 2014;97(5):1597–603.
122. Herberg U, Gatzweiler E, Breuer T, et al. Ventricular pressure-volume loops obtained by 3D real-time echocardiography and mini pressure wire-a feasibility study. Clin Res Cardiol 2013;102(6):427–38.

Optimizing Perioperative Blood and Coagulation Management During Cardiac Surgery

Michael Isaäc Meesters, MD, PhD, DESA[a],*,
Christian von Heymann, MD, PhD, DEAA[b]

KEYWORDS

- Cardiac surgery • Cardiopulmonary bypass • Hemostasis • Bleeding • Coagulation
- Transfusion

KEY POINTS

- Bleeding and transfusion in cardiac surgery are common and associated with poorer outcomes.
- Hemostasis in cardiac surgery with cardiopulmonary bypass is complex and influenced by major surgical trauma, cardiopulmonary bypass–associated coagulopathy, anticoagulation management, and additional perioperative factors.
- Patient blood management aims to improve outcomes by the prediction, prevention, monitoring, and treatment of bleeding and transfusion.
- Patient blood management includes many options to improve outcome and should be combined in a multidisciplinary approach.

INTRODUCTION

Major blood loss remains common in cardiac surgery with an incidence of up to 15%.[1,2] Bleeding leads to anemia and blood product transfusion, and can lead to the need for rethoracotomy, which are all independently associated with an adverse outcome (**Fig. 1**).[3,4] Patient blood management is the bundle of measures to

Disclosure Statement: M.I. Meesters does not have any disclosures. C. von Heymann discloses that he has received honoraria for lectures and consultancy work, travel reimbursements and research grants related to the topic of this article from CSL Behring, Novo Nordisk, Ferring GmbH, and Shire over the last 3 years.
^a Department of Anesthesiology, University Medical Center Utrecht, Heidelberglaan 100, Utrecht 3584 CX, the Netherlands; ^b Department of Anaesthesia, Intensive Care Medicine, Emergency Medicine and Pain Therapy, Vivantes Klinikum im Friedrichshain, Landsberger Allee 49, Berlin 10249, Germany
* Corresponding author.
E-mail address: m.meesters.md@gmail.com

Anesthesiology Clin 37 (2019) 713–728
https://doi.org/10.1016/j.anclin.2019.08.006   **anesthesiology.theclinics.com**
1932-2275/19/© 2019 The Authors. Published by Elsevier Inc. This is an open access article under the CC BY-NC-ND license (http://creativecommons.org/licenses/by-nc-nd/4.0/).

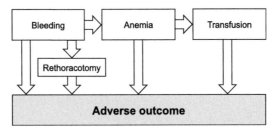

Fig. 1. The relationship between bleeding, rethoracotomy, anemia, transfusion, and outcome.

encounter bleeding and prevent unnecessary transfusion aiming to improve patient outcome.[5] This article focuses on these blood conservation strategies in cardiac surgery. For the understanding of patient blood management in this setting, the pathophysiology of coagulopathy during these procedures, including the effect of cardiopulmonary bypass (CPB), is first discussed. Thereafter, the most important patient blood management strategies are reviewed.

PATHOPHYSIOLOGY OF COAGULOPATHY IN CARDIAC SURGERY

During cardiac surgery with CPB, the coagulation system faces major alterations. First, patients undergo major surgical trauma including sternotomy, venesection, and arterial and venous cannulation, which all lead to hemostasis activation.[6] Second, blood flows over the large surface of the tubing of the heart lung machine, which despite heparinization is highly thrombogenic.[7]

During CPB several mechanisms lead to coagulopathy, as shown in **Fig. 2**. First, fibrinogen binds to the nonbiological surface of the extracorporeal circuit, which causes platelet activation.[8] Second, leukocytes that come in contact with the

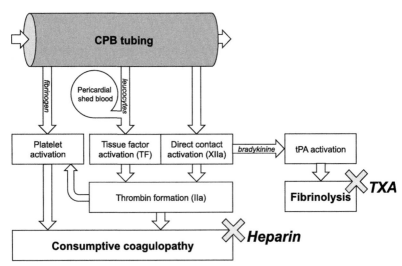

Fig. 2. Hemostasis activation during CPB leading to consumptive coagulopathy and fibrinolysis. IIa, coagulation factor IIa (eg, thrombin, XIIa is coagulation factor XIIa); TF, tissue factor; tPA, tissue plasminogen activator; TXA, tranexamic acid or other antifibrinolytic agent.

pericardial cavity and CPB are activated and express tissue factor, activating the extrinsic coagulation cascade.[9] Furthermore, the tubing of the heart lung machine causes activation of factor XII, which initiates the intrinsic coagulation cascade.[10] Both coagulation pathways lead to thrombin formation and the consumption of coagulation factors (consumptive coagulopathy). Thrombin is a potent platelet activator that causes further thrombocyte degranulation, enhancing hemostasis activation.[11]

Heparin is administrated during bypass to prevent consumptive coagulopathy and the formation of (micro)-thrombi, with subsequent organ infarction. Also, the extracorporeal circulation is nowadays usually covered with a biocompatible heparin coating to damp the hemostatic and immunologic response during bypass.[12]

Activation of the intrinsic coagulation cascade further leads to the formation of active kallikrein that, in turn, enhances the formation of bradykinin.[13] Bradykinin activates tissue plasminogen activator, cleaving plasminogen to plasmin, which breaks down freshly formed clots, for example, fibrinolysis.[14] Usually bradykinin is inactivated in the pulmonary circulation; however, during extracorporeal circulation the lung circulation is bypassed leading to accumulation of bradykinin. This is the cause for massive fibrinolysis in cardiac surgery, which is usually counteracted by the administration of an antifibrinolytic drug (ie, tranexamic acid or ε-aminocaproic acid).

After CPB, the anticoagulant effect of heparin needs to be reversed to restore hemostasis and prevent postoperative bleeding. Protamine is used for this purpose, which binds and inactivates heparin in a 1:1 ratio. However, over the last decades it has become more apparent that protamine itself has several anticoagulant properties.[15] When in excess, protamine inhibits platelet function, causes coagulation factor dysfunction, and enhances fibrinolysis. Therefore, adequate protamine management is important for optimal clot formation after bypass.[16]

Finally, other perioperative disturbances in cardiac surgery can lead to coagulopathy and need to be optimized to prevent a nonsurgical cause of bleeding. Inadequate tissue perfusion leads to anaerobic metabolism and lactate acid formation, which causes acidosis. Acidosis impairs clot formation and adequate hemodynamic management, especially in the cardiac patient with left ventricular dysfunction, is therefore important to optimize hemostasis.[17] However, when excessive fluid administration is used to improve tissue perfusion the prohemostatic components are diluted, impairing hemostasis.[18] Therefore (excessive) hemodilution should be prevented. Furthermore, red blood cell transfusion can lead to better tissue oxygenation, but also to the dilution of coagulation factors. Additionally, packed red blood cell transfusion can cause hypocalcemia by the concurrent administration of citrate.[17] Because calcium (coagulation factor IV) is an important factor in the activation of clotting factors in the coagulation cascade, a calcium debit should be supplemented to prevent coagulopathy. Finally, hypothermia inhibits enzyme activity (reversibly) and, therefore, temperature management is important to optimize clotting after surgery.[17] The most important factors affecting hemostasis in cardiac surgery are summarized in **Box 1**.

PATIENT BLOOD MANAGEMENT

The goal of patient blood management is to reduce bleeding and unnecessary blood transfusion, with the subsequent aim to prevent unfavorable outcomes. This is a multimodal approach comprising the identification of the patients at risk (prediction) as well as the prevention, monitoring, and treatment of microvascular bleeding caused by coagulopathy. **Fig. 3** provides an overview of the individual major patient blood management modalities in cardiac surgery. Each intervention attributes to a small

---

Box 1
Perioperative factors influencing hemostasis in cardiac surgery with CPB

- Major surgical trauma
  - Sternotomy
  - Venesection
  - Arterial and venous cannulation
- CPB-associated coagulopathy
  - Consumptive coagulopathy
  - (Hyper)fibrinolysis
- Anticoagulation management
  - Heparin
  - Protamine
- Additional perioperative factors
  - Acidosis
  - Hemodilution
  - Hypocalcemia
  - Hypothermia

---

improvement in outcome, and when combined these interventions lead to a major decrease in blood loss and transfusion requirements.[19,20] Importantly, all components must be combined in a multidisciplinary approach involving the anesthesiologist, cardiac surgeon, perfusionist, intensivist, and hematologist.

The first step in patient blood management should be the identification of patients at risk for bleeding and transfusion, for example, prediction. Based on this assessment an individual patient blood management strategy can be planned. In patients at high risk for major blood loss and/or transfusion, additional techniques might be appropriate to decrease this risk. These techniques comprise the prevention of unnecessary transfusion and the prevention of coagulopathy. After surgery the amount of blood loss needs to be closely observed and when bleeding is excessive patient's hemostatic potential needs to be monitored. Based on these test results, several treatment modalities aim to improve hemostasis, preventing further hemorrhage and transfusion.

PATIENT BLOOD MANAGEMENT

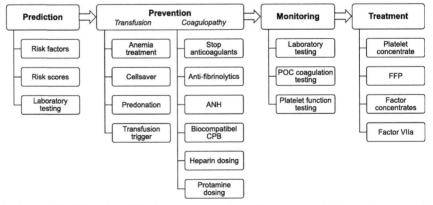

Fig. 3. Multimodal patient blood management in cardiac surgery. ANH, acute normovolemic hemodilution; FFP, fresh frozen plasma; POC, point of care.

Prediction

Risk scores

Many studies identified risk factors for bleeding and transfusion, which include patient-related factors (advancing age, female sex, low body surface area, poor left ventricular function, renal or hepatic impairment) and surgery-related factors (more complex or emergency surgery and a longer duration of CPB).[21,22] Although these risk factors give the clinician an idea about high-risk patients, they have a poor individual predictive value. Therefore, several studies developed scores to better discriminate which patients are at risk. Well evaluated scores include the TRACKS, TRUST, WILL-BLEED, and Papworth Bleeding Risk Score.[23–26] The predictive value of these scores is fair to good (area under the curve of receiver operator characteristic analysis of 0.70–0.80) and can easily be incorporated into daily practice to identify patients at risk for major bleeding and transfusion.

Hemostasis testing for prediction

Although it is common practice to perform routine hemostasis testing before cardiac surgery (prothrombin time, activated partial thromboplastin time, and platelet count) the predictive value of these tests is poor.[27] Only for fibrinogen there is a significant although weak to moderate association with bleeding.[28] As viscoelastometry emerged as an alternative to classical laboratory measurements, it is believed that the predictive value of this method is better. However, a recent systematic review shows that thromboelastometry has a poor positive predictive value for identifying patients at risk for bleeding and/or transfusion in cardiac surgery, although the negative predictive value is good.[29] Platelet function testing in contrast has a much higher positive predictive value, although its clinical applicability to guide interventions remains uncertain.[30,31]

Prevention of Transfusion

Treatment of preoperative anemia

Several studies have identified preoperative anemia as a major risk factor for perioperative transfusion, morbidity and short-term as well as long-term mortality.[32] Moreover, anemia before cardiac surgery is common, with an incidence of 1 in 3 patients.[33] In the cardiac surgical population, anemia is most frequently due to iron deficiency caused by chronic diseases (50%) followed by anemia owing to chronic renal impairment (16%).[34] The increase of the red blood cell mass in these iron-deficient patients can be achieved by the preoperative supplementation of iron with or without the addition of erythropoietin.[35]

Recently, several studies have investigated whether the treatment of preoperative anemia in cardiac surgery results in fewer blood transfusions and improves outcome.[36] So far, there are insufficient robust data to give a high-level recommendation on this matter. Yet, several studies showed positive results of even short-term anemia treatment before cardiac surgery.[37,38] The recent European guideline therefore recommends preoperative hemoglobin optimization by iron infusion with or without erythropoietin in selected patients.[5] Still, the definitive role of preoperative anemia treatment using iron with or without erythropoietin in cardiac surgery remains to be elucidated.

Cell salvage

A well-proven method to decrease red blood cell transfusion in cardiac surgery is the (structural) use of cell salvage.[39] The technique washes blood sucked from the surgical field and/or remaining in the heart lung machine after weaning from CPB. After the processing, solely erythrocytes are retransfused with 2 subsequent benefits. First, patients receive their own red blood cells, increasing the hemoglobin level, preventing anemia and allogenic blood transfusion. Second, after processing, the activated coagulation factors and blood cells are not retransfused, preventing consumptive coagulopathy and inflammation. However, large volumes of salvaged blood transfusion may dilute coagulation factors and platelets, which may increase the risk for dilutional coagulopathy.[40] Therefore, it is suggested to limit the transfusion of large amounts of cell salvaged blood. Still, routine use of cell salvage and the prevention of direct retransfusion of cardiotomy suction blood reduces patient's allogenic transfusion requirements.[39]

Autologous (pre)donation

A less frequently used method to prevent allogenic blood product transfusion is autologous (pre)donation of whole blood before cardiac surgery. In the weeks before surgery, a patient's blood is (repeatedly) withdrawn and stored. This induced anemia leads to increased erythropoiesis, restoring patient's hemoglobin level. Blood loss during surgery can then be substituted by the patient's own predonated blood, preventing the need for allogenic blood transfusion. However, this method is infrequently used because there are several downsides to the technique. First, surgery frequently needs to be postponed to recover from phlebotomy. Second, the stored blood is only temporarily preservable, risking the shed of the donated blood. Finally, patients with aortic stenosis and/or coronary insufficiency, together the most frequent indications for cardiac surgery, are frequently precluded because predonation and the induction of anemia may worsen their condition before surgery. In addition, the safety, criteria and indication for predonation have not yet been clarified. These downsides therefore largely limit its application and resulted in its sporadic use.

Transfusion trigger

In the last decades several large randomized controlled trials were published in search for the optimal red blood cell transfusion trigger in cardiac surgery, aiming to decrease blood product transfusion. First, the TRACS trial compared a hematocrit trigger of 30% with a hematocrit of 24% and found no difference in outcome.[41] The Titer2 trial compared a hemoglobin transfusion trigger of 90 g/L with 75 g/L and likewise found no major differences between the groups.[42] However, at 90 days a borderline statistically higher mortality was found in the restrictive group. In contrast, the more recent TRICS III trial did not find any differences between transfusion thresholds of 90 g/L and 75 g/L in the short- and long-term analysis.[43,44] These results suggest that a restrictive transfusion trigger is safe in patients undergoing cardiac surgery.

Despite these large, high-quality trails, the optimal transfusion threshold for packed red blood cell transfusion remains a matter of debate. This debate is understandable when we look at the rationale for packed red blood cell transfusion, for which we have to go back to the basic physiologic principle of the delivery of oxygen (DO_2). When the DO_2 meets its oxygen demands (VO_2) mitochondria conduct aerobe metabolization as a source of energy. However, when the tissue oxygenation drops below the VO_2, anaerobic metabolization starts, inducing an oxygen debt and lactate acidosis.

$$DO_2 = CO \times CaO_2$$

$$DO_2 = CO \times [(Hb \times 1.39 \times SaO_2) + (Po_2 \times 0.003)]$$

The formula for oxygen delivery is:
DO_2 = oxygen delivery, CO = cardiac output, CaO_2 = arterial oxygen capacity, Hb = hemoglobin level, SaO_2 = arterial oxygen saturation, Po_2 = arterial oxygen tension.

Red blood cells are transfused to prevent tissue hypoxemia. However, tissue oxygenation depends on the patient's cardiac output, hemoglobin level, and arterial oxygen saturation, as shown by the DO_2 formula. Herein lies the difficulty for the optimal transfusion trigger. A patient with a normal cardiac reserve might have sufficient oxygen delivery with a hemoglobin level of 3.0 mmol/L when the circulating volume is appropriate. However, a patient with a decreased left ventricular function and a low arterial saturation might need a hemoglobin concentration of 5.0 mmol/L for adequate tissue oxygenation. Furthermore, the optimal transfusion trigger will be different when cooled and under anesthesia (with lower oxygen demands) compared with the increased oxygen demands when rehabilitating in the ward. These factors are difficult to incorporate into clinical trials. Most randomized controlled trials therefore randomized patients to 2 hemoglobin levels. However, it is advocated to incorporate signs of tissue oxygenation ($ScvO_2$, lactate, heart rate, etc) into the rationale for the transfusion of red blood cells and thereby individualize the transfusion trigger.[5]

Prevention of Coagulopathy

Stop anticoagulation
An important part of patient blood management is the preoperative cessation of anticoagulants. Guidelines exist for the optimal timing for interruption of antithrombotic drugs.[5,45] However, when anticoagulants are stopped the bleeding risk decreases and the thrombotic risk increases. Some drugs are given to prevent low risk incidence thrombotic events whereas others have a high risk of thrombosis when stopped. Therefore, it is important to keep the overall outcome (eg, morbidity and mortality) in mind when stopping anticoagulants before surgery and individually weigh the risk of reduction of transfusion and thrombotic complications.[46]

Antifibrinolytics
It is common practice to use antifibrinolytics to prevent clot breakdown. Formerly, aprotinin was used for this purpose with pleiotropic positive effects on hemostasis, including the prevention of fibrinolysis. However, owing to safety concerns aprotinin has been withdrawn from the market in 2007 as it was associated with kidney failure and increased mortality, although it was superior in hemostasis optimization. After critical reappraisal of the risks, aprotinin has recently been readmitted to the European market.[47] However, its use has largely been replaced by tranexamic acid (and ε-aminocapron acid).[48,49] However, when tranexamic acid is administrated in high dosage, there is an increased incidence of postoperative seizures, associated with poorer outcomes.[49,50] A dosage more than 50 mg/kg^{-1} is, therefore, not recommended.

Acute normovolemic hemodilution
An easier alternative to preoperative autologous predonation is acute normovolemic hemodilution. The patient's whole blood is withdrawn directly before CPB and replaced with crystalloids to intercept the hemodynamic consequences. After weaning from bypass, the patient's own blood is retransfused. The advantage of this method is that the stored autologous whole blood is not exposed to the coagulopathic effects of the extracorporeal circulation, preserving its hemostatic potential. The technique is mainly used in patients with high preoperative hemoglobin levels and is associated with a decrease in bleeding and transfusion.[51] However, some patients cannot withstand an acute decrease in hemoglobin level or circulating volume. This limits its use in patients with cardiovascular compromise.

A similar method is available for the harvesting patient's thrombocytes before bypass by acute preoperative platelet pheresis. By returning the preserved platelets to the patient after bypass, thrombocytopathy can be prevented. Although this method might lead to a decrease in blood product transfusion, the evidence for this technique is scarce, outdated, and of poor quality.[52]

Anticoagulation during cardiopulmonary bypass

Heparin is administrated in cardiac surgery to prevent the formation of (micro)thrombi caused by the CPB. However, there is poor evidence for the optimal anticoagulation regimen and even at target anticoagulation levels thrombin formation can still be observed.[53] The typical activated clotting time target is 400 to 480 seconds, for which the rationale dates back to the 1970s.[54,55] Although some more recent studies show advantages of lower anticoagulation regimes (activated clotting time target 180–250 seconds), this practice has not found way into daily practice.[56,57] So, despite advances in the development of biocompatible and heparin-coated circuits, the problem of how to monitor the efficacy of heparinization during CPB persists.[12,58,59]

Protamine dosing

In the last decade, interest in protamine emerged as it became clear that protamine overdosing impairs hemostasis, as mentioned.[15] In 1994, Despotis and colleagues[60] showed that, although the activated clotting time remains above the desired target, the heparin concentration decreases during bypass. This leads to overdosing when the protamine dose is based on the full initial heparin dose administrated. However, for many years this has been common practice because high protamine dosing was thought to be harmless. More recently, many studies have investigated the effect of protamine dosing based on a pharmacokinetic model of heparin. This practice has led to a major decrease in the amount of protamine administrated and decreased bleeding and transfusion.[16,61] It is therefore recommended to decrease protamine dosing to a dosing ratio less than 1:1 based on the initial heparin dose to prevent postoperative coagulopathy.

Monitoring

Bleeding in cardiac surgery has many causes and various diagnostic algorithms exist to identify its source and guide its treatment. First, it is important to distinguish a surgical bleed (the origin of bleeding in up to 70% of the cases) from a nonsurgical origin because they require different therapy.[2] For the latter, also known as coagulopathic bleeding or oozing, still many causes remain in cardiac surgery, including decreased thrombin formation (coagulation factor deficiency, residual heparin or protamine overdosing), hypofibrinogenemia, thrombocytopenia, platelet dysfunction, or excessive fibrinolysis (**Fig. 4**).[62] Obviously, multiple causes can occur simultaneously.

Clinically, it can be difficult to distinguish a surgical from a nonsurgical cause of bleeding and both can occur concurrently. Furthermore, when blood loss persists coagulopathy can be induced or aggravated by the dilution, consumption and loss of prohemostatic components (ie, platelets and coagulation factors). Therefore, when a nonsurgical cause of bleeding is suspected, it is important to promptly reverse the coagulopathic state to prevent further hemorrhage and transfusion.

Laboratory coagulation tests can be used to investigate the cause of bleeding. However, owing to their long turnaround times, treatment will be delayed and the test results do not reflect the present coagulation status. This leads to the blind administration of prohemostatic components and risks the patient for inadequate or excessive treatment.[63] To overcome this limitation several point-of-care devices have emerged to rapidly investigate patient's hemostasis status.

Point-of-care coagulation testing is a popular method to identify coagulopathic causes of bleeding, described in detail elsewhere.[64] In the last decades, many studies

A less known product is coagulation factor XIII concentrate, which stabilizes a freshly formed fibrin network. CPB diminishes the concentration of this factor and bleeding can be reduced when it is supplemented in the case of an FXIII plasma activity of less than 70%.[86,87] However, only few centers have the option to rapidly measure its activity and its use is therefore limited in common practice.

In the beginning of this century recombinant factor VIIa emerged a "magic bullet" for coagulopathy-induced bleeding. However, when the data of its trials were systematically investigated, it became apparent that activated factor VII increased the risk of severe thromboembolic events.[88] Therefore, its use should be reserved for patients in which all other treatment options fail.

SUMMARY

Bleeding and transfusion remain common in cardiac surgery and are associated with adverse outcomes. Bleeding is frequently due to, or aggravated by, coagulopathy, which is caused by the complex interaction between the CPB, major surgical trauma, anticoagulation management and additional perioperative factors. Patient blood management strategies emerged to improve outcome by the prediction, prevention, monitoring, and treatment of bleeding and transfusion. Each part of this chain has several individual modalities and when combined improves outcome. It is important to implement patient blood management in a multidisciplinary approach, involving the anesthesiologist, cardiac surgeon, perfusionist, intensivist, hematologist and cardiologist for it to lead to optimal results.

REFERENCES

1. Karkouti K, Wijeysundera DN, Beattie WS, et al. Variability and predictability of large-volume red blood cell transfusion in cardiac surgery: a multicenter study. Transfusion 2007;47(11):2081–8.

2. Colson PH, Gaudard P, Fellahi J-L, et al. Active bleeding after cardiac surgery: a prospective observational multicenter study. PLoS One 2016;11(9):e0162396. Garcia de Frutos P, ed.

3. Murphy GJ, Reeves BC, Rogers CA, et al. Increased mortality, postoperative morbidity, and cost after red blood cell transfusion in patients having cardiac surgery. Circulation 2007;116(22):2544–52.

4. Ranucci M, Baryshnikova E, Castelvecchio S, et al, Surgical and Clinical Outcome Research (SCORE) Group. Major bleeding, transfusions, and anemia: the deadly triad of cardiac surgery. Ann Thorac Surg 2013;96(2):478–85.

5. Boer C, Meesters MI, Milojevic M, et al. 2017 EACTS/EACTA guidelines on patient blood management for adult cardiac surgery. J Cardiothorac Vasc Anesth 2018; 53(1):79–111.

6. Gravlee GP, Whitaker CL, Mark LJ, et al. Baseline activated coagulation time should be measured after surgical incision. Anesth Analg 1990;71(5):549–53.

7. Gorbet MB, Sefton MV. Biomaterial-associated thrombosis: roles of coagulation factors, complement, platelets and leukocytes. Biomaterials 2004;25(26): 5681–703.

8. Tsai W-B, Grunkemeier JM, McFarland CD, et al. Platelet adhesion to polystyrene-based surfaces preadsorbed with plasmas selectively depleted in fibrinogen, fibronectin, vitronectin, or von Willebrand's factor. J Biomed Mater Res 2002; 60(3):348–59.

9. Shibamiya A, Tabuchi N, Chung J, et al. Formation of tissue factor-bearing leukocytes during and after cardiopulmonary bypass. Thromb Haemost 2004;92(1):124–31.

10. Burman JF, Chung HI, Lane DA, et al. Role of factor XII in thrombin generation and fibrinolysis during cardiopulmonary bypass. Lancet 1994;344(8931):1192–3.

11. De Candia E. Mechanisms of platelet activation by thrombin: a short history. Thromb Res 2012;129(3):250–6.

12. Ranucci M, Balduini A, Ditta A, et al. A systematic review of biocompatible cardiopulmonary bypass circuits and clinical outcome. Ann Thorac Surg 2009;87(4):1311–9.

13. Campbell DJ, Dixon B, Kladis A, et al. Activation of the kallikrein-kinin system by cardiopulmonary bypass in humans. Am J Physiol Regul Integr Comp Physiol 2001;281(4):R1059–70.

14. Balaguer JM, Yu C, Byrne JG, et al. Contribution of endogenous bradykinin to fibrinolysis, inflammation, and blood product transfusion following cardiac surgery: a randomized clinical trial. Clin Pharmacol Ther 2013;93(4):326–34.

15. Boer C, Meesters MI, Veerhoek D, et al. Anticoagulant and side-effects of protamine in cardiac surgery: a narrative review. Br J Anaesth 2018;120(5):914–27.

16. Meesters MI, Veerhoek D, de Jong JR, et al. A pharmacokinetic model for protamine dosing after cardiopulmonary bypass. J Cardiothorac Vasc Anesth 2016;30(5):1190–5.

17. De Robertis E, Kozek-Langenecker SA, Tufano R, et al. Coagulopathy induced by acidosis, hypothermia and hypocalcaemia in severe bleeding. Minerva Anestesiol 2015;81(1):65–75.

18. Chandler WL. Effects of hemodilution, blood loss, and consumption on hemostatic factor levels during cardiopulmonary bypass. J Cardiothorac Vasc Anesth 2005;19(4):459–67.

19. Vonk ABA, Meesters MI, van Dijk WB, et al. Ten-year patterns in blood product utilization during cardiothoracic surgery with cardiopulmonary bypass in a tertiary hospital. Transfusion 2013;54(10pt2):2608–16.

20. Ranucci M, Baryshnikova E, Pistuddi V, et al. The effectiveness of 10 years of interventions to control postoperative bleeding in adult cardiac surgery. Interact Cardiovasc Thorac Surg 2017;24(2):196–202.

21. Ferraris VA, Brown JR, Despotis GJ, et al. 2011 Update to the Society of Thoracic Surgeons and the Society of Cardiovascular Anesthesiologists blood conservation clinical practice guidelines. Ann Thorac Surg 2011;91(3):944–82.

22. Lopes CT, Santos dos TR, Brunori EHFR, et al. Excessive bleeding predictors after cardiac surgery in adults: integrative review. J Clin Nurs 2015;24(21–22):3046–62.

23. Ranucci M, Castelvecchio S, Frigiola A, et al. Predicting transfusions in cardiac surgery: the easier, the better: the Transfusion Risk and Clinical Knowledge score. Vox Sang 2009;96(4):324–32.

24. Alghamdi AA, Davis A, Brister S, et al. Development and validation of Transfusion Risk Understanding Scoring Tool (TRUST) to stratify cardiac surgery patients according to their blood transfusion needs. Transfusion 2006;46(7):1120–9.

25. Biancari F, Brascia D, Onorati F, et al. Prediction of severe bleeding after coronary surgery: the WILL-BLEED Risk Score. Thromb Haemost 2017;117(03):445–56.

26. Vuylsteke A, Pagel C, Gerrard C, et al. The Papworth Bleeding Risk Score: a stratification scheme for identifying cardiac surgery patients at risk of excessive early postoperative bleeding. Eur J Cardiothorac Surg 2011;39(6):924–30.

27. Haas T, Fries D, Tanaka KA, et al. Usefulness of standard plasma coagulation tests in the management of perioperative coagulopathic bleeding: is there any evidence? Br J Anaesth 2015;114(2):217–24.
28. Gielen C, Dekkers O, Stijnen T, et al. The effects of pre- and postoperative fibrinogen levels on blood loss after cardiac surgery: a systematic review and meta-analysis. Interact Cardiovasc Thorac Surg 2014;18(3):292–8.
29. Meesters MI, Burtman D, van de Ven PM, et al. Prediction of postoperative blood loss by thromboelastometry in adult cardiac surgery: cohort study & systematic review. J Cardiothorac Vasc Anesth 2018;32(1):141–50.
30. Corredor C, Wasowicz M, Karkouti K, et al. The role of point-of-care platelet function testing in predicting postoperative bleeding following cardiac surgery: a systematic review and meta-analysis. Anaesthesia 2015;70(6):715–31.
31. Petricevic M, Kopjar T, Biocina B, et al. The predictive value of platelet function point-of-care tests for postoperative blood loss and transfusion in routine cardiac surgery: a systematic review. Thorac Cardiovasc Surg 2015;63(1):2–20.
32. Heymann von C, Kaufner L, Sander M, et al. Does the severity of preoperative anemia or blood transfusion have a stronger impact on long-term survival after cardiac surgery? J Thorac Cardiovasc Surg 2016;152(5):1412–20.
33. Klein AA, Collier TJ, Brar MS, et al. The incidence and importance of anaemia in patients undergoing cardiac surgery in the UK - the first Association of Cardiothoracic Anaesthetists national audit. Anaesthesia 2016;71(6):627–35.
34. Hung M, Ortmann E, Besser M, et al. A prospective observational cohort study to identify the causes of anaemia and association with outcome in cardiac surgical patients. Heart 2015;101(2):107–12.
35. Anker SD, Comin Colet J, Filippatos G, et al. Ferric carboxymaltose in patients with heart failure and iron deficiency. N Engl J Med 2009;361(25):2436–48.
36. Hogan M, Klein AA, Richards T. The impact of anaemia and intravenous iron replacement therapy on outcomes in cardiac surgery. Eur J Cardiothorac Surg 2015;47(2):218–26.
37. Yoo Y-C, Shim J-K, Kim J-C, et al. Effect of single recombinant human erythropoietin injection on transfusion requirements in preoperatively anemic patients undergoing valvular heart surgery. Anesthesiology 2011;115(5):929–37.
38. Weltert L, Rondinelli B, Bello R, et al. A single dose of erythropoietin reduces perioperative transfusions in cardiac surgery: results of a prospective single blind randomized controlled trial. Transfusion 2015;55(7):1644–54.
39. Carless PA, Henry DA, Moxey AJ, et al. Cell salvage for minimising perioperative allogeneic blood transfusion. Carless PA, ed. Cochrane Database Syst Rev 2010;(4):CD001888.
40. Shen S, Zhang J, Wang W, et al. Impact of intra-operative cell salvage on blood coagulation in high-bleeding-risk patients undergoing cardiac surgery with cardiopulmonary bypass: a prospective randomized and controlled trial. J Transl Med 2016;14(1):228.
41. Hajjar LA, Vincent J-L, Galas FRBG, et al. Transfusion requirements after cardiac surgery: the TRACS randomized controlled trial. JAMA 2010;304(14):1559–67.
42. Murphy GJ, Pike K, Rogers CA, et al. Liberal or restrictive transfusion after cardiac surgery. N Engl J Med 2015;372(11):997–1008.
43. Mazer CD, Whitlock RP, Fergusson DA, et al. Restrictive or liberal red-cell transfusion for cardiac surgery. N Engl J Med 2017;377(22):2133–44.
44. Mazer CD, Whitlock RP, Fergusson DA, et al. Six-month outcomes after restrictive or liberal transfusion for cardiac surgery. N Engl J Med 2018;379(13):1224–33.

45. Sousa Uva M, Head SJ, Milojevic M, et al. 2017 EACTS Guidelines on perioperative medication in adult cardiac surgery. Eur J Cardiothorac Surg 2018; 53(1):5–33.

46. Meesters MI, Boer C. Cessation of antithrombotic therapy before surgery: weighing thrombosis and bleeding risks. Neth Heart J 2014;22(9):370–1.

47. Available at: https://www.ema.europa.eu/en/medicines/human/referrals/anti fibrinolytic-medicines. Accessed December, 2018.

48. Adler Ma SC, Brindle W, Burton G, et al. Tranexamic acid is associated with less blood transfusion in off-pump coronary artery bypass graft surgery: a systematic review and meta-analysis. J Cardiothorac Vasc Anesth 2011;25(1):26–35.

49. Myles PS, Smith JA, Forbes A, et al. Tranexamic acid in patients undergoing coronary-artery surgery. N Engl J Med 2017;376(2):136–48.

50. Lin Z, Xiaoyi Z. Tranexamic acid-associated seizures: a meta-analysis. Seizure 2016;36:70–3.

51. Barile L, Fominskiy E, Di Tomasso N, et al. Acute normovolemic hemodilution reduces allogeneic red blood cell transfusion in cardiac surgery: a systematic review and meta-analysis of randomized trials. Anesth Analg 2017;124(3):743–52.

52. Rubens FD, Fergusson D, Wells PS, et al. Platelet-rich plasmapheresis in cardiac surgery: a meta-analysis of the effect on transfusion requirements. J Thorac Cardiovasc Surg 1998;116(4):641–7.

53. Shore-Lesserson L, Baker RA, Ferraris V, et al. STS/SCA/AmSECT clinical practice guidelines: anticoagulation during cardiopulmonary bypass. J Extra Corpor Technol 2018;50(1):5–18.

54. Bull BS, Korpman RA, Huse WM, et al. Heparin therapy during extracorporeal circulation. I. Problems inherent in existing heparin protocols. J Thorac Cardiovasc Surg 1975;69(5):674–84.

55. Young JA, Kisker CT, Doty DB. Adequate anticoagulation during cardiopulmonary bypass determined by activated clotting time and the appearance of fibrin monomer 1978;26(3):231–40.

56. Segesser von LK, Weiss BM, Pasic M, et al. Risk and benefit of low systemic heparinization during open heart operations. Ann Thorac Surg 1994;58(2):391–8.

57. Aldea GS, O'Gara P, Shapira OM, et al. Effect of anticoagulation protocol on outcome in patients undergoing CABG with heparin-bonded cardiopulmonary bypass circuits. Ann Thorac Surg 1998;65(2):425–33.

58. Mangoush O, Purkayastha S, Haj-Yahia S, et al. Heparin-bonded circuits versus nonheparin-bonded circuits: an evaluation of their effect on clinical outcomes. Eur J Cardiothorac Surg 2007;31(6):1058–69.

59. Zangrillo A, Garozzo FA, Biondi-Zoccai G, et al. Miniaturized cardiopulmonary bypass improves short-term outcome in cardiac surgery: a meta-analysis of randomized controlled studies. J Thorac Cardiovasc Surg 2010;139(5):1162–9.

60. Despotis GJ, Summerfield AL, Joist JH, et al. Comparison of activated coagulation time and whole blood heparin measurements with laboratory plasma anti-Xa heparin concentration in patients having cardiac operations. J Thorac Cardiovasc Surg 1994;108(6):1076–82.

61. Kjellberg G, Holm M, Fux T, et al. Calculation algorithm reduces protamine doses without increasing blood loss or the transfusion rate in cardiac surgery: results of a randomized controlled trial. J Cardiothorac Vasc Anesth 2019;33(4):985–92.

62. Ranucci M. Hemostatic and thrombotic issues in cardiac surgery. Semin Thromb Hemost 2015;41(1):84–90.

63. Meesters MI, Koning NJ, Romijn JWA, et al. Clinical decision versus thromboelas-tometry based fresh frozen plasma transfusion in cardiac surgery. Br J Anaesth 2017;118(3):458–9.
64. Bolliger D, Tanaka KA. Point-of-care coagulation testing in cardiac surgery. Semin Thromb Hemost 2017;43(4):386–96.
65. Serraino GF, Murphy GJ. Routine use of viscoelastic blood tests for diagnosis and treatment of coagulopathic bleeding in cardiac surgery: updated systematic re-view and meta-analysis. Br J Anaesth 2017;118(6):823–33.
66. Dai Y, Lee A, Critchley LAH, et al. Does thromboelastography predict postoper-ative thromboembolic events? A systematic review of the literature. Anesth Analg 2009;108(3):734–42.
67. Zaffar N, Joseph A, Mazer CD, et al. Justification de la transfusion de plaquettes pendant la circulation extracorporelle: une étude observationnelle. Can J Anaesth 2013;60(4):345–54.
68. Kong R, Trimmings A, Hutchinson N, et al. Consensus recommendations for us-ing the Multiplate(®) for platelet function monitoring before cardiac surgery. Int J Lab Hematol 2015;37(2):143–7.
69. Desborough MJR, Smethurst PA, Estcourt LJ, et al. Alternatives to allogeneic platelet transfusion. Br J Haematol 2016;175(3):381–92.
70. Velik-Salchner C, Haas T, Innerhofer P, et al. The effect of fibrinogen concentrate on thrombocytopenia. J Thromb Haemost 2007;5(5):1019–25.
71. Caudill JSC, Nichols WL, Plumhoff EA, et al. Comparison of coagulation factor XIII content and concentration in cryoprecipitate and fresh-frozen plasma. Transfu-sion 2009;49(4):765–70.
72. Shaz BH. Bye-bye TRALI: by understanding and innovation. Blood 2014;123(22):3374–6.
73. Peng Z, Pati S, Potter D, et al. Fresh frozen plasma lessens pulmonary endothelial inflammation and hyperpermeability after hemorrhagic shock and is associated with loss of syndecan 1. Shock 2013;40(3):195–202.
74. Kozar RA, Peng Z, Zhang R, et al. Plasma restoration of endothelial glycocalyx in a rodent model of hemorrhagic shock. Anesth Analg 2011;112(6):1289–95.
75. Murad MH, Stubbs JR, Gandhi MJ, et al. The effect of plasma transfusion on morbidity and mortality: a systematic review and meta-analysis. Transfusion 2010;50(6):1370–83.
76. Desborough M, Sandu R, Brunskill SJ, et al. Fresh frozen plasma for cardiovascular surgery. Desborough M, ed. Cochrane Database Syst Rev 2015;(7):CD007614.
77. Bolliger D, Tanaka KA. Fibrinogen—is it a universal haemostatic agent? Br J Anaesth 2016;117(5):548–50.
78. Hiippala ST, Myllylä GJ, Vahtera EM. Hemostatic factors and replacement of ma-jor blood loss with plasma-poor red cell concentrates. Anesth Analg 1995;81(2):360–5.
79. Li J-Y, Gong J, Zhu F, et al. Fibrinogen concentrate in cardiovascular surgery. Anesth Analg 2018;127(3):612–21.
80. Fassl J, Lurati Buse G, Filipovic M, et al. Perioperative administration of fibrinogen does not increase adverse cardiac and thromboembolic events after cardiac sur-gery. Br J Anaesth 2015;114(2):225–34.
81. Ortmann E, Besser MW, Sharples LD, et al. An exploratory cohort study comparing prothrombin complex concentrate and fresh frozen plasma for the treatment of coagulopathy after complex cardiac surgery. Anesth Analg 2015;121(1):26–33.

82. Fitzgerald J, Lenihan M, Callum J, et al. Use of prothrombin complex concentrate for management of coagulopathy after cardiac surgery: a propensity score matched comparison to plasma. Br J Anaesth 2018;120(5):928–34.

83. Percy CL, Hartmann R, Jones RM, et al. Correcting thrombin generation ex vivo using different haemostatic agents following cardiac surgery requiring the use of cardiopulmonary bypass. Blood Coagul Fibrinolysis 2015;26(4):357–67.

84. Schenk B, Goerke S, Beer R, et al. Four-factor prothrombin complex concentrate improves thrombin generation and prothrombin time in patients with bleeding complications related to rivaroxaban: a single-center pilot trial. Thromb J 2018; 16(1):1.

85. Crescenzi G, Landoni G, Biondi-Zoccai G, et al. Desmopressin reduces transfusion needs after surgery: a meta-analysis of randomized clinical trials. Anesthesiology 2008;109(6):1063–76.

86. Gödje O, Gallmeier U, Schelian M, et al. Coagulation factor XIII reduces postoperative bleeding after coronary surgery with extracorporeal circulation. Thorac Cardiovasc Surg 2006;54(1):26–33

87. Karkouti K, Heymann von C, Jespersen CM, et al. Efficacy and safety of recombinant factor XIII on reducing blood transfusions in cardiac surgery: a randomized, placebo-controlled, multicenter clinical trial. J Thorac Cardiovasc Surg 2013;146(4):927–39.

88. Simpson E, Lin Y, Stanworth S, et al. Recombinant factor VIIa for the prevention and treatment of bleeding in patients without haemophilia. Stanworth S, ed. Cochrane Database Syst Rev 2012;(3):CD005011.

Prevention of Cardiac Surgery-Associated Acute Kidney Injury
A Review of Current Strategies

Kirolos A. Jacob, MD, PhD[a],*, David E. Leaf, MD, MMSc[b]

KEYWORDS

- Acute kidney injury • Prevention • Perioperative care • Inflammation
- Cardiac surgery • Randomized controlled trial

KEY POINTS

- Most large randomized controlled trials in cardiac surgery-associated acute kidney injury have been negative.
- Encouraging results have been shown with administration of glucocorticoids preoperatively, leukocyte filtration, and inhaled nitric oxide intraoperatively, and implementation of a postoperative Kidney Disease: Improving Global Outcomes bundle of care.
- Future trials should use more precise phenotyping of patients to more accurately identify subgroups of patients most likely to benefit from various interventions.

INTRODUCTION

Cardiac surgery is one of the most common surgical procedures performed worldwide.[1] Technological advances and protocolized perioperative patient care have resulted in major improvements in clinical outcomes, including mortality. Despite these improvements, multiple postoperative complications, including atrial fibrillation, myocardial infarction, and stroke, remain common after cardiac surgery, and are associated with significant morbidity and mortality.[2]

Acute kidney injury (AKI) is a common and often devastating complication of cardiac surgery. The reported incidence of cardiac surgery-associated AKI (CS-AKI) depends on the characteristics of the patient population, as well as on the definition used for

Conflict of Interest: None declared.
[a] Department of Cardiothoracic Surgery, University Medical Center Utrecht, Mail Stop E03.511, PO Box 85500, Utrecht 3508 GA, the Netherlands; [b] Division of Renal Medicine, Brigham and Women's Hospital, 75 Francis Street, Medial Research Building Room MR416B, Boston, MA 02115, USA
* Corresponding author.
E-mail address: k.a.jacob@umcutrecht.nl

Anesthesiology Clin 37 (2019) 729–749
https://doi.org/10.1016/j.anclin.2019.08.007   **anesthesiology.theclinics.com**
1932-2275/19/© 2019 The Authors. Published by Elsevier Inc. This is an open access article under the CC BY-NC-ND license (http://creativecommons.org/licenses/by-nc-nd/4.0/).

AKI. Mild forms of CS-AKI occur in up to 30% of patients undergoing cardiac surgery,[3] whereas CS-AKI requiring dialysis occurs in only approximately 1% of patients, but is associated with a markedly increased risk of death.[4–6] Patients who recover from an episode of CS-AKI remain at greatly increased risk of incident and progressive chronic kidney disease.[3,7–9]

Various consensus-based definitions have been proposed for AKI, and are summarized in **Table 1**. Known risk factors for CS-AKI include advancing age, diabetes mellitus, preoperative chronic kidney disease (often defined as an estimated glomerular filtration rate of <60 mL/min/1.73 m^2), and type of surgery, with open chamber procedures and reoperations corresponding with a higher risk of AKI. Among these risk factors, chronic kidney disease likely has the greatest prognostic value.[4,7,10]

Numerous studies have attempted to determine the factors and mechanisms that cause CS-AKI. Pathways that have been proposed include the systemic inflammatory response, hemolysis-induced injury, as well as ischemia–reperfusion injury caused by oxidative stress perioperatively.[3,7,11–13] It is likely that a combination of more than one of these factors, together with patient-related predisposing risk factors, is responsible for CS-AKI in any given patient.

Table 1
Consensus-based definitions have been proposed for AKI

Classification	Definitions of AKI Incidence and Severity	
	Based on Changes in SCr	**Based on Changes in UOP**
RIFLE	Definition: Increase in SCr ≥1.5× or decrease in GFR ≥25% within 7 d Risk (R): Increase in SCr ≥1.5× or decrease in GFR ≥25% Injury (I): Increase in SCr ≥2× or decrease in GFR ≥50% Failure (F): Increase in SCr ≥3× or decrease in GFR ≥75%, or SCr >4 mg/dL with an acute increase >0.5 mg/dL	Definition: UOP <0.5 mL/kg per hour for ≥6 h Risk (R): UOP <0.5 mL/kg per hour for ≥6 h Injury (I): UOP <0.5 mL/kg per hour for ≥12 h Failure (F): UOP <0.3 mL/kg per hour for ≥24 h or anuria for ≥12 h
AKIN	Definition: Increase in SCr ≥0.3 mg/dL or ≥1.5x within <48h Stage 1: Increase in SCr ≥0.3 mg/dL or ≥1.5× Stage 2: Increase in SCr ≥2× Stage 3: Increase in SCr ≥3×, or SCr >4 mg/dL with an acute increase >0.5 mg/dL, or RRT	Definition: UOP <0.5 mL/kg per hour for ≥6 h Stage 1: UOP <0.5 mL/kg per hour for ≥6 h Stage 2: UOP <0.5 mL/kg per hour for ≥12 h Stage 3: UOP <0.3 mL/kg per hour for ≥24 h or anuria for ≥12 h
KDIGO	Definition: Increase in SCr ≥0.3 mg/dL within 48 h or ≥50% within 7 d Stage 1: Increase in SCr ≥0.3 mg/dL or ≥1.5× Stage 2: Increase in SCr ≥2× Stage 3: Increase in SCr ≥3×, or SCr >4 mg/dL, or RRT	Definition: UOP <0.5 mL/kg per hour for ≥6 h Stage 1: UOP <0.5 mL/kg per hour for ≥6 h Stage 2: UOP <0.5 mL/kg per hour for ≥12 h Stage 3: UOP <0.3 mL/kg per hour for ≥24 h or anuria for ≥12 h

RIFLE was adopted in 2004 by the Acute Dialysis Quality Initiative. AKIN was adopted in 2007 by the Acute Kidney Injury Network. KDIGO was adopted in 2012 by the KDIGO AKI Work Group.

Abbreviations: KDIGO, Kidney Disease Improving Global Outcomes; RIFLE, Risk, Injury, Failure, Loss, and End-stage renal disease; SCr, serum creatinine; UOP, urine output.

Although CS-AKI is an important problem on its own, it is also an excellent model for studying novel therapeutic agents and strategies for AKI prevention in humans in general. Accordingly, many randomized controlled trials (RCTs) have been performed to investigate strategies for prevention of CS-AKI. In this review, we summarize these various strategies, including their rationale and their findings.

METHODS

We searched Medline via Pubmed and the Cochrane Database of Systematic Reviews via Ovid for RCTs investigating strategies targeting CS-AKI in patients undergoing cardiac surgery. We restricted our search to, double-blind RCTs published since January 1, 2000, that enrolled a minimum of 100 adult patients (>18 years of age). Studies focused on contrast-induced nephropathy, and those studying patients undergoing emergency cardiac surgery were excluded. We categorized the therapeutic strategies into 3 groups according to the time period of therapeutic intervention: preoperative, intraoperative, and postoperative.

The following information was extracted from each article: study design (including blinding and use of placebo), mean age, sample size, type of surgery (coronary artery bypass grafting, valve, or combined surgery), AKI definition used, intervention, and outcome.

PREOPERATIVE INTERVENTIONS

A variety of preoperative interventions have been studied for prevention of CS-AKI, including corticosteroids, remote ischemic preconditioning (RIPC), N-acetylcysteine (NAC), and statins. Major RCTs conducted in this area that included 100 or more patients are summarized in **Table 2**.

Corticosteroids

Rationale
Cardiac surgery and cardiopulmonary bypass (CPB) invariably cause an acute systemic inflammatory response syndrome (SIRS).[11,14] Release of key cytokines, including IL-6, IL-8, complement C3/C4, and tumor necrosis factor-α are characteristic of SIRS and may contribute importantly to postoperative AKI.[7,11,15,16] Corticosteroids are potent anti-inflammatory drugs. In the cardiac surgery setting, corticosteroids have been extensively investigated in preventing both renal and extrarenal postoperative complications.

Findings
A 2011 Cochrane database systematic review on the use of steroids in cardiac surgery included 54 relatively small RCTs (total of 3615 patients). It concluded that corticosteroids had no beneficial effect on CS-AKI.[17] After this review, 2 large RCTs were conducted: The DExamethasone in Cardiac Surgery (DECS) (N = 4494),[18] and the Steroids In caRdiac Surgery (SIRS) (N = 7507).[19] Both studies concluded that steroids had no protective effect on AKI postoperatively. The DECS trial used the Failure stage of the Risk, Injury, Failure, Loss, and End-stage renal disease criteria for diagnosing AKI and the SIRS trial used Kidney Disease: Improving Global Outcomes (KDIGO) stage 3.[18,19] A recent meta-analysis that included both of these large RCTs found that steroids had no beneficial effect on prevention of CS-AKI in more than 16,000 cardiac surgical patients. Specifically, KDIGO stage 3 AKI occurred with an incidence of 2.7% (172 of 6330 patients) in the steroid group and in 3.3% (207 of 6336 patients) in the control group (relative risk, 0.83; 95% confidence interval,

Table 2
RCTs of preoperative therapeutic interventions for prevention of CS-AKI

Trial	Multicenter	Double Blinded	No. of Patients	Cardiac Surgery Type	Intervention	AKI Definition	Major Findings
Yared et al,[92] 2000, USA	No	Yes	235	CABG, valve	Dexamethasone	RRT	Dexamethasone did not decrease the incidence of CS- AKI (P = .25)
Dieleman et al,[18] 2012, Netherlands	Yes	Yes	4494	CABG, valve, combined	Dexamethasone	RIFLE stage F	Dexamethasone did not decrease the incidence of CS- AKI (RR, 0.7; 95% CI, 0.44–1.14)
Whitlock et al,[19] 2015, Int	Yes	Yes	7507	CABG, valve, combined	Methyl- prednisolone	KDIGO stage 3	Methylprednisolone did not decrease the incidence of CS-AKI (RR, 0.91; 95% CI, 0.79–1.05)
Rahman et al,[93] 2010, UK	No	Yes	162	CABG	RIPC	≥0.5 mg/dL SCr increase	RIPC did not decrease the incidence of CS- AKI (P = .56)
Zimmerman et al,[28] 2011, USA	No	Yes	118	CABG, valve, combined	RIPC	KDIGO (any stage)	RIPC decreased the incidence of CS-AKI (RR, 0.43; 95% CI, 0.24–0.76)
Candilio et al,[94] 2015, UK	No	Yes	178	CABG, valve	RIPC	RIFLE stage F	RIPC did not decrease the incidence of CS- AKI (P = .06)
Hausenloy et al,[26] 2015, UK	Yes	Yes	1612	CABG	RIPC	KDIGO (any stage)	RIPC did not decrease the incidence of CS-AKI (P = .98)
Meybohm et al,[27] 2015, Germany	Yes	Yes	1385	CABG, valve, combined	RIPC	≥200% SCr increase or RRT	RIPC did not decrease the incidence of CS-AKI (RR, 0.82; 95% CI, 0.52–1.30)
Zarbock et al,[95] 2015, Germany	Yes	Yes	240	CABG, valve, combined	RIPC	KDIGO (any stage)	RIPC decreased the incidence of CS-AKI in all KDIGO stages (P = .02)
Burns et al,[36] 2005, Canada	No	Yes	295	CABG	NAC	≥0.5 mg/dL SCr increase or ≥25% SCr increase, RRT	NAC did not decrease the incidence of CS-AKI (RR, 1.03; 95% CI, 0.72–1.46) or RRT (P = .26)

Study				Surgery	Intervention	CS-AKI definition	Outcome
Sisillo et al,[96] 2008, Italy	No	Yes	254	CABG, valve, combined	NAC	≥25% SCr increase	NAC did not decrease the incidence of CS-AKI (RR, 1.60; 95% CI, 0.98–2.63)
Mannacio et al,[97] 2008, Italy	No	Yes	200	CABG	Rosuvastatin	Postoperative SCr of ≥2.5 mg/dL	Rosuvastatin did not decrease the incidence of CS-AKI (RR, 0.33; 95% CI, 0.03–3.19)
Billings et al,[39] 2016, USA	No	Yes	615	CABG, valve, combined	Atorvastatin	≥0.5 mg/dL SCr increase or RRT	Atorvastatin did not decrease the incidence of CS-AKI (RR, 1.06; 95% CI, 0.78–1.46)
Park et al,[40] 2016, Korea	No	Yes	200	Valve	Atorvastatin	AKIN (any stage)	Atorvastatin did not decrease the incidence of CS-AKI according to all AKIN stages ($P = .404$ and $P = .817$, respectively)
Zheng et al,[41] 2016, China	Yes	Yes	1922	CABG, valve, combined	Rosuvastatin	KDIGO (any stage)	Rosuvastatin increased the incidence of CS-AKI (21% vs 17.5%; $P = .005$)
Haase et al,[48] 2009, Germany	No	Yes	100	CABG, valve, combined	Bicarbonate	≥25% SCr increase	Bicarbonate decreased the incidence of CS-AKI (RR, 0.43; 95% CI, 0.19–0.98)
Haase et al,[49] 2013, Germany	Yes	Yes	350	CABG, valve, combined	Bicarbonate	≥0.5 mg/dL SCr increase or ≥25% SCr increase	Bicarbonate increased the incidence of CS-AKI (RR 1.60; 95% CI 1.04–2.45)
McGuinness et al,[98] 2013, Australia	Yes	Yes	427	CABG, valve, combined	Bicarbonate	≥0.5 mg/dL SCr increase or ≥25% SCr increase	Bicarbonate did not decrease the incidence of CS-AKI ($P = .58$)

Abbreviations: AKIN, Acute Kidney Injury Network; CABG, coronary artery bypass grafting; CI, confidence interval; Int, international; KDIGO, Kidney Disease Improving Global Outcome; NAC, N-acetylcysteine; RIFLE, Risk, Injury, Failure, Loss, and End-stage renal disease; RR, relative risk; SCr, serum creatinine.

0.68–1.01; $P = .07$; $I^2 = 0$%).[20] Of note, a major limitation in the definition used for AKI in the DECS trial was the failure to consider renal replacement therapy (RRT), which could have resulted in misclassification. A post hoc analysis of the DECS trial that assessed AKI requiring RRT found that dexamethasone was indeed effective in preventing CS-AKI (relative risk, 0.44; 95% confidence interval, 0.19–0.96).[21] This study illustrates the need for careful consideration of appropriate end points in RCTs that assess AKI prevention, and particularly the need for inclusion of RRT in the definition of AKI.[22]

Bottom line
Taken in aggregate, there is currently insufficient evidence to recommend routine prophylactic administration of steroids to patients undergoing cardiac surgery for prevention of AKI. Furthermore, a one-size-fits-all approach with respect to steroids (as well as other interventions) fails to take into account the heterogeneity of patient and surgical factors that predispose to AKI. Carefully conducted subgroup analyses may reveal key characteristics that identify patients most likely to benefit from steroids and other interventions.

Remote Ischemic Preconditioning

Rationale
RIPC involves brief induction of ischemia and reperfusion to distal tissues, usually by using a sphygmomanometer in the upper arm or leg. This ischemia–reperfusion could result in protection from future ischemia–reperfusion injury, because the first episode of ischemia–reperfusion leads to the release and activation of anti-inflammatory cytokines and oxidative stress scavengers. RIPC has shown promising results in animal models as well as various clinical settings.[23–25] Therefore, unsurprisingly, RIPC has been advocated as a strategy for prevention of CS-AKI.

Findings
Multiple RCTs have been conducted to investigate the effect of RIPC on CS-AKI, and have shown inconsistent results.[23,26–28] One trial conducted in 120 patients found that RIPC decreased the incidence of CS-AKI, as diagnosed by KDIGO stage 1.[28] However, the 2 largest trials (each included >1500 patients) concluded that RIPC did not affect the incidence of more severe CS-AKI (KDIGO stage 3).[26,27] Two meta-analyses concluded that RIPC compared with a sham intervention did not lead to differences in postoperative serum creatinine levels, incidence of AKI, need for RRT, or probability of death.[29,30]

Bottom line
RIPC, at least for the time being, cannot be recommended for prevention of CS-AKI.

N-Acetylcysteine

Rationale
NAC is a precursor of intracellular glutathione, a tripeptide antioxidant that scavenges reactive oxygen species. NAC has been shown to prevent or attenuate AKI in animal models.[31–33] Early studies in humans also suggested a protective effect of NAC in the setting of contrast nephropathy,[34] although a more recent study of 4993 patients found no effect on major adverse kidney events at 90 days.[35]

Findings
Several small RCTs have evaluated the efficacy of NAC in preventing CS-AKI. The largest study randomly assigned 148 individuals to NAC and 147 individuals to

placebo, and found that NAC did not prevent postoperative renal dysfunction.[36] Recent meta-analyses have also failed to demonstrate a significant protective effect of NAC in preventing CS-AKI.[37,38]

Bottom line
Use of NAC for the prevention of CS-AKI is not supported by current evidence.

Statins

Rationale
The 3-hydroxy-3-methyl-glutaryl-CoA reductase inhibitors, also known as statins, attenuate inflammation and oxidative stress, 2 of the possible underlying mechanisms responsible for CS-AKI.

Findings
Three recent large RCTs found that high-dose perioperative administration of atorvastatin compared with placebo did not decrease the incidence of CS-AKI, either in patients naive to statins or in patients already taking statins.[39–41] Several meta-analyses of RCTs have also been performed to evaluate the effects of statins given in the preoperative and postoperative period on the incidence of CS-AKI, and none have shown beneficial effects of these drugs.[42–44] Noteworthy, a meta-analysis by Putzu and colleagues[45] found that preoperative statins were associated with a possible increased risk of AKI postoperatively.

Bottom line
These results do not support the initiation of statin therapy to prevent CS-AKI.

Sodium Bicarbonate

Rationale
At neutral or alkaline pH, free ferric ions precipitate as insoluble ferric hydroxide, which is excreted as an inert complex in the urine. A higher urinary pH also reduces the generation of injurious hydroxyl radicals and lipid peroxidation.[46] In a murine model of acute renal failure induced by bilateral renal artery occlusion, animals that received sodium bicarbonate to increase the renal tubular pH were protected against tubular injury.[47] Thus, urinary alkalinization with sodium bicarbonate might protect against CS-AKI.

Findings
One RCT that enrolled 100 patients found that the administration of sodium bicarbonate attenuated the severity of CS-AKI, as indicated by a smaller increase in urinary neutrophil gelatinase-associated lipocalin postoperatively.[48,49] A study by the same group a couple of years later in 350 patients showed that bicarbonate administration resulted in a greater incidence of CS-AKI.[49] Hence, whether administering intravenous sodium bicarbonate prevents CS-AKI remains uncertain, however, because published RCTs have yielded discordant results. Moreover, 3 meta-analyses, the largest of which included more than 1000 patients from 5 RCTs, did not demonstrate any benefit of sodium bicarbonate administration.[50–52]

Bottom line
The use of perioperative administration of sodium bicarbonate for the prevention of CS-AKI is questionable. Larger studies are needed to determine its potential efficacy. It is possible that sodium bicarbonate could be particularly helpful to a subpopulation

of patients undergoing cardiac surgery who have longer CPB times, and thus more hemolysis and release of free hemoglobin (Hb) and iron.[13,53]

INTRAOPERATIVE MEASURES

A variety of intraoperative interventions have been studied for prevention of CS-AKI, including off-pump surgery, leukocyte filtration, inotropes and volatile anesthetics. Major RCTs conducted in this area that included 100 or more patients are summarized in **Table 3**.

On-Pump Versus Off-Pump Coronary Artery Bypass Grafting

Rationale
The use of the CPB results in a systemic inflammatory response influencing the function of multiple organs throughout the body, including the kidneys, lungs, and the heart itself. Contact of blood with foreign surfaces such as the CPB circuit, the use of cardiotomy suction, blood–air interface, and surgical trauma and stress are regarded as the main pathophysiologic determinants of this condition.[14] Consequently, the effect of on-pump versus off-pump CPB on postoperative outcomes, including AKI, has been an area of active investigation.

Findings
The 3 largest RCTs to date (the CORONARY, GOPCABE, and ROOBY studies) that investigated on-pump versus off-pump CPB enrolled nearly 10,000 patients in total.[54–56] The CORONARY study enrolled 4752 patients and found no significant difference in the incidence of postoperative AKI requiring RRT between patients undergoing on-pump versus off-pump CPB.[54] A detailed analysis showed that off-pump surgery did decrease the incidence of mild AKI at 30-days (defined as a relative increase in serum creatinine of >50% or an absolute increase of $\geq$0.3 mg/dL), but the beneficial effects on renal function did not persist at 1 year of follow-up.[57] Further, neither the ROOBY nor the GOPCABE study showed any renoprotective effects of off-pump compared with on-pump CABG surgery.[55,56]

Bottom line
There are conflicting findings regarding the efficacy of off-pump CABG on decreasing the risk of CS-AKI, but consistent findings regarding lack of efficacy in preventing moderate to severe CS-AKI.

Leukocyte Filtration

Rationale
There is evidence from both animal and human studies that neutrophils and other leukocytes accumulate in the kidneys in the setting of AKI and play an important role in mediating tubular injury.[58] The application of leukocyte filters and cytokine filtration techniques has therefore been researched in several studies of CS-AKI prevention.

Findings
A recent meta-analysis of 6 RCTs that enrolled a total of 374 patients concluded that leukocyte filters did indeed protect against CS-AKI (odds ratio, 0.18; 95% confidence interval, 0.05–0.64).[6] However, caution is necessary in interpreting these results, because the sample sizes of the studies were relatively small, and the definitions used for CS-AKI varied from study to study.

Table 3
RCTs of intraoperative therapeutic interventions for prevention of CS-AKI

Trial	Multicenter	Double Blinded	No. of Patients	Cardiac Surgery Type	Intervention	AKI Definition	Primary Outcome
Shroyer et al,[55] 2009, USA	Yes	No	2203	CABG	Off-pump surgery	RRT	Off-pump CABG did not decrease the incidence of RRT (RR, 0.90; 95% CI, 0.37–2.20)
Lamy et al,[54] 2012, Int	Yes	No	4752	CABG	Off-pump surgery	RIFLE stages R, I and F, and RRT	Off-pump CABG did not decrease the incidence of RRT (HR, 1.04; 95% CI, 0.61-1.76). Off-pump CABG did decrease the incidence of RIFLE stage R (HR, 0.87; 95% CI, 0.76–0.98)
Diegeler et al,[56] 2013, Germany	Yes	No	2539	CABG	Off-pump surgery	RRT	Off-pump CABG did not decrease the incidence of RRT (HR, 0.80; 95% CI, 0.49-1.29)
Lemma et al,[99] 2012, Italy	Yes	No	693	CABG	Off-pump surgery	RIFLE stage I	Off-pump CABG did not decrease the incidence of CS-AKI ($P = .15$)
Mentzer et al,[100] 2007, USA	No	Yes	303	CABG	BNP	Peak increase in SCr	BNP decreased the incidence of CS-AKI ($P<.001$)
Sezai et al,[101] 2011, Japan	No	Yes	504	CABG	ANP	≥0.3 mg/dL SCr increase or RRT	ANP decreased the incidence of CS-AKI ($P = .001$)
Cogliati et al,[102] 2007, Italy	No	Yes	193	CABG, valve, combined	Fenoldopam	Postoperative SCr >2 mg/dL or ≥0.7 mg/dL SCr increase	Fenoldopam decreased the incidence of CS-AKI ($P = .004$)
Bove et al,[65] 2014, Italy	Yes	Yes	667	CABG, valve, combined	Fenoldopam	RRT	Fenoldopam did not decrease the incidence of RRT ($P = .47$)

(continued on next page)

Table 3
(continued)

Trial	Multicenter	Double Blinded	No. of Patients	Cardiac Surgery Type	Intervention	AKI Definition	Primary Outcome
Lahtinen et al,[103] 2011, Finland	No	Yes	200	CABG, valve, combined	Levosimendan	≥50% SCr increase or RRT	Levosimendan did not decrease the incidence of CS-AKI (RR, 1.02; 95% CI, 0.37–2.84)
Landoni et al,[68] 2017, Int	Yes	Yes	506	CABG, valve, combined	Levosimendan	RIFLE stages R, I, F and RRT	Levosimendan did not decrease the incidence of any RIFLE stage or RRT (P = .18; .98; .49, and .27, respectively)
Mehta et al,[69] 2017, Int	Yes	Yes	882	CABG, valve, combined	Levosimendan	RRT	Levosimendan did not decrease the incidence of RRT (RR, 0.54; 95% CI, 0.24–1.24)
Lei & Berra,[72] 2018, China	No	Yes	244	Multiple valve	NO	KDIGO stage 1	NO decreased the incidence of CS-AKI (RR, 0.78; 95% CI, 0·62–0.97)

Abbreviations: ANP, atrial natriuretic peptide; BNP, brain natriuretic peptide; CABG, coronary artery bypass grafting; CI, confidence interval; HR, hazard ratio; Int, international; KDIGO, Kidney Disease Improving Global Outcome; NO, nitric oxide; RIFLE, Risk, Injury, Failure, Loss, and End-stage renal disease; RR, relative risk; SCr, serum creatinine.

Bottom line
Additional research is needed to evaluate the efficacy of leukocyte filters for the prevention of CS-AKI.

Vasodilators and Inotropes

Rationale
Renal vasodilators, including natriuretic peptide, fenoldopam, and levosimendan, have been found to increase renal blood flow in a rat model.[59] Natriuretic peptide consists of atrial natriuretic peptide, brain natriuretic peptide, and C-type natriuretic peptide. Atrial natriuretic peptide and brain natriuretic peptide, administered as human analogues, may have renoprotective properties, including anti-inflammatory effects and the reduction of renal ischemia–reperfusion injury via upregulation of intrarenal angiotensin II.[60] Fenoldopam, a dopamine 1 receptor partial agonist, may reverse renal hypoperfusion and have anti-inflammatory effects in humans.[61] Levosimendan is an adenosine triphosphate–sensitive potassium channel opener that could improve renal perfusion in the vasoplegic state after cardiac surgery by inducing mesangial cell relaxation. In animal models, administration of levosimendan before injury significantly improved renal tubular ischemia–reperfusion injury.[59]

Findings
Two meta-analyses assessed pooled data from 9 small RCTs of intraoperative administration of natriuretic peptides for prevention of CS-AKI. These trials, which enrolled nearly 1000 patients, found a significantly decreased incidence of postoperative AKI in patients who received natriuretic peptides.[51,62,63] A meta-analysis of RCTs performed in patients undergoing cardiac surgery and other major surgery indicated that fenoldopam led to a lower risk of AKI, but not RRT or death.[64] However, these studies also had small sample sizes and were of variable quality. Recently, a large multicenter, double-blind, RCT failed to show any renoprotective effects or survival benefits of fenoldopam infusion in patients undergoing cardiac surgery. Fenoldopam was even related to increased rates of hypotension.[65] Meta-analyses of small sized RCTs concluded that levosimendan resulted in a significant decrease in the incidence of AKI after cardiac surgical procedures.[63,66,67] However, the 2 largest RCTs conducted to date, failed to report any beneficial effects of levosimendan in preventing severe AKI (defined as need for RRT) in patients undergoing cardiac surgery.[68,69]

Bottom line
Natriuretic peptides seem to have some protective effects on CS-AKI, but large RCTs are still needed to confirm this effect. There is no definite evidence that fenoldopam nor levosimendan protects against postoperative AKI.

Nitric Oxide

Rationale
During hemolysis in cardiac surgery, Hb is released into the circulation in the form of oxyhemoglobin (Oxy-Hb). Nitric oxide (NO) is a potent vasodilator, which relaxes vascular smooth muscle, and NO depletion by plasma Oxy-Hb produces vasoconstriction, impairs tissue perfusion, and causes inflammation in animal models.[70] Consequently, plasma Oxy-Hb facilitates development of AKI by intrarenal oxidative reactions.[71] The administration of exogenous NO gas oxidizes plasma Oxy-Hb to methemoglobin and might thus prevent CS-AKI.

Findings

In a randomized clinical trial in China of 217 adults with rheumatic valve disease undergoing elective, multiple valve replacement surgery, administration of 80 parts per million of NO during and after prolonged CPB reduced the incidence of CS-AKI and improved renal function at a follow-up of 1 year after surgery.[72]

Bottom line

NO intraoperatively seems to decrease the incidence of AKI in a Chinese population undergoing cardiac surgery. More trials are necessary to establish its use in Caucasians and those with calcific vessel or valve disease.

POSTOPERATIVE MEASURES

A variety of postoperative interventions have been studied for prevention of CS-AKI, including a KDIGO-based bundle of care, several resuscitation strategies, restrictive packed red blood cell (pRBC) transfusions, and strict glycemic control. Major RCTs conducted in this area that included 100 or more patients are summarized in **Table 4**.

Kidney Disease: Improving Global Outcomes–Based Bundle of Care

Rationale

Because of the multifactorial nature of CS-AKI, it is likely that a combination of interventions, rather than a single intervention, is needed to result in meaningful reductions in the incidence of CS-AKI.

Findings

The PrevAKI RCT was a single-center trial that investigated the use of KDIGO guidelines in the prevention of postoperative AKI in high-risk patients who were identified using a urinary (TIMP-2)/(IGFBP7) ratio of greater than 0.3.[73] The investigators assessed the effect of a KDIGO bundle of care, consisting of optimization of volume status and hemodynamics, avoidance of nephrotoxic drugs, and prevention of hyperglycemia, among patients undergoing cardiac surgery. Implementation of the KDIGO bundle of care decreased the incidence and severity of AKI after cardiac surgery in these high-risk patients.[73]

Bottom line

The results from this single-center trial are promising. However, an adequately powered multicenter trial is needed to confirm whether implementation of a KDIGO-based bundle of care is effective in reducing CS-AKI.

Fluid Management Strategies

Rationale

Fluid management in the perioperative setting is complex and controversial. Fluid overload and hypovolemia are each associated with worse outcomes, including AKI, among patients undergoing cardiac surgery.

Findings

A multicenter, double-blind, double-crossover RCT known as the SPLIT Trial assessed the use of a buffered crystalloid solution compared with saline in 2278 patients who were admitted to the intensive care unit and who required fluid therapy (50% of these were cardiac surgery patients). They found similar rates of postoperative AKI in both fluid management strategies.[74] These results require additional investigation, however, because saline resuscitation in other settings, including critical

Table 4
RCTs of postoperative therapeutic interventions for prevention of CS-AKI

Trial	Multicenter	Double Blinded	No. of Patients	Cardiac Surgery Type	Intervention	AKI Definition	Primary Outcome
Meersch et al,[73] 2017, Germany	No	No	276	CABG, valve, combined	KDIGO-based approach	KDIGO stage 1–3	The KDIGO-based approach decreased the incidence of CS-AKI (OR, 0.48; 95% CI, 0.29–0.80)
Young et al,[74] 2015, Australia	Yes	Yes	2278	NS	Crystalloid vs saline resuscitation	RIFLE stage R, I, F	Crystalloids vs saline did not decrease the incidence of AKI (RR, 1.04; 95% CI, 0.80–1.36)
Hajjar et al,[104] 2010, Brazil	Yes	No	502	CABG, valve, combined	Restrictive (Ht ≥24%) threshold for pRBC transfusion	RRT	Restrictive vs liberal threshold for pRBC transfusion did not decrease the incidence of RRT (P = .99)
Murphy et al,[105] 2015, UK	Yes	No	2007	CABG, valve, combined	Restrictive (Hb <7.5 g/dL) threshold for pRBC transfusion	AKIN stages 1–3	Restrictive vs liberal threshold for pRBC transfusion did not decrease the incidence of CS-AKI (P>.05)
Mazer et al,[81] 2017, Int	Yes	No	5243	CABG, valve, combined	Restrictive (Hb <7.5 g/dL) threshold for pRBC transfusion	RRT	Restrictive vs liberal threshold for pRBC transfusion did not decrease the incidence of RRT (HR,0.84; 95% CI, 0.60–1.19)
Steiner et al,[83] 2015, USA	Yes	No	1098	CABG, valve, combined	Fresh (≤10 d) vs old pRBC (≥21 d)	SCr change	Fresh vs old pRBC did not decrease the incidence of CS-AKI (P = .72)
Desai et al,[86] 2012, USA	No	No	189	CABG	Tight (90–120 mg/dL) vs liberal (121–180 mg/dL) glucose ranges	RIFLE stage F	Tight vs liberal glucose control did not decrease the incidence of CS-AKI (absolute difference 2.2%; 95% CI, −5% to 8%)
Umpierrez et al,[87] 2015, USA	Yes	No	302	CABG, valve	Tight (100–140 mg/dL) vs liberal (141–180 mg/dL) glucose ranges	≥50% SCr increase	Tight vs liberal glucose control did not decrease the incidence of CS-AKI (P = .08).

Abbreviations: CABG, coronary artery bypass grafting; CI, confidence interval; HR, hazard ratio; Ht, hematocrit; Int, international; KDIGO, Kidney Disease Improving Global Outcome; NS, not specified; OR, odds ratio; RIFLE, Risk, Injury, Failure, Loss, and End-stage renal disease; RR, relative risk; SCr, serum creatinine.

illness, has been shown to result in higher rates of AKI as compared with balanced solutions.[75]

Noteworthy, concerns have been raised regarding administration of higher molecular weight hydroxyethyl starches as part of fluid resuscitation in various settings, including cardiac surgery, because this approach seems to be associated with a higher incidence of AKI requiring RRT.[76,77]

Bottom line

Additional studies are needed to investigate the effects of resuscitation using normal saline versus balanced solutions (eg, Ringer's lactate) on the incidence of CS-AKI. Hydroxyethyl starches are contradicted in cardiac surgery.

Packed Red Blood Cell Transfusions

Rationale

Anemia and transfusion of pRBCs are each associated with an increased risk of CS-AKI,[78,79] but direct causal relationships in this setting cannot be determined from observational studies owing to confounding by severity of illness. Thus, optimal transfusion thresholds can only be determined from RCTs. Additionally, a large retrospective cohort study (n = 2872) found that transfusion of older pRBCs is associated with worse outcomes postoperatively following cardiac surgery, including in-hospital, renal failure and sepsis.[80]

Findings

The TRICs-III study is a recently published RCT that assessed the effects of a restrictive versus liberal threshold for transfusion of pRBCs in 5243 adults undergoing cardiac surgery. The restrictive transfusion group received pRBCs if their Hb concentration decreased to less than 7.5 g/dL, whereas the liberal transfusion group received pRBCs if their Hb concentration decreased to less than 9.5 g/dL. The investigators found that the incidence of AKI requiring RRT was similar in both groups.[81] A recent meta-analysis found similar results.[82] Of note, only 1 RCT (the RECESS trial) investigated the effects of storage time of pRBCs on outcomes after cardiac surgery.[83] This trial, which included 1098 patients, found that transfusion of pRBCs stored for 10 or fewer days was not superior to transfusion of pRBCs stored for 21 or more days with respect to severe organ dysfunction.[83]

Bottom line

The use of a restrictive versus liberal threshold for perioperative pRBC transfusion does not affect the incidence of CS-AKI. Additionally, the storage duration of pRBCs does not seem to affect the incidence of CS-AKI.

Glycemic Control

Rationale

Perioperative hyperglycemia is associated with increased mortality, surgical complications, and AKI.[84] Mechanisms by which hyperglycemia could predispose patients to a greater susceptibility to AKI are not entirely clear; however, hyperglycemia is known to induce oxidative stress and also to inhibit sodium-glucose co-transporters in the renal proximal tubules.[85]

Findings

Two RCTs (N = 189 and N = 302) assessed the effect of tight (100–140 mg/dL) versus liberal (141–180 mg/dL) glycemic control. These studies found no difference in the incidence of CS-AKI.[86,87]

Bottom line

Liberal glycemic control has the same effects on CS-AKI as tight glycemic control. Consequently, this has prompted the Society for Thoracic Surgeons to issue guidelines for blood glucose management after cardiac surgery, recommending targeting blood glucose levels of less than 180 mg/dL.[88]

DISCUSSION

CS-AKI remains a complex and challenging problem. Numerous trials of various preoperative, intraoperative, and postoperative preventive measures have been attempted, yet the majority of RCTs were negative. Preliminary data suggest that a KDIGO-based bundle of care, which includes optimization of volume status and hemodynamics, avoidance of nephrotoxic drugs, and prevention of hyperglycemia, might help to decrease the incidence of CS-AKI.[3,73] These strategies are low-cost and relatively easy to implement in clinical practice. Although these strategies are promising, larger studies are still needed to confirm these findings.

The use of anti-inflammatory interventions such as steroids, RIPC, statins, NAC, and urinary alkalization seems to be ineffective in preventing CS-AKI in the general cardiac surgery population. Post hoc analyses, however, have shown that certain subgroups of patients may benefit from some of these interventions, for example, corticosteroids.[21] Of all intraoperative measures that have been investigated, none except leukocyte filtration and inhaled NO has proven to be of benefit in protecting against CS-AKI. Yet, the positive findings related to these 2 interventions are based on RCTs that had small sample sizes; thus, additional research is needed to confirm these findings.

One important reason why the majority of RCTs may have been negative is because they assessed interventions aimed at a general cardiac surgical population. Future RCTs should include more precise phenotyping of patients to determine which patients are at the greatest risk of developing AKI, and as such would likely benefit most from the intervention, rather than a one-size-fits-all approach. Phenotyping could be performed through the use of clinical characteristics (eg, preoperative estimated glomerular filtration rate , diabetes mellitus), blood and urine biomarkers (eg, urinary [TIMP-2]/[IGFBP7] ratio, urinary neutrophil gelatinase-associated lipocalin, or plasma fibroblast growth factor-23),[10,13,89] immune characteristics,[90] or (epi)genetic markers.[91]

SUMMARY

Thousands of patients have been enrolled in clinical trials assessing various therapeutic strategies for prevention of CS-AKI, and the vast majority of these studies have been negative. More comprehensive phenotyping of patients may yield higher success rates in future trials, and could be accomplished through a variety of approaches. Finally, implementation of a KDIGO bundle of care the and administration of inhaled NO intraoperatively represent promising therapeutic strategies. However, the efficacy of these strategies in preventing CS-AKI requires confirmation in larger, multicenter trials before they can be recommended for widespread implementation.

REFERENCES

1. Roger VL, Go AS, Lloyd-Jones DM, et al. Heart disease and stroke statistics–2011 update: a report from the American Heart Association. Circulation 2011; 123(4):e18–209.

2. D'Agostino RS, Jacobs JP, Badhwar V, et al. The Society of Thoracic Surgeons adult cardiac surgery database: 2019 update on outcomes and quality. Ann Thorac Surg 2019;107(1):24–32.
3. Wang Y, Bellomo R. Cardiac surgery-associated acute kidney injury: risk factors, pathophysiology and treatment. Nat Rev Nephrol 2017;13(11):697–711.
4. Chertow GM, Burdick E, Honour M, et al. Acute kidney injury, mortality, length of stay, and costs in hospitalized patients. J Am Soc Nephrol 2005;16(11): 3365–70.
5. Rosner MH, Okusa MD. Acute kidney injury associated with cardiac surgery. Clin J Am Soc Nephrol 2006;1(1):19–32.
6. Scrascia G, Guida P, Rotunno C, et al. Anti-inflammatory strategies to reduce acute kidney injury in cardiac surgery patients: a meta-analysis of randomized controlled trials. Artif Organs 2014;38(2):101–12.
7. Mariscalco G, Lorusso R, Dominici C, et al. Acute kidney injury: a relevant complication after cardiac surgery. Ann Thorac Surg 2011;92(4):1539–47.
8. Ranucci M, Pavesi M, Mazza E, et al. Risk factors for renal dysfunction after coronary surgery: the role of cardiopulmonary bypass technique. Perfusion 1994; 9(5):319–26.
9. Wijeysundera DN, Karkouti K, Dupuis JY, et al. Derivation and validation of a simplified predictive index for renal replacement therapy after cardiac surgery. JAMA 2007;297(16):1801–9.
10. Parikh CR, Coca SG, Thiessen-Philbrook H, et al. Postoperative biomarkers predict acute kidney injury and poor outcomes after adult cardiac surgery. J Am Soc Nephrol 2011;22(9):1748–57.
11. Asimakopoulos G. Systemic inflammation and cardiac surgery: an update. Perfusion 2001;16(5):353–60.
12. Okusa MD. The inflammatory cascade in acute ischemic renal failure. Nephron 2002;90(2):133–8.
13. Leaf DE, Rajapurkar M, Lele SS, et al. Increased plasma catalytic iron in patients may mediate acute kidney injury and death following cardiac surgery. Kidney Int 2015;87(5):1046–54.
14. Paparella D, Yau TM, Young E. Cardiopulmonary bypass induced inflammation: pathophysiology and treatment. An update. Eur J Cardiothorac Surg 2002; 21(2):232–44.
15. Moat NE, Shore DF, Evans TW. Organ dysfunction and cardiopulmonary bypass: the role of complement and complement regulatory proteins. Eur J Cardiothorac Surg 1993;7(11):563–73.
16. Wan S, LeClerc JL, Vincent JL. Inflammatory response to cardiopulmonary bypass: mechanisms involved and possible therapeutic strategies. Chest 1997;112(3):676–92.
17. Dieleman JM, van Paassen J, van Dijk D, et al. Prophylactic corticosteroids for cardiopulmonary bypass in adults. Cochrane Database Syst Rev 2011;(5):CD005566.
18. Dieleman JM, Nierich AP, Rosseel PM, et al. Intraoperative high-dose dexamethasone for cardiac surgery: a randomized controlled trial. JAMA 2012;308(17): 1761–7.
19. Whitlock RP, Devereaux PJ, Teoh KH, et al. Methylprednisolone in patients undergoing cardiopulmonary bypass (SIRS): a randomised, double-blind, placebo-controlled trial. Lancet 2015;386(10000):1243–53.
20. Dvirnik N, Belley-Cote EP, Hanif H, et al. Steroids in cardiac surgery: a systematic review and meta-analysis. Br J Anaesth 2018;120(4):657–67.

21. Jacob KA, Leaf DE, Dieleman JM, et al. Intraoperative high-dose dexamethasone and severe AKI after cardiac surgery. J Am Soc Nephrol 2015;26(12): 2947–51.
22. Leaf DE, Waikar SS. End points for clinical trials in acute kidney injury. Am J Kidney Dis 2017;69(1):108–16.
23. Choi YS, Shim JK, Kim JC, et al. Effect of remote ischemic preconditioning on renal dysfunction after complex valvular heart surgery: a randomized controlled trial. J Thorac Cardiovasc Surg 2011;142(1):148–54.
24. Gassanov N, Nia AM, Caglayan E, et al. Remote ischemic preconditioning and renoprotection: from myth to a novel therapeutic option? J Am Soc Nephrol 2014;25(2):216–24.
25. Kharbanda RK, Nielsen TT, Redington AN. Translation of remote ischaemic preconditioning into clinical practice. Lancet 2009;374(9700):1557–65.
26. Hausenloy DJ, Candilio L, Evans R, et al. Remote ischemic preconditioning and outcomes of cardiac surgery. N Engl J Med 2015;373(15):1408–17.
27. Meybohm P, Bein B, Brosteanu O, et al. A multicenter trial of remote ischemic preconditioning for heart surgery. N Engl J Med 2015;373(15):1397–407.
28. Zimmerman RF, Ezeanuna PU, Kane JC, et al. Ischemic preconditioning at a remote site prevents acute kidney injury in patients following cardiac surgery. Kidney Int 2011;80(8):861–7.
29. Menting TP, Wever KE, Ozdemir-van Brunschot DM, et al. Ischaemic preconditioning for the reduction of renal ischaemia reperfusion injury. Cochrane Database Syst Rev 2017;(3):CD010777.
30. Pierce B, Bole I, Patel V, et al. Clinical outcomes of remote ischemic preconditioning prior to cardiac surgery: a meta-analysis of randomized controlled trials. J Am Heart Assoc 2017;6(2) [pii:e004666].
31. Baliga R, Ueda N, Walker PD, et al. Oxidant mechanisms in toxic acute renal failure. Am J Kidney Dis 1997;29(3):465–77.
32. Lee JH, Jo YH, Kim K, et al. Effect of N-acetylcysteine (NAC) on acute lung injury and acute kidney injury in hemorrhagic shock. Resuscitation 2013;84(1): 121–7.
33. Campos R, Shimizu MH, Volpini RA, et al. N-acetylcysteine prevents pulmonary edema and acute kidney injury in rats with sepsis submitted to mechanical ventilation. Am J Physiol Lung Cell Mol Physiol 2012;302(7):L640–50.
34. Tepel M, van der Giet M, Schwarzfeld C, et al. Prevention of radiographic-contrast-agent-induced reductions in renal function by acetylcysteine. N Engl J Med 2000;343(3):180–4.
35. Weisbord SD, Gallagher M, Jneid H, et al. Outcomes after angiography with sodium bicarbonate and acetylcysteine. N Engl J Med 2018;378(7):603–14.
36. Burns KE, Chu MW, Novick RJ, et al. Perioperative N-acetylcysteine to prevent renal dysfunction in high-risk patients undergoing CABG surgery: a randomized controlled trial. JAMA 2005;294(3):342–50.
37. Adabag AS, Ishani A, Bloomfield HE, et al. Efficacy of N-acetylcysteine in preventing renal injury after heart surgery: a systematic review of randomized trials. Eur Heart J 2009;30(15):1910–7.
38. Mei M, Zhao HW, Pan QG, et al. Efficacy of N-acetylcysteine in preventing acute kidney injury after cardiac surgery: a meta-analysis study. J Invest Surg 2018; 31(1):14–23.
39. Billings FT, Hendricks PA, Schildcrout JS, et al. High-Dose perioperative atorvastatin and acute kidney injury following cardiac surgery: a randomized clinical trial. JAMA 2016;315(9):877–88.

40. Park JH, Shim JK, Song JW, et al. Effect of atorvastatin on the incidence of acute kidney injury following valvular heart surgery: a randomized, placebo-controlled trial. Intensive Care Med 2016;42(9):1398–407.

41. Zheng Z, Jayaram R, Jiang L, et al. Perioperative rosuvastatin in cardiac surgery. N Engl J Med 2016;374(18):1744–53.

42. Kuhn EW, Slottosch I, Wahlers T, et al. Preoperative statin therapy for patients undergoing cardiac surgery. Cochrane Database Syst Rev 2015;(8):CD008493.

43. Liakopoulos OJ, Choi YH, Haldenwang PL, et al. Impact of preoperative statin therapy on adverse postoperative outcomes in patients undergoing cardiac surgery: a meta-analysis of over 30,000 patients. Eur Heart J 2008;29(12):1548–59.

44. Yuan X, Du J, Liu Q, et al. Defining the role of perioperative statin treatment in patients after cardiac surgery: a meta-analysis and systematic review of 20 randomized controlled trials. Int J Cardiol 2017;228:958–66.

45. Putzu A, Capelli B, Belletti A, et al. Perioperative statin therapy in cardiac surgery: a meta-analysis of randomized controlled trials. Crit Care 2016;20(1):395.

46. Caulfield JL, Singh SP, Wishnok JS, et al. Bicarbonate inhibits N-nitrosation in oxygenated nitric oxide solutions. J Biol Chem 1996;271(42):25859–63.

47. Atkins JL. Effect of sodium bicarbonate preloading on ischemic renal failure. Nephron 1986;44(1):70–4.

48. Haase M, Haase-Fielitz A, Bellomo R, et al. Sodium bicarbonate to prevent increases in serum creatinine after cardiac surgery: a pilot double-blind, randomized controlled trial. Crit Care Med 2009;37(1):39–47.

49. Haase M, Haase-Fielitz A, Plass M, et al. Prophylactic perioperative sodium bicarbonate to prevent acute kidney injury following open heart surgery: a multicenter double-blinded randomized controlled trial. PLoS Med 2013;10(4): e1001426.

50. Bailey M, McGuinness S, Haase M, et al. Sodium bicarbonate and renal function after cardiac surgery: a prospectively planned individual patient meta-analysis. Anesthesiology 2015;122(2):294–306.

51. Kim JH, Kim HJ, Kim JY, et al. Meta-analysis of sodium bicarbonate therapy for prevention of cardiac surgery-associated acute kidney injury. J Cardiothorac Vasc Anesth 2015;29(5):1248–56.

52. Tie HT, Luo MZ, Luo MJ, et al. Sodium bicarbonate in the prevention of cardiac surgery-associated acute kidney injury: a systematic review and meta-analysis. Crit Care 2014;18(5):517.

53. Leaf DE, Swinkels DW. Catalytic iron and acute kidney injury. Am J Physiol Renal Physiol 2016;311(5):F871–6.

54. Lamy A, Devereaux PJ, Prabhakaran D, et al. Off-pump or on-pump coronary-artery bypass grafting at 30 days. N Engl J Med 2012;366(16):1489–97.

55. Shroyer AL, Grover FL, Hattler B, et al. On-pump versus off-pump coronary-artery bypass surgery. N Engl J Med 2009;361(19):1827–37.

56. Diegeler A, Borgermann J, Kappert U, et al. Off-pump versus on-pump coronary-artery bypass grafting in elderly patients. N Engl J Med 2013;368(13): 1189–98.

57. Garg AX, Devereaux PJ, Yusuf S, et al. Kidney function after off-pump or on-pump coronary artery bypass graft surgery: a randomized clinical trial. JAMA 2014;311(21):2191–8.

58. Bolisetty S, Agarwal A. Neutrophils in acute kidney injury: not neutral any more. Kidney Int 2009;75(7):674–6.

59. Yakut N, Yasa H, Bahriye Lafci B, et al. The influence of levosimendan and ilo-prost on renal ischemia-reperfusion: an experimental study. Interact Cardiovasc Thorac Surg 2008;7(2):235–9.
60. Mitaka C, Si MK, Tulafu M, et al. Effects of atrial natriuretic peptide on inter-organ crosstalk among the kidney, lung, and heart in a rat model of renal ischemia-reperfusion injury. Intensive Care Med Exp 2014;2(1):28.
61. Gillies MA, Kakar V, Parker RJ, et al. Fenoldopam to prevent acute kidney injury after major surgery-a systematic review and meta-analysis. Crit Care 2015; 19:449.
62. Nigwekar SU, Navaneethan SD, Parikh CR, et al. Atrial natriuretic peptide for preventing and treating acute kidney injury. Cochrane Database Syst Rev 2009;(4):CD006028.
63. Chen X, Huang T, Cao X, et al. Comparative efficacy of drugs for preventing acute kidney injury after cardiac surgery: a network meta-analysis. Am J Cardi-ovasc Drugs 2018;18(1):49–58.
64. Zangrillo A, Biondi-Zoccai GG, Frati E, et al. Fenoldopam and acute renal failure in cardiac surgery: a meta-analysis of randomized placebo-controlled trials. J Cardiothorac Vasc Anesth 2012;26(3):407–13.
65. Bove T, Zangrillo A, Guarracino F, et al. Effect of fenoldopam on use of renal replacement therapy among patients with acute kidney injury after cardiac sur-gery: a randomized clinical trial. JAMA 2014;312(21):2244–53.
66. Zhou C, Gong J, Chen D, et al. Levosimendan for prevention of acute kidney injury after cardiac surgery: a meta-analysis of randomized controlled trials. Am J Kidney Dis 2016;67(3):408–16.
67. Niu ZZ, Wu SM, Sun WY, et al. Perioperative levosimendan therapy is associated with a lower incidence of acute kidney injury after cardiac surgery: a meta-anal-ysis. J Cardiovasc Pharmacol 2014;63(2):107–12.
68. Landoni G, Lomivorotov VV, Alvaro G, et al. Levosimendan for hemodynamic support after cardiac surgery. N Engl J Med 2017;376(21):2021–31.
69. Mehta RH, Leimberger JD, van Diepen S, et al. Levosimendan in patients with left ventricular dysfunction undergoing cardiac surgery. N Engl J Med 2017; 376(21):2032–42.
70. Minneci PC, Deans KJ, Zhi H, et al. Hemolysis-associated endothelial dysfunc-tion mediated by accelerated NO inactivation by decompartmentalized oxyhe-moglobin. J Clin Invest 2005;115(12):3409–17.
71. Deuel JW, Schaer CA, Boretti FS, et al. Hemoglobinuria-related acute kidney injury is driven by intrarenal oxidative reactions triggering a heme toxicity response. Cell Death Dis 2016;7:e2064.
72. Lei C, Berra L. Nitric oxide decreases acute kidney injury and stage 3 chronic kidney disease after cardiac surgery. Am J Respir Crit Care Med 2018; 198(10):1279–87.
73. Meersch M, Schmidt C, Hoffmeier A, et al. Prevention of cardiac surgery-associated AKI by implementing the KDIGO guidelines in high risk patients identified by biomarkers: the PrevAKI randomized controlled trial. Intensive Care Med 2017;43(11):1551–61.
74. Young P, Bailey M, Beasley R, et al. Effect of a buffered crystalloid solution vs saline on acute kidney injury among patients in the intensive care unit: the SPLIT randomized clinical trial. JAMA 2015;314(16):1701–10.
75. Semler MW, Self WH, Wanderer JP, et al. Balanced crystalloids versus saline in critically Ill adults. N Engl J Med 2018;378(9):829–39.

76. Krajewski ML, Raghunathan K, Paluszkiewicz SM, et al. Meta-analysis of high-versus low-chloride content in perioperative and critical care fluid resuscitation. Br J Surg 2015;102(1):24–36.

77. Myburgh JA, Finfer S, Bellomo R, et al. Hydroxyethyl starch or saline for fluid resuscitation in intensive care. N Engl J Med 2012;367(20):1901–11.

78. Khan UA, Coca SG, Hong K, et al. Blood transfusions are associated with urinary biomarkers of kidney injury in cardiac surgery. J Thorac Cardiovasc Surg 2014;148(2):726–32.

79. Kindzelski BA, Corcoran P, Siegenthaler MP, et al. Postoperative acute kidney injury following intraoperative blood product transfusions during cardiac surgery. Perfusion 2018;33(1):62–70.

80. Koch CG, Li L, Sessler DI, et al. Duration of red-cell storage and complications after cardiac surgery. N Engl J Med 2008;358(12):1229–39.

81. Mazer CD, Whitlock RP, Fergusson DA, et al. Restrictive or liberal red-cell transfusion for cardiac surgery. N Engl J Med 2017;377(22):2133–44.

82. Chen QH, Wang HL, Liu L, et al. Effects of restrictive red blood cell transfusion on the prognoses of adult patients undergoing cardiac surgery: a meta-analysis of randomized controlled trials. Crit Care 2018;22(1):142.

83. Steiner ME, Ness PM, Assmann SF, et al. Effects of red-cell storage duration on patients undergoing cardiac surgery. N Engl J Med 2015;372(15):1419–29.

84. Szekely A, Levin J, Miao Y, et al. Impact of hyperglycemia on perioperative mortality after coronary artery bypass graft surgery. J Thorac Cardiovasc Surg 2011; 142(2):430–7.e1.

85. Han HJ, Lee YJ, Park SH, et al. High glucose-induced oxidative stress inhibits Na+/glucose cotransporter activity in renal proximal tubule cells. Am J Physiol Renal Physiol 2005;288(5):F988–96.

86. Desai SP, Henry LL, Holmes SD, et al. Strict versus liberal target range for perioperative glucose in patients undergoing coronary artery bypass grafting: a prospective randomized controlled trial. J Thorac Cardiovasc Surg 2012; 143(2):318–25.

87. Umpierrez G, Cardona S, Pasquel F, et al. Randomized controlled trial of intensive versus conservative glucose control in patients undergoing coronary artery bypass graft surgery: GLUCO-CABG trial. Diabetes Care 2015;38(9):1665–72.

88. Lazar HL, McDonnell M, Chipkin SR, et al. The Society of Thoracic Surgeons practice guideline series: blood glucose management during adult cardiac surgery. Ann Thorac Surg 2009;87(2):663–9.

89. Leaf DE, Christov M, Juppner H, et al. Fibroblast growth factor 23 levels are elevated and associated with severe acute kidney injury and death following cardiac surgery. Kidney Int 2016;89(4):939–48.

90. Holmannova D, Kolackova M, Kunes P, et al. Impact of cardiac surgery on the expression of CD40, CD80, CD86 and HLA-DR on B cells and monocytes. Perfusion 2016;31(5):391–400.

91. Leaf DE, Body SC, Muehlschlegel JD, et al. Length polymorphisms in heme oxygenase-1 and AKI after cardiac surgery. J Am Soc Nephrol 2016;27(11): 3291–7.

92. Yared JP, Starr NJ, Torres FK, et al. Effects of single dose, postinduction dexamethasone on recovery after cardiac surgery. Ann Thorac Surg 2000;69(5): 1420–4.

93. Rahman IA, Mascaro JG, Steeds RP, et al. Remote ischemic preconditioning in human coronary artery bypass surgery: from promise to disappointment? Circulation 2010;122(11 Suppl):S53–9.

94. Candilio L, Malik A, Ariti C, et al. Effect of remote ischaemic preconditioning on clinical outcomes in patients undergoing cardiac bypass surgery: a randomised controlled clinical trial. Heart 2015;101(3):185–92.
95. Zarbock A, Schmidt C, Van Aken H, et al. Effect of remote ischemic preconditioning on kidney injury among high-risk patients undergoing cardiac surgery: a randomized clinical trial. JAMA 2015;313(21):2133–41.
96. Sisillo E, Ceriani R, Bortone F, et al. N-acetylcysteine for prevention of acute renal failure in patients with chronic renal insufficiency undergoing cardiac surgery: a prospective, randomized, clinical trial. Crit Care Med 2008;36(1):81–6.
97. Mannacio VA, Iorio D, De Amicis V, et al. Effect of rosuvastatin pretreatment on myocardial damage after coronary surgery: a randomized trial. J Thorac Cardiovasc Surg 2008;136(6):1541–8.
98. McGuinness SP, Parke RL, Bellomo R, et al. Sodium bicarbonate infusion to reduce cardiac surgery-associated acute kidney injury: a phase II multicenter double-blind randomized controlled trial. Crit Care Med 2013;41(7):1599–607.
99. Lemma MG, Coscioni E, Tritto FP, et al. On-pump versus off-pump coronary artery bypass surgery in high-risk patients: operative results of a prospective randomized trial (on-off study). J Thorac Cardiovasc Surg 2012;143(3):625–31.
100. Mentzer RM Jr, Oz MC, Sladen RN, et al. Effects of perioperative nesiritide in patients with left ventricular dysfunction undergoing cardiac surgery: the NAPA trial. J Am Coll Cardiol 2007;49(6):716–26.
101. Sezai A, Hata M, Niino T, et al. Results of low-dose human atrial natriuretic peptide infusion in nondialysis patients with chronic kidney disease undergoing coronary artery bypass grafting: the NU-HIT (Nihon University working group study of low-dose HANP Infusion Therapy during cardiac surgery) trial for CKD. J Am Coll Cardiol 2011;58(9):897–903.
102. Cogliati AA, Vellutini R, Nardini A, et al. Fenoldopam infusion for renal protection in high-risk cardiac surgery patients: a randomized clinical study. J Cardiothorac Vasc Anesth 2007;21(6):847–50.
103. Lahtinen P, Pitkanen O, Polonen P, et al. Levosimendan reduces heart failure after cardiac surgery: a prospective, randomized, placebo-controlled trial. Crit Care Med 2011;39(10):2263–70.
104. Hajjar LA, Vincent JL, Galas FR, et al. Transfusion requirements after cardiac surgery: the TRACS randomized controlled trial. JAMA 2010;304(14):1559–67.
105. Murphy GJ, Pike K, Rogers CA, et al. Liberal or restrictive transfusion after cardiac surgery. N Engl J Med 2015;372(11):997–1008.

Heart Failure in Adult Patients with Congenital Heart Disease

Valérie M. Smit-Fun, MD*, Wolfgang F. Buhre, MD, PhD

KEYWORDS

- Adult congenital heart disease • Grown-up congenital heart disease • Heart failure
- Fontan circulation • Single ventricle

KEY POINTS

- Almost 90% of children born with a congenital heart disease survive into adulthood and achieve an average age of almost 60 years.
- With increasing age the care for adult patients with congenital heart disease becomes more challenging as residual cardiac defects, superimposed by acquired disease, result in complex morbidity.
- Heart failure has a high prevalence in adults with congenital heart disease and is the main cause of mortality; knowledge of pathophysiology and prevention of complications is essential.
- Care for adults with congenital heart disease is not restricted to highly specialized centers, although it is recommended to manage patients with complex morbidity in specialized centers with multidisciplinary expert teams.

INTRODUCTION

Owing to advances in cardiac surgery, intensive care, and diagnostic capabilities, 88% of children born with a congenital heart disease (CHD) survive into adulthood.[1–3] Besides arrhythmias, (end-stage) heart failure is the primary source of morbidity and mortality. In accordance with the increasing number of adult patients with CHD (ACHD)[a], the need for noncardiac surgical and interventional procedures is increasing, both in the elective and acute settings. Therefore, there is a practical need for anesthesiologists to be familiar with the pathophysiologic considerations. In this review,

Disclosure Statement: None.
Department of Anaesthesiology and Pain Medicine, Maastricht University Medical Center, PO Box 5800, Maastricht 6202 AZ, The Netherlands
* Corresponding author.
E-mail address: v.smit.fun@mumc.nl

[a] There are some inconsistencies regarding the nomenclature. In some countries the term "grown-up congenital heart disease" is used (GUCH). The reference to this patient population as "adults with congenital heart disease" (ACHD) is more common.

Anesthesiology Clin 37 (2019) 751–768
https://doi.org/10.1016/j.anclin.2019.08.005
anesthesiology.theclinics.com

we describe the actual knowledge about heart failure in this heterogeneous patient population. Special attention is given to patients with a Fontan circulation, for example, the cohort with a single ventricle circulation and passive pulmonary circulation. Furthermore, general considerations regarding the increasingly present obstetric and surgical patient populations with ACHD are discussed. There are only a couple of controlled clinical trials available, and, thus, our knowledge is based primarily on single-center experiences, case series, and small-scale observational clinical studies.

CONGENITAL HEART DEFECTS

Structural heart disease is the most common congenital disorder in newborns. The pathophysiology of CHD is heterogeneous and consists of a great range of cardiac anomalies. The 8 most common CHD subtypes and their birth prevalence[4] are shown in **Fig. 1**.

The complexity of the congenital defect, the possibility of surgical correction or definitive palliation largely determine morbidity and mortality in patients with CHD.

Usually, the Bethesda Classification of Congenital Heart Disease is used to describe the severity of CHD in terms of complexity. The definition was developed at a consensus meeting in 2000, and is still applicable and widely used. In 2018, Stout and colleagues[5] published the actual guideline for the management of ACHD including

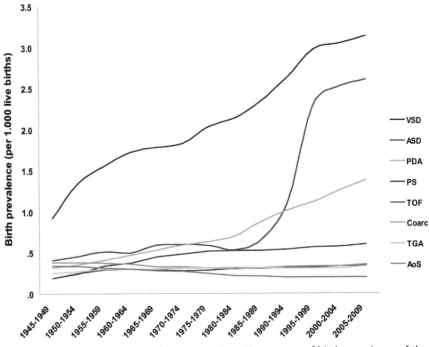

Fig. 1. Birth prevalence of CHD subtypes over time. Time course of birth prevalence of the 8 most common CHD subtypes from 1945 until 2010. AoS, aortic stenosis; ASD, atrial septal defect; Coarc, coarctation; PDA, patent ductus arteriosus; PS, pulmonary stenosis; TGA, transposition of the great arteries; TOF, tetralogy of Fallot; VSD, ventricular septal defect. (*From* van der Linde D, Konings EE, Slager MA, et al. Birth Prevalence of Congenital Heart Disease Worldwide: a systematic review and meta-analysis. J Am Coll Cardiol 2011;58(21):2245; with permission.)

the classification of disease and the relation to the New York Heart Association (NYHA) functional classification of heart failure (**Box 1**). According to complexity, 3 groups of patients with CHD are identified: those with simple defects, moderately complex defects, and complex defects. Approximately 3% of live births with CHD are complex defects and 15% are moderately complex defects.

EPIDEMIOLOGY

The incidence of CHD is 3 to 20 per 1000 live births, resulting in a prevalence of 6.9 in North America, 8.2 in Europe, and 9.3 per 1000 live births in Asia.[4,6] In infants and children, complexity and surgical results have been shown to be the primary determinants of mortality.[1–3] Owing to advances in cardiac surgery, intensive care, and diagnostic capabilities, 88% of patients survive into adulthood.[1–3] The reported average age for patients with ACHD in 2007 was 57 years.[2,7] Data from Afilalo and colleagues[8] showed that the aged population older than 65 years is still substantial with a similar prevalence as in the adult population of 3 per thousand elderly.

Despite surgical correction, patients with CHD carry a life-long risk for cardiovascular complications arising from residual defects and the clinical course of the disease. Moreover, for some patients no corrective approach is possible resulting in a stage of definitive palliation.

Agarwal and colleagues[9] studied trends in resource use from 2003 to 2012 and noted a significant increase in the number of ACHD related emergent and nonemergent hospital admissions, with almost 30% presenting to small- and medium-sized hospitals, whereby 25% represented complex ACHD. In 2012, compared with 2003, there was a considerable increase in the prevalence of traditional cardiovascular risk factors (hypertension, diabetes, smoking, obesity, chronic kidney disease, and peripheral arterial disease), a significant increase in length of stay, and a considerable increase in cost of admission for both simple and complex patients with ACHD. In this study cohort, in-hospital mortality remained relatively constant.

Heart failure is responsible for approximately 13% of hospitalizations, with other main reasons being valve disease (15%) and cerebrovascular accidents (26%).[7,9] Hospital admission caused by heart failure is associated with a 5-fold increase in mortality[10] and is the main cause of death in ACHD (20%).[11] Patients admitted with heart failure are significantly older and generally have more complex ACHD.[7]

HEART FAILURE IN ADULT CONGENITAL HEART DISEASE
Causes of Heart Failure in Patients with Congenital Heart Disease

In patients with acquired cardiac disease, heart failure mainly results from left ventricle (LV) systolic or diastolic dysfunction caused by ischemia, valve disease, or even cardiomyopathy. In ACHD heart failure the underlying mechanism is more heterogenous and includes chronic pressure and/or volume (over)loading, inadequate myocardial preservation during prior surgeries, myocardial fibrosis, surgical injury to a coronary artery, pulmonary hypertension, and neurohormonal activation. Furthermore, a subset of patients can develop symptoms of heart failure in the time course after initial successful surgical correction of a congenital anomaly. In a variety of settings the right ventricle (RV) acts as the systemic ventricle which ultimately can lead to an increased incidence of RV systemic failure.

Thus, in patients with ACHD, RV failure is a common phenomenon with an incidence of up to 70% in selected patient populations. Moreover, some patients suffer from residual shunt, which can lead to increased pulmonary blood flow in case of a left-to-right shunt, thus, resulting in pulmonary hypertension, ultimately leading to RV

Box 1
AP classification of ACHD

CHD anatomy[a]

I: Simple
   Native disease
   - Isolated small ASD
   - Isolated small VSD
   - Mild isolated pulmonic stenosis
   Repaired conditions
   - Previously ligated or occluded ductus arteriosus
   - Repaired secundum ASD or sinus venosus defect without significant residual shunt or chamber enlargement
   - Repaired VSD without significant residual shunt or chamber enlargement

II: Moderate complexity repaired
   Repaired or unrepaired conditions
   - Aorto–left ventricular fistula
   - Anomalous pulmonary venous connection, partial or total
   - Atrioventricular septal defects (partial or complete, including primum ASD)
   - Coarctation of the aorta
   - Ebstein anomaly (disease spectrum includes mild, moderate, and severe variations)
   - Infundibular right ventricular outflow obstruction
   - Ostium primum ASD
   - Moderate and large persistently patent ductus arteriosus
   - Pulmonary valve regurgitation (moderate or greater)
   - Pulmonary valve stenosis (moderate or greater)
   - Sinus of Valsalva fistula/aneurysm
   - Sinus venosus defect
   - Subvalvar or supravalvar aortic stenosis
   - Repaired tetralogy of Fallot
   - Ventricular septal defect with associated abnormality and/or moderate or greater shunt

III: Great complexity (or complex)
   - Cyanotic congenital heart defect (unrepaired or palliated, all forms)
   - Double-outlet ventricle
   - Fontan procedure
   - Mitral atresia
   - Single ventricle (including double inlet left ventricle, tricuspid atresia, hypoplastic left heart, any other anatomic abnormality with a functionally single ventricle)
   - Pulmonary atresia (all forms)
   - TGA (classic or d-TGA; cc-TGA or l-TGA)
   - Truncus arteriosus
   - Other abnormalities of atrioventricular and ventriculoarterial connection (ie, crisscross heart, isomerism, heterotaxy syndromes, ventricular inversion)

Physiologic stage A

NYHA FC I symptoms
   - No hemodynamic or anatomic sequelae
   - No arrhythmias
   - Normal exercise capacity
   - Normal renal/hepatic/pulmonary function

Physiologic stage B

NYHA FC II symptoms
   - Mild hemodynamic sequelae (mild aortic enlargement, mild ventricular enlargement, mild ventricular dysfunction)
   - Mild valvular disease
   - Trivial or small shunt (not hemodynamically significant)
   - Arrhythmia not requiring treatment
   - Abnormal objective cardiac limitation to exercise

Physiologic stage C

NYHA FC III symptoms
- Significant (moderate or greater) valvular disease; moderate or greater ventricular dysfunction (systemic, pulmonic, or both)
- Moderate aortic enlargement
- Venous or arterial stenosis
- Mild or moderate hypoxemia/cyanosis
- Hemodynamically significant shunt
- Arrhythmias controlled with treatment
- Pulmonary hypertension (less than severe)
- End-organ dysfunction responsive to therapy

Physiologic stage D

NYHA FC IV symptoms
- Severe aortic enlargement
- Arrhythmias refractory to treatment
- Severe hypoxemia (almost always associated with cyanosis)
- Severe pulmonary hypertension
- Eisenmenger syndrome
- Refractory end-organ dysfunction

CHD Anatomy + Physiologic stage = ACHD AP classification.
Abbreviations: AP, anatomic and physiologic; ASD, atrial septal defect; cc-TGA, congenitally corrected transposition of the great arteries; d-TGA, dextro-transposition of the great arteries; FC, functional class; l-TGA, levo-transposition of the great arteries; TGA, transposition of the great arteries; VSD, ventricular septal defect.

[a] This list is not meant to be comprehensive; other conditions may be important in individual patients.

Adapted from Stout KK, Daniels CJ, Aboulhosn JA, et al. 2018 AHA/ACC Guideline for the Management of Adults With Congenital Heart Disease: Executive Summary: A Report of the American College of Cardiology/American Heart Association Task Force on Clinical Practice Guidelines. J Am Coll Cardiol 2019;73(12):1504; with permission.

dysfunction secondary to pressure overload.[12–15] The prevalence of ACHD-heart failure is highest in patients with complex anatomy, including single ventricle physiology, transposition of the great arteries (TGA), tetralogy of Fallot (TOF), and pulmonary hypertension.[13]

Patients with ACHD are generally younger when developing heart failure and often the decrease in cardiac function is accompanied by tachyarrhythmias of a different origin. Basically, advanced rhythm therapy can contribute to treating heart failure appropriately.

Diastolic Heart Failure

During the past years, there has been an increasing focus on LV heart failure with preserved systolic LV (diastolic) function, or diastolic heart failure. In the population of patients with ACHD, information on diastolic LV failure is relatively sparse.

Diagnosis of Heart Failure in Adult Patients with Congenital Heart Disease

Signs and symptoms

Heart failure is a clinical diagnosis. It is defined as a syndrome of signs and symptoms of cardiac congestion caused by a structural and/or functional cardiac abnormality, resulting in reduced cardiac output and/or elevated intracardiac pressures at rest or during stress.[5,16,17]

Patients with ACHD themselves tend to underreport their cardiac symptoms because they are used to living with cardiac disease. At the time of symptom recognition, the extent of ventricular dysfunction and valve disease may be severe and irreversible. Considering the high mortality of ACHD heart failure, it is recommended to pay specific attention to signs of developing heart failure and perform diagnostic tests during follow-up to initiate therapy in an early stage of ACHD-heart failure.

Diagnostic and therapeutic recommendations in guidelines are based on the majority of heart failure, which is usually caused by LV systolic or diastolic dysfunction in patients without CHD. However, heart failure in CHD is more often a consequence of RV disease, valve dysfunction, shunting or pulmonary hypertension. The evaluation and treatment of heart failure in CHD should therefore be based on the specific structural and functional circulatory lesion. Recently, a task force of the American Heart Association and the American College of Cardiologists published the first guideline for the management of ACHD.[5]

Diagnosis

In general, patients with ACHD should be treated by specialist cardiologists. Within the last years, cardiac centers have established specialized ambulatory care units dedicated to these patients. Within such centers, a wide range of technical and clinical diagnostics is available. The basic assumptions for diagnosing heart failure is the combination of clinical examination, functional capacity testing, and technical investigations combined with biomarker monitoring.

Functional capacity Cardiopulmonary exercise testing is often considered the gold standard for quantitative assessment of functional capacity. It correlates well with NYHA functional classification, functional capacity, and anaerobic threshold during cardiopulmonary exercise testing. A subnormal peak Vo_2 during cardiopulmonary exercise testing has been demonstrated in asymptomatic ACHD, highlighting the need for the evaluation of heart failure even in the absence of symptoms.[18]

The NYHA Functional Classification (see **Box 1**) is commonly used to describe the functional capacity in heart failure[18] and correlates well with the severity of heart failure and strategies for treatment, and ultimately predicts mortality.[5,18] It was however questionable whether this was also applicable for patients with ACHD. Recently, Bredy and colleagues[18] demonstrated that the NYHA functional class correlated strongly with predictive capacity of exercise testing and with the Bethesda classification in ACHD.

Cardiac imaging Echocardiography is a noninvasive technique for monitoring disease progression and provides assessment of intracardiac anatomy and overall cardiac function at rest and during exercise. Specific guidelines for echocardiographic evaluation of RV pressures and volumes in ACHD are available.[19]

Cardiac magnetic resonance imaging has the ability to provide quantitative assessment of blood flow, valvular regurgitation, chamber volumes and ventricular function. Also, anatomic and functional cardiac assessment during pharmacologic stress testing is possible with a stress MRI. In the presence of contraindications to cardiac magnetic resonance imaging, a cardiac computed tomography scan is an alternative with the ability to quantify ventricular volumes and assess ventricular function.

Cardiac biomarkers At baseline, elevated levels of atrial natriuretic peptide, brain-type natriuretic peptide, N-terminal pro-brain-type natriuretic peptide (NT-proBNP), endothelin-1, norepinephrine, renin, and aldosterone have been found in ACHD. Several studies have shown a relationship between the degree of cardiac biomarker elevations, NYHA functional class, and systemic ventricular function.[3,12] The degree of elevation varies between ACHD lesions.

Management of Heart Failure in Adult Patients with Congenital Heart Disease

General considerations

Guidelines published by the American College of Cardiology/American Heart Association/Heart Failure Society of America and the European Society of Cardiology on the management of heart failure in acquired heart disease are readily available. These recommendations emphasize the use of neurohormonal blockade with angiotensin-converting enzyme inhibitors, angiotensin receptor blockers (ARB), and beta-blockers, which have proven morbidity and mortality benefits in heart failure.[17] Management of this complex ACHD population has largely been extrapolated from literature that is based on adults with acquired heart disease. Very recently, the American College of Cardiology/American Heart Association guidelines for the management of ACHD in general were published, but recommendations for the specific management of heart failure in ACHD are scarce. For further reading on heart failure in ACHD, 2 major publications from Stout and colleagues[14] and Budts and colleagues[20] are recommended.

Subtypes of heart failure in adult patients with congenital heart disease

Systolic dysfunction of the systemic left ventricle Systolic dysfunction in the systemic LV results from coronary artery disease, systolic dysfunction of the LV as a consequence of volume loading (aortic regurgitation, mitral regurgitation, and residual ventricular septal defect) or pressure loading (aortic stenosis, and coarctation of the aorta) (**Table 1**).[3,5,12,14,15,17] Diagnosis and treatment is in line with the general American College of Cardiology/American Heart Association heart failure guidelines for patients without ACHD.[16]

Systolic dysfunction of the systemic right ventricle In some types of ACHD, the anatomic right ventricle acts as the ventricle serving the systemic circulation. Classical examples are congenitally corrected TGA, as well as surgically corrected TGA (d-TGA) after the Mustard or Senning atrial switch operations (**Table 2**). RV failure has been shown to develop in 67% of patients with congenitally corrected TGA by the age of 45 years, and in 12% of patients with d-TGA 12 years after the atrial switch procedure. Overall, heart failure is the leading cause of death in up to 66% of patients with a systemic RV.[3,12,14]

The effectiveness of guideline-directed medical therapy in decreasing morbidity or mortality in systemic RV failure is unclear. Some studies with angiotensin-converting enzyme inhibitor treatment have noted a trend toward improved peak Vo_2 and a decrease in levels of NT-proBNP, but evidence for significant improvements in exercise peak Vo_2, tricuspid regurgitation, RV size, or RV systolic function is lacking. Studies involving ARBs have demonstrated a lack of benefit. Increased catecholamine levels in patients with systemic RV and increases in concentrations of epinephrine and norepinephrine correlate with increased cardiothoracic ratio and RV diastolic dimensions. In small studies the use of beta-blockers have demonstrated improvements in quality of life and NYHA functional class. Treatment with higher doses of beta-blockers in patients with d-TGA and cardiac pacemakers failed to demonstrate improvement in RV size and systolic function, but showed significant improvements in NYHA functional class.[3,5,12-15,17]

Tachycardia-mediated cardiomyopathy is an important cause of systemic RV failure. In patients after an atrial switch procedure for d-TGA, the incidence of arrhythmia increases over time, from nearly 78% arrhythmia-free survival at 10 years to only 36%

Table 1
Failure of the systemic LV

Contributing cardiac lesions and mechanisms	Coronary artery disease
	Volume loading
	  Aortic regurgitation
	  Mitral regurgitation
	  Ventricular septal defect
	  Patent ductus arteriosus
	Pressure loading
	  Subaortic stenosis
	  Valvar aortic stenosis
	  Supravalvar aortic stenosis
	  Coarctation of the aorta

Symptoms	Pulmonary edema, dependent edema, persistent cough, orthopnea, decline in functional capacity

Diagnostic method	Laboratory: cardiopulmonary exercise testing: determine exercise capacity, symptoms, electrocardiogram changes or arrhythmias
	Imaging
	  Echocardiography: assessment of LV size and function and severity of LV outflow tract obstructions
	  MRI: assessment of supravalvular aortic stenosis and coarctation of the aorta

Management	Pharmacologic
	  If persistent heart failure after intervention as a result of dysfunctional myocardium owing to LV diastolic dysfunction or adverse LV remodeling, than treat according to existing heart failure guidelines for acquired heart disease.
	  Hypertension in coarctation of aorta: beta-blockade more effective than ARB
	Mechanical support
	  Cardiac resynchronization therapy
	  Implantable cardioverter-defibrillator
	  Ventricular assist device
	Surgical
	  Corrective measure of valvular or LV outflow tract obstruction (catheter-based intervention, surgical) according to guidelines.
	  Balloon valvulotomy (first line therapy in children, adolescents, young adults)
	  Resection of endocardial fibroelastosis to ameliorate diastolic dysfunction (limited experience)

at 25 years after the procedure. In these patients, intense monitoring of heart rhythm is justified. It remains unknown if modern electrophysiology approaches may result in improved outcome in these patients.[3,5,12–14]

Right ventricular dysfunction RV dysfunction is most common in patients with Tetralogy of Fallot, but can develop in a variety of other cardiac lesions caused by right-sided volume and/or pressure overload (**Table 3**). Pulmonary stenosis and pulmonary hypertension are the most common pressure-loading lesions that have the potential to result in subpulmonic RV failure. A number of CHD types are characterized by outflow obstruction of the RVOT with increasing risk of RV failure.[3,12,14]

Table 2
Failure of the systemic right ventricle

Contributing cardiac lesions and mechanisms	Congenitally corrected TGA D-TGA
Symptoms	Pulmonary edema, dependent edema, persistent cough, orthopnea, decline in functional status, chronotropic incompetence, atrial and ventricular tachyarrhythmia
Diagnostic method	Annual clinical evaluation, more frequent as necessary Laboratory, brain-type natriuretic peptide: level correlates with deterioration in clinical status, declining RV ejection fraction, decreasing exercise capacity, worsening TR. Cut off value not defined. Imaging, periodic (RV function, TR): Echocardiography MRI/cardiac MRI (RV size and function, TR severity, myocardial fibrosis) Stress cardiac MRI (inability to increase RV ejection fraction predictive for cardiac events)
Management	Pharmacologic Conclusive data are lacking. Beware of preexisting sinus node dysfunction, heart block, baffle stenosis, nondistensible atria, restrictive RV physiology Angiotensin-converting enzyme inhibitors/ARB: no improvement in ejection fraction Vo_2, CI Beta-blockade: shown to improve RV function and symptoms, less systemic TR, improve functional status, positive effect RV remodeling, protection against arrhythmia Mechanical support Implantable cardioverter-defibrillator: consider for primary prevention, although only after or in conjunction with beta-blockers to mitigate arrhythmias CRT: management of brady- and tachyarrhythmia. Benefit unknown; modest improvement in RVEF and NYHA suggested Surgical Treat residual such as outflow obstruction or valvular regurgitation before significant valvular dysfunction. Ventricular assist device and CHD transplantation: systolic RV failure who fail medical therapy and without residual lesions.

Abbreviations: CRT, cardiac resynchronization therapy; TR, tricuspid regurgitation.

Echocardiography is the most common used diagnostic measure in these patients. In addition, cardiac MRI is sometimes indicated. Assessment of peak exercise capacity helps to document the course of the disease.[3,5,14,15,17]

Surgical or percutaneous intervention aimed at correcting these volume/pressure loading conditions offer the best chance of improving ventricular function, but the timing of such interventions is a matter of debate. Pharmacologic therapy with pulmonary vasodilators (phosphodiesterase-5 inhibitors, endothelin-receptor antagonists, or prostacyclin analogs) form the basis of pulmonary hypertension management, and diuretics can be effective for symptom management in the setting of significant RV volume loading. ARBs have not proven beneficial in improving ventricular function,

Table 3 Failure of the right ventricle	

Contributing cardiac lesions and mechanisms	Volume loading
	  Pulmonary regurgitation (ie, repaired TOF)
	  Ebstein anomaly
	  Atrial septal defect (ASD)
	  Anomalous pulmonary venous return
	  Extra cardiac arteriovenous malformation
	Pressure loading
	  Sub pulmonary stenosis
	  Valvar pulmonary stenosis
	  Supra valvar pulmonary stenosis
	  Pulmonary hypertension/Eisenmenger

Symptoms	Erythrocytosis, progressive cyanosis/desaturation during exertion
Diagnostic method	Echocardiography: RV volume and function, LV end-diastolic pressure and function (predictors of VT and SCD) MRI/cardiac MRI: ventricle volumes and function (extent of LGE adds predictive value for development of clinical arrhythmia) Electrophysiological study: risk stratification, particularly with symptoms of syncope (inducibility of monomorphic and polymorphic VT is predictive of subsequent clinical events) Cardiac catheterization: to assess pulmonary vascular hemodynamics for adults with septal or great artery shunts and clinical symptoms, signs, or echocardiographic findings suggestive of pulmonary hypertension

Management	Pharmacologic
	  Angiotensin-converting enzyme inhibitors/ARB: no improvement in RV or LV function, exercise capacity or degree of pulmonary regurgitation. Significant improvement in RV and LV long-axis shortening. Improvement in LV volume and EF.
	  Beta-blockade increasingly used based on description of increased SNS activity after TOF repair. No improvement in NYHA functional class, exercise capacity or RV or LV size or function, but increase in brain-type natriuretic peptide.
	  Endothelin-receptor antagonists and phosphodiesterase type 5: beneficial long-term effect on patients with Eisenmenger syndrome
	Mechanical support
	  Implantable cardioverter-defibrillator implantation: for secondary prevention of VT and SCD (6%–14%). Good indications: elevated LVEDP, nonsustained VT, VT inducibility, elevated RVSP. For primary prevention when multiple risk factors for SCD are present.
	  CRT: favorable in LV systolic dysfunction (small studies), apply guidelines for CRT from acquired heart disease. It has yet to be determined whether patients with RV dysfunction benefit, manage on a case-by-case basis.
	Surgical
	  Percutaneous or surgical pulmonary valve replacement: indicated in patients with severe PR, severe RV dilatation, evidence of RV systolic dysfunction, decreased exercise tolerance attributable to PR, ideally before manifestation of heart failure.

Abbreviations: CRT, cardiac resynchronization therapy; TOF, tetralogy of Fallot.

exercise capacity, NT-proBNP levels, or clinical symptoms of right-sided heart failure. Similarly, there is a lack of evidence showing any benefits with the use of angiotensin-converting enzyme inhibitors and beta-blockers in right-sided heart failure.[3,5,14,15,17]

HEART FAILURE IN SPECIFIC LESIONS
Heart Failure in Patients with Fontan Procedure

There are a number of anatomic variations resulting in a single ventricle physiology (**Table 4**). In the newborn, the primary goal of surgical therapy is to establish sufficient

Table 4 Failure of Fontan circulation	
Contributing cardiac lesions and mechanisms	Fontan failure with reduced ejection fraction Fontan failure with preserved ejection fraction
Symptoms	Protein-losing enteropathy, plastic bronchitis, portal hypertension, peripheral edema, thrombus/pulmonary embolism/stroke, cyanosis, atrial and ventricular arrhythmia
Diagnostic method	Regular clinical evaluation: heart failure should be anticipated in the long-term care Important to assess potentially reversible causes of heart failure such as ventricular dysfunction, arrhythmias, thrombus in the Fontan pathways, protein-losing enteropathy, valvular dysfunction, residual right-to-left shunt, inflow or outflow obstruction including a restrictive atrial or ventricular septal defect that can impede cardiac output, elevated systemic vascular resistance, elevated systemic venous pressures and pulmonary vascular resistance, plastic bronchitis Electrocardiogram: monitoring for bradycardia or sinus node dysfunction Stress testing: for assessing symptoms suggestive of myocardial ischemia and heart failure MRI or computed tomography scan: evaluation of common long-term complications of atrial or arterial switch Cardiac catheterization: invasive anatomic and hemodynamic assessment, coronary patency
Management	Pharmacologic Angiotensin-converting enzyme inhibitors: no significant differences in SVR, resting CI, diastolic function, exercise capacity, ventricular size, Ross heart failure class, brain-type natriuretic peptide levels, ejection fraction or mortality (evidence: few studies, nonadult) Beta-blockade: negative or neutral effect on symptoms or clinical parameters Diuretics and digoxin: widely used (evidence: not empirical) Pulmonary vasodilator therapy: mixed results (improved peak Vo$_2$ during exercise, increased pulmonary and systemic blood flow at peak exercise, doppler derived myocardial performance index, systolic arterial and ventricular elastance, ventilatory efficiency (evidence: small studies) Endothelin antagonists: unknown (evidence: studies ongoing) Mechanical support CRT: maintenance of atrioventricular synchrony (evidence: case series) Surgical -

Abbreviations: CRT, cardiac resynchronization therapy; SVR, systemic vascular resistance.

pulmonary blood flow to reach an acceptable level of oxygenation. This target is usually reached via surgical creation of a shunt to improve pulmonary blood flow. Thereafter, a surgical connection between the superior and inferior vena cava and the pulmonary artery is created. This so-called Fontan circulation is based on a passive flow of blood through the pulmonary circulation, strictly depending on the pressure gradient between central venous and left atrial pressure.

Over time, up to 40% of patients with a Fontan circulation develop heart failure.[21] The underlying mechanisms are variable. Fontan failure can occur with depressed ejection fraction or with normal ejection fraction (primary diastolic failure). Diastolic failure of the single ventricle is commonly accompanied by valve insufficiency, and arrhythmias are regularly observed. Hebson and colleagues[22] showed that patients with circulatory failure regularly develop elevated central venous and pulmonary capillary wedge pressures with low systemic vascular resistance and a preserved cardiac index. This hemodynamic profile is comparable with that of patients suffering from portal hypertension. However, in a Fontan circulation the ability to augment cardiac output above a certain threshold is limited. The increased postsinusoidal pressure in the inferior vena cava leads to liver fibrosis and to a portal hypertensive type circulatory derangement, resulting in vasoconstriction of the renal vasculature, sodium/water retention, edema and ascites. Patients with a systemic right ventricle face both limitations of a systemic right ventricle and failing Fontan pathophysiology.

If a failing Fontan circulation is present, a complete cardiac workup is recommended to identify correctable hemodynamic disturbance.[3,22] However, pharmacologic heart failure treatment is rather difficult. The maintenance of ventricular contractility, treatment of arrhythmias and optimized balance between preload and afterload remain the most relevant targets.

The Fontan circulation depends on low pulmonary vascular resistance. A sustained increase in pulmonary vascular resistance, and thus afterload, should be treated. Studies with phosphodiesterase type 5 inhibitors such as sildenafil have shown some benefit (increase in peak pulmonary blood flow, peak Vo_2, cardiac index, and stroke volume during exercise). Similar results have emerged in studies using bosentan (an endothelin-receptor antagonist). More recently, studies involving newer generation pulmonary vasodilators in Fontan patients have been initiated.[3,5,13–15,17]

To preserve ventricular contractility and an adequate preload, aggressive treatment of any arrhythmia is recommended. In the event of dyssynchronous contraction of the functional systemic ventricle, pacemaker therapy should be considered. Diuretics are effective for inappropriate fluid retention, such as edema, pleural effusion, and ascites. After initiation of beta-blockade in children and adolescents with a failing Fontan circulation, decreased requirements for diuretics were demonstrated in addition to increased ventricular ejection fraction.[3,14] The effect of beta-blockers on the systemic vascular resistance has shown to be neutral in large studies.[22] Neurohormonal blockade in Fontan failure has not shown benefit. The use of angiotensin-converting enzyme/ARB was not associated with improvements in cardiac index, exercise capacity, or diastolic filling patterns.[23]

Heart Failure in Patients after Surgery for Transposition of the Great Arteries

In patients with congenital TGA, the arterial switch operation is nowadays the standard of care. After the arterial switch, the LV acts as the systemic ventricle (anatomic correction). However, if a switch operation is not possible, the Senning or Mustard procedure (atrial switch) is performed.

Recently, Couperus and colleagues[24] described the long-term follow-up of up to more than 30 years after atrial correction in 76 adult patients with TGA. Survival was

82% at 39.7 years postoperatively and exceeded 50 years in 4 patients. The most common complication was supraventricular tachycardia in more than 50% of patients. Heart failure was observed in 19% of patients 30 years after surgery. RV function was depressed in 31 (46%) patients, and NYHA class was II or greater in 34 patients (48%). Bradyarrhythmia, supraventricular tachycardia, and ventricular arrhythmia were associated with depressed RV and functional capacity. Ventricular arrhythmias, heart failure and surgical reinterventions were common during late follow-up. Heart failure therapy in these patients is therefore primarily based on antiarrhythmic therapy and preservation of RV function.

PERIOPERATIVE CARE FOR ADULT PATIENTS WITH CONGENITAL HEART DISEASE–RELATED HEART FAILURE

The number of adults with CHD now surpasses the number of children with CHD,[25] leading to the fact that adults with complex CHD managed for noncardiac surgery are not restricted to highly specialized centers. Agarwal and colleagues[9] reported that 27.1% of ACHD admissions to small-sized hospitals represented complex ACHD. In the United States, general anesthesia knowledge and training standards for ACHD are lacking, resulting in a low level of knowledge and comfort with providing perioperative and obstetric care for patients with ACHD, even in academic centers.[26]

Cardiac and noncardiac surgical procedures in patients with CHD carry an increased risk for perioperative adverse events. Factors judged to have a major contribution to adverse events were the nature of CHD (50%), preoperative assessment or optimization (40%), intraoperative anesthetic care (55%), and postoperative monitoring/care (50%).[27]

Preoperative Risk Assessment

The risk of patients with ACHD generally depends on 4 factors: the underlying nature of CHD, the individual course of this CHD, associated noncardiac morbidity, and the type of the noncardiac surgical procedure. Because of the complexity of morbidity and the individual course of disease, individualized preoperative risk assessment is necessary. This process includes assessment, optimization, and care by a multidisciplinary team with a detailed understanding of the patient's cardiac defect, functional status, and anticipation of the perioperative stresses[5,28] (**Box 2**).

Heart Failure

Clinical performance may be misleading as a relevant part of the ACHD may present with good physical performance. Proven predictive tools for evaluation of the ventricular function are echocardiography and the use of biomarkers such as NT-proBNP. An NT-proBNP of greater than 33.3 mmol/L is strongly associated with cardiac events, death, or heart failure, independent of echocardiography findings.[29] The risk of patients with a high level of NT-proBNP could be further differentiated by adding hs-TnT and growth differentiation factor 15. Patients with elevated levels of all 3 biomarkers are at highest risk of cardiac events, death, and heart failure.[29] Low biomarker levels were accurately associated with a low risk of heart failure and death.[29] These findings could enable accurate preoperative identification of patients at high perioperative cardiac risk and allow for the timely initiation or expansion of risk-reducing strategies.

Arrhythmias

Almost 50% of all ACHD will develop atrial tachyarrhythmias during their lifetime.[30] Factors such as underlying anatomy, age, and surgical repair technique have an

---

Box 2
Recommendations for preoperative risk assessment in ACHD

1. Basic preoperative assessment for patients with ACHD should include systemic arterial oximetry, an electrocardiogram, chest radiographs, transthoracic echocardiography, and blood tests for full blood count and coagulation screen. (LOE: C)

2. It is recommended that when possible, the preoperative evaluation and surgery for patients with ACHD be performed in a regional center specializing in congenital cardiology, with experienced surgeons and cardiac anesthesiologists. (LOE: C)

3. Certain high-risk patient populations should be managed at centers for the care of patients with ACHD under all circumstances, unless the operative intervention is an absolute emergency. High-risk categories include patients with the following:
   a. Prior Fontan procedure.
   b. Severe pulmonary arterial hypertension.
   c. Cyanotic CHD.
   d. Complex CHD with residua such as heart failure, valve disease, or the need for anticoagulation.
   e. Patients with CHD and malignant arrhythmias. (LOE: C)

4. Consultation with ACHD experts regarding the assessment of risk is recommended for patients with CHD who will undergo noncardiac surgery. (LOE: C)

5. Consultation with a cardiac anesthesiologist is recommended for moderate- and high-risk patients. (LOE: C)

Abbreviation: LOE, level of evidence.

Adapted from Warnes CA, Williams RG, Bashore TM, et al. ACC/AHA 2008 guidelines for the management of adults with congenital heart disease: a report of the American College of Cardiology/American Heart Association Task Force on Practice Guidelines (Writing Committee to Develop Guidelines on the Management of Adults With Congenital Heart Disease). Developed in Collaboration With the American Society of Echocardiography, Heart Rhythm Society, International Society for Adult Congenital Heart Disease, Society for Cardiovascular Angiography and Interventions, and Society of Thoracic Surgeons. J Am Coll Cardiol 2008;52(23):e143-e263; with permission.

---

impact on prevalence and arrhythmia substrate. Atrial tachyarrhythmia, mostly in the form of intra-atrial reentrant tachycardia and atrial fibrillation, are more frequent than ventricular tachyarrhythmias. The presence of atrial tachyarrhythmia significantly increases the risk of heart failure and stroke.[31] For perioperative management, common scores for thromboembolic risk calculation, like CHADS2 and CHA2DS2-VASc, are not predictive for thromboembolic risk in patients with ACHD.[30,31] The complexity of CHD, however, was independently associated with thromboembolic events.[32] Antiarrhythmic therapy with class IC antiarrhythmic agents and amiodarone is effective in almost 50% of the patients, although systemic side effects and proarrhythmic properties being of concern.[30,32] Electrical cardioversion with appropriate anticoagulation is safe and effective.[30,32] Catheter ablation procedures and the MAZE procedure for drug-refractory atrial fibrillation may be beneficial in selected patients, but experience is limited.[32] Antiarrhythmic therapy is effective in suppressing ventricular arrhythmias, but has not been associated with improved survival.[28]

PREGNANCY

The overall incidence of maternal CHD is 0.6%[33] and accounts for 60% to 80% of abnormalities in pregnant women with structural heart disease.[34] The incidence of cardiac complications in pregnancies associated with CHD is estimated to be around

11%, but may be as high as 20%.[33,35] Heart failure is the most common cardiac complication during pregnancy with 2 peaks of onset. The first peak is between 23 and 30 weeks, when most of the hemodynamic changes have taken place and the second peak around delivery. If heart failure affects a woman with CHD during pregnancy, maternal mortality today is around 4.8%.[33–35]

Women with CHD should receive pregnancy counseling with input from an ACHD cardiologist to determine maternal cardiac, obstetric and fetal risks, and long-term risks to the mother. Then an individualized plan of care should be developed. During pregnancy, women with CHD (especially those with complex forms of ACHD) should be managed collaboratively by cardiologists, obstetricians, and anesthesiologists who are all experienced in ACHD.[5]

To assess the maternal cardiovascular risk, the Canadian Cardiac Disease in Pregnancy and Zwangerschap bij Aangeboren HARtAfwijkingen (ZAHARA) scores are used, along with the modified World Health Organization classification of maternal cardiovascular risk.[36] Pregnancy is generally contraindicated in women at high risk of maternal morbidity and mortality, which includes women with pulmonary arterial hypertension, severe left-sided obstructive lesions, significant systemic ventricular dysfunction (ejection fraction of <30%) and NYHA functional class III or IV.[5,36]

Medical management involves optimizing heart failure medications, in particular the discontinuation of agents toxic to the fetus while titrating nontoxic heart failure medications.[37] If well-managed, vaginal delivery with adequate analgesia is well-tolerated in most obstetric patients with CHD.[37]

For intrapartum monitoring, telemetry, oxygen saturation monitoring, and invasive hemodynamic monitoring should be considered on an individualized basis.[36,37] Postpartum monitoring of the patient with CHD with heart failure or at high risk for heart failure requires telemetry monitoring for at least 24 hours postpartum, as well as careful clinical monitoring for evidence of decompensated heart failure and development of arrhythmia. The risk for recurrent or worsening heart failure can occur up to 8 weeks after delivery.[37]

NONMEDICAL THERAPY FOR REFRACTORY HEART FAILURE

In refractory and end-stage heart failure, mechanical circulatory support remains one of the final treatment options. There is a wide spectrum of techniques ranging from acute implementation of temporary venovenous or venoarterial extracorporeal membrane oxygenation to continuous treatment with implantable mechanical assist devices as a bridge to recovery or even as a bridge to heart transplantation. It is estimated that 10% to 20% of patients with ACHD will require heart transplantation at some point in their life.[38]

In 2018, Esteve-Ruiz and co-workers presented the results of a series of 10 patients with ACHD undergoing heart transplantation. All of these patients suffered from failing Fontan circulation or another form of single ventricle pathology. Nine of the 10 patients were transplanted electively, whereas 1 patient required extracorporeal membrane oxygenation preoperatively. Compared with patients with heart failure from non-CHD, both short-term mortality and postoperative stay in the intensive care unit were increased. After 1 year, outcomes were comparable between the 2 groups.[39] However, these series of individual patient cases is too small to draw definitive conclusions on whether or not heart transplantation is suitable in patients with ACHD. In an analysis by Goldberg and colleagues, patients with ACHD represented 2.5% of all patients placed on the US heart transplantation list.[40]

Although there is no evidence-based consensus on the role of heart transplantation in patients with ACHD, the use of ventricular assist devices in these patients is an established standard of care. In experienced centers, the mortality of ventricular assist device implantation in patients with ACHD is comparable to mortality in non-patients with ACHD, although this only holds true for patients with a 2-ventricle anatomy. There are no systematic studies addressing the use of mechanical support systems in patients with single ventricle physiology (Fontan circulation), although some information is available from case series or individual case reports.

SUMMARY

Owing to advances in care, almost 90% of children born with a CHD grow up into adulthood and many achieve elderly age. Although many cardiac birth defects can be surgically well-managed, residual anomalies eventually give rise to complications and increase the risk of severe morbidity and mortality. Because of their heterogeneity and the complexity of the pathophysiologic profile, care for these patients is very challenging. With the increasing number of adults with CHD and the increasing complexity with aging of these patients, there is a growing need for multidisciplinary care programs and guidelines. However, most guidelines are based on studies with patients without CHD and should be extrapolated with care when used for patients with CHD, taking into account the individual pathophysiology. In the follow-up of adults with CHD and in the perioperative care of these patients, special attention should be paid to signs and symptoms of developing heart failure and to prevention of deteriorating heart function and arrhythmias for these are major causes of adverse cardiac events and mortality. Also, pregnant women with ACHD who may clinically seem to have normal heart function are at increased risk, mainly owing to hematologic and cardiovascular changes related to pregnancy. Challenges for the near future are to improve knowledge on optimal diagnostics and pharmacologic treatment, adequate timing of interventions, and education of health care teams.

REFERENCES

1. Mitchell SC, Korones SB, Berendes HW. Congenital heart disease in 56,109 births incidence and natural history. Circulation 1971;43(3):323–32.
2. van der Bom T, Bouma BJ, Meijboom FJ, et al. The prevalence of adult congenital heart disease, results from a systematic review and evidence based calculation. Am Heart J 2012;164(4):568–75.
3. Opina AD, Franklin WJ. Management of heart failure in adult congenital heart disease. Prog Cardiovasc Dis 2018;61(3–4):308–13.
4. van der Linde D, Konings EEM, Slager MA, et al. Birth prevalence of congenital heart disease worldwide. J Am Coll Cardiol 2011;58(21):2241–7.
5. Stout KK, Daniels CJ, Aboulhosn JA, et al. 2018 AHA/ACC guideline for the management of adults with congenital heart disease. A report of the American College of Cardiology/American Heart Association Task Force on Clinical Practice Guidelines. Circulation 2019;139(14):e698–800.
6. Hoffman JIE, Kaplan S, Liberthson RR. Prevalence of congenital heart disease. Am Heart J 2004;147(3):425–39.
7. Moussa NB, Karsenty C, Pontnau F, et al. Characteristics and outcomes of heart failure-related hospitalization in adults with congenital heart disease. Arch Cardiovasc Dis 2017;110(5):283–91.
8. Afilalo J, Therrien J, Pilote L, et al. Geriatric congenital heart disease. J Am Coll Cardiol 2011;58(14):1509–15.

9. Agarwal S, Sud K, Menon V. Nationwide hospitalization trends in adult congenital heart disease across 2003–2012. J Am Heart Assoc 2016;5(1) [pii:e002330].

10. Zomer A, Vaartjes I, van der Velde E. Heart failure admissions in adults with congenital heart disease; risk factors and prognosis. Int J Cardiol 2013;168: 2487–93.

11. Verheugt CL, Uiterwaal CSPM, van der Velde ET, et al. Mortality in adult congenital heart disease. Eur Heart J 2010;31(10):1220–9.

12. Bolger AP, Gatzoulis MA. Towards defining heart failure in adults with congenital heart disease. Int J Cardiol 2004;97:15–23.

13. Krieger EV, Valente AM. Heart failure treatment in adults with congenital heart disease: where do we stand in 2014? Heart 2014;100(17):1329–34.

14. Stout KK, Broberg CS, Book WM, et al. Chronic heart failure in congenital heart disease: a scientific statement from the American Heart Association. Circulation 2016;133(8):770–801.

15. Warnes CA, Williams RG, Bashore TM, et al. ACC/AHA 2008 guidelines for the management of adults with congenital heart disease. J Am Coll Cardiol 2008; 52(23):e143–263.

16. Ponikowski P, Voors AA, Anker SD, et al. 2016 ESC guidelines for the diagnosis and treatment of acute and chronic heart failure: the task force for the diagnosis and treatment of acute and chronic heart failure of the European Society of Cardiology (ESC) Developed with the special contribution of the Heart Failure Association (HFA) of the ESC. Eur Heart J 2016;37(27):2129–200.

17. Yancy CW, Jessup M, Bozkurt B, et al. 2017 ACC/AHA/HFSA focused update of the 2013 ACCF/AHA guideline for the management of heart failure. J Card Fail 2017;23(8):628–51.

18. Bredy C, Ministeri M, Kempny A, et al. New York Heart Association (NYHA) classification in adults with congenital heart disease: relation to objective measures of exercise and outcome. Eur Heart J Qual Care Clin Outcomes 2018;4(1):51–8.

19. Rudski LG, Lai WW, Afilalo J, et al. Guidelines for the echocardiographic assessment of the right heart in adults: a report from the American Society of Echocardiography. J Am Soc Echocardiogr 2010;23(7):685–713.

20. Budts W, Roos-Hesselink J, Rädle-Hurst T, et al. Treatment of heart failure in adult congenital heart disease: a position paper of the Working Group of Grown-Up Congenital Heart Disease and the Heart Failure Association of the European Society of Cardiology. Eur Heart J 2016;37(18):1419–27.

21. Norozi K, Wessel A, Alpers V, et al. Incidence and risk distribution of heart failure in adolescents and adults with congenital heart disease after cardiac surgery. Am J Cardiol 2006;97:1238–43.

22. Hebson CL, McCabe NM, Elder RW, et al. Hemodynamic phenotype of the failing Fontan in an adult population. Am J Cardiol 2013;112(12):1943–7.

23. Ohuchi H. Adult patients with Fontan circulation: what we know and how to manage adults with Fontan circulation? J Cardiol 2016;68:181–9.

24. Couperus LE, Vliegen HW, Zandstra TE, et al. Long-term outcome after atrial correction for transposition of the great arteries. Heart 2019;105(10):790–6.

25. Gilboa SM, Devine OJ, Kucik JE, et al. Congenital heart defects in the United States: estimating the magnitude of the affected population in 2010. Circulation 2016;134(2):101–9.

26. Maxwell BG, Williams GD, Ramamoorthy C. Knowledge and attitudes of anesthesia providers about noncardiac surgery in adults with congenital heart disease: survey of anesthesiologists caring for adults. Congenit Heart Dis 2014; 9(1):45–53.

27. Maxwell BG, Posner KL, Wong JK, et al. Factors contributing to adverse perioperative events in adults with congenital heart disease: a structured analysis of cases from the closed claims project: adverse perioperative events in ACHD. Congenit Heart Dis 2015;10(1):21–9.

28. Lovell AT. Anaesthetic implications of grown-up congenital heart disease. Br J Anaesth 2004;93(1):129–39.

29. Baggen VJM, van den Bosch AE, Eindhoven JA, et al. Prognostic value of N-Terminal Pro-B-Type natriuretic peptide, Troponin-T, and growth-differentiation factor 15 in adult congenital heart disease. Circulation 2017;135(3):264–79.

30. Bouchardy J, Therrien J, Pilote L, et al. Atrial arrhythmias in adults with congenital heart disease. Circulation 2009;120(17):1679–86.

31. Baehner T, Ellerkmann RK. Anesthesia in adults with congenital heart disease. Curr Opin Anaesthesiol 2017;30(3):418–25.

32. Hernández-Madrid A, Paul T, Abrams D, et al. Arrhythmias in congenital heart disease: a position paper of the European Heart Rhythm Association (EHRA), Association for European Paediatric and Congenital Cardiology (AEPC), and the European Society of Cardiology (ESC) Working Group on Grown-up Congenital heart disease, endorsed by HRS, PACES, APHRS, and SOLAECE. Europace 2018;20(11):1719–53.

33. Warrick CM, Hart JE, Lynch AM, et al. Prevalence and descriptive analysis of congenital heart disease in parturients: obstetric, neonatal, and anesthetic outcomes. J Clin Anesth 2015;27(6):492–8.

34. Westhoff-Bleck M, Hilfiker-Kleiner D, Pankuweit S, et al. Cardiomyopathies and congenital heart disease in pregnancy. Geburtshilfe Frauenheilkd 2018;78(12): 1256–61.

35. van Hagen IM, Boersma E, Johnson MR, et al. Global cardiac risk assessment in the Registry Of Pregnancy And Cardiac disease: results of a registry from the European Society of Cardiology: Cardiac risk assessment in the ROPAC. Eur J Heart Fail 2016;18(5):523–33.

36. Canobbio MM, Warnes CA, Aboulhosn J, et al. Management of pregnancy in patients with complex congenital heart disease: a scientific statement for healthcare professionals from the American Heart Association. Circulation 2017;135(8): e50–87.

37. Bradley EA, Saraf A, Book W. Heart failure in women with congenital heart disease. Heart Fail Clin 2019;15(1):87–96.

38. Schweiger M, Lorts A, Conway J. Mechanical circulatory support challenges in pediatric and (adult) congenital heart disease. Curr Opin Organ Transplant 2018;23(3):301–7.

39. Esteve-Ruiz I, Grande-Trillo A, Rangel-Sousa D, et al. Complex congenital heart disease: is heart transplantation an option? Transplant Proc 2018;50(2):655–7.

40. Goldberg SW, Fisher SA, Wehman B, et al. Adults with congenital heart disease and heart transplantation: optimising outcomes. J Heart Lung Transplant 2014; 33(9):873–7.

Mitochondrial Dysfunction in Cardiac Surgery

Anne D. Cherry, MD

KEYWORDS

- Mitochondria • Cardiac surgery • Myocardial metabolism
- Ischemia/reperfusion injury • Cardioprotection • Cardiopulmonary bypass
- Inflammation

KEY POINTS

- Mitochondria are key to cellular energy production, but are also vital to reactive oxygen species signaling, calcium hemostasis, and regulation of cell death.
- Cardiac surgical patients with chronic comorbidities (diabetes, heart failure, advanced age, cardiomyopathies) may have preexisting mitochondrial dysfunction or be more sensitive to perioperative injury.
- Mitochondrial dysfunction from ischemia/reperfusion injury and inflammatory responses to cardiopulmonary bypass and surgical tissue trauma impact myocardial contractility and predispose to arrhythmias.
- Strategies for perioperative mitochondrial protection or recovery after injury include well-established cardioprotective protocols as well as a number of targeted therapies that remain under investigation.

INTRODUCTION

The human heart has one of highest metabolic requirements in the body: even in a resting physiologic state it must work to circulate approximately 5 to 8 L/min of blood against systemic vascular afterload. In addition, overall cardiac mechanical efficiency is only 20% to 25%,[1] with cellular maintenance and heat production accounting for the balance of energetic requirements. A dense network of mitochondria, which contain the machinery of oxidative phosphorylation, is needed to maintain the balance of cellular ATP utilization and production in the setting of such a high energetic demand. Indeed, cardiac myocytes have one of highest mitochondrial volume densities of any cell in the body, with mitochondria occupying almost one-third of the cell volume.[2]

Disclosure Statement: None.
Funding: This document was written with the support of: (1) NIH 5T32GM008600 (PI Warner). (2) American Society of Transplantation: Transplantation and Immunology Research Network (AST TIRN) Basic Science Faculty Development Research Grant (PI Cherry). (3) American Society of Anesthesiologists: Foundation for Anesthesia Education and Research (FAER) Mentored Research Training Grant (PI Cherry).
Department of Anesthesiology, Duke University, DUMC Box 3094, Durham, NC 27712, USA
E-mail address: ANNE.CHERRY@DUKE.EDU

This network is highly vulnerable to injury, and therefore impaired function, due to a combination of patient factors and stressors encountered in the context of cardiac surgery. A discussion of normal and pathologic cardiac mitochondrial function, specific perioperative stressors, and protective strategies for cardiac surgical patients follows.

THE ROLES OF CARDIAC MITOCHONDRIA IN HEALTH AND DISEASE

Under normoxic conditions, cardiac ATP production is accomplished primarily through oxidation of fatty acids and, to a lesser degree, carbohydrates.[3] Ketone bodies, lactate, and amino acids can also be used as substrate, but they contribute little to maintaining the ATP/ADP balance at baseline.[4] However, cardiac metabolism is dynamic, and adapts in response to both chronic and acute pathologic perturbations.

Chronic pathologies most relevant to cardiac surgical patients include heart failure and diabetes. In heart failure, there is an increase in glucose utilization and a decrease in fatty acid oxidation, which has been compared to a shift back toward fetal cardiac metabolism.[5] As a result, in the long-term failing hearts demonstrate an overall reduction in energy reserves as reflected by the phosphocreatinine (PCr)/ATP ratio. Clinically, a decline in the PCr/ATP ratio predicts mortality in heart failure, suggesting that such a metabolic shift is ultimately maladaptive.[6] In diabetes on the other hand, fatty acid uptake and oxidation is increased, and glucose metabolism is decreased, with an overall decrease in metabolic efficiency and increased oxidative stress. In addition, despite the increased fatty acid oxidation, there is a relative abundance of lipid substrate. These factors lead to accumulation of toxic metabolic intermediates and contractile failure, which has been termed "lipotoxic cardiomyopathy."[7] Clinically, impaired mitochondrial function and dynamics are associated with contractile dysfunction[8,9] and an increased risk of arrhythmia and sudden cardiac death[10] in type 2 diabetic patients.

Acutely, ischemia and reperfusion are the most well-studied pathologies that impact cardiac surgical patients. Within seconds of the onset of ischemia, high-energy phosphate reserves are exhausted and anaerobic glycolysis becomes the only source of ATP. As a consequence, intracellular H+ accumulates, pH decreases, and contractile function is impaired.[11] With reperfusion, oxidative phosphorylation is restored rapidly, but mechanical efficiency is diminished due to disproportionately increased fatty acid oxidation with continued upregulation of anaerobic glycolysis. The preexisting and ongoing accumulation of intracellular H+ is normalized, but at the expense of increased intracellular Ca^{2+} (via the H^+/Na^+ and $2Na^+/Ca^{2+}$ exchangers). Intracellular Ca^{2+} overload increases the risk of mitochondrial permeability transition pore (MPTP) opening and activation of cell death.[12,13]

In all, maintaining the cellular ATP supply is one of the fundamental roles of mitochondria. The chronic and acute perturbations discussed demonstrate how dynamic cardiac metabolism can be, and illuminate therapeutic opportunities for improving mitochondrial efficiency and limiting damage in the setting of cardiac surgery (please see the "Opportunities for intervention"section).

In addition to their central role in energy supply, mitochondria are important to several other cellular processes, including reactive oxygen species (ROS) signaling, calcium hemostasis, and regulation of apoptosis and necrosis pathways. First, mitochondria are a source of intracellular ROS, which are normal byproducts of the electron transport chain (ETC) complex in oxidative phosphorylation. Although ROS can contribute to oxidative stress, it is important not to overlook that at low levels, ROS activate crucial intracellular signaling pathways (termed redox signaling,[14,15] which may underlie the mechanisms of ischemic pre,[16] post,[17] and remote ischemic preconditioning[18]). ROS are balanced by antioxidant systems, preventing damage to cellular components. However, ROS production is tied to the rate of respiration, and increases disproportionately when there are perturbations in respiratory chain complex activity or cofactor availability. Ischemia and reperfusion are examples of such perturbations, in which ROS production is increased first due to inadequate substrate availability,[19] followed by increased electron leakage by ETC complexes and decreased ROS scavenging (antioxidant) capacity during the hyperoxic period of reperfusion.[20]

Second, mitochondria play a role in Ca^{2+} hemostasis[21]; mitochondrial Ca^{2+} uptake serves as a buffer for cytoplasmic levels, and increased Ca^{2+} within the mitochondrial matrix activates ATP synthesis. As mentioned, this capacity can be overwhelmed in pathologic states, and Ca^{2+} overload can contribute to mitochondrial activation of cell death. In addition, excessive levels of ROS, such as those produced in the reperfusion phase of ischemia/reperfusion (I/R) injury,[22] heart failure,[23] and other cardiomyopathies[24] result in damage to lipids, proteins, mitochondrial DNA (mtDNA), and ETC complexes themselves, perpetuating oxidative stress. When there is overwhelming oxidative stress or mitochondrial Ca^{2+} overload, as can occur during reperfusion, mitochondrial "metabolic checkpoints"[25] activate cell death programming. Well-known mitochondrial pathways of cell death activation include the following:

a. Permeabilization of the mitochondrial outer membrane, with release of cytochrome c and other mitochondrial proteins into the cytosol, leading to caspase activation.
b. Induction of the mitochondrial permeability transition, with uncoupling of oxidative phosphorylation, mitochondrial swelling, rupture, and release of cytochrome c.[25]

Ultimately these can lead to apoptosis or regulated necrosis[26] depending on the degree and mechanism of stress.

MITOCHONDRIAL DYSFUNCTION IN CARDIAC SURGERY PATIENTS

It is clear that mitochondria have important impacts on myocardial function through their roles in energy and calcium balance, ROS signaling, and regulation of cell death. Cardiac surgical patients may present with preexisting mitochondrial dysfunction due to prior insult or chronic pathology,[27] as discussed. In addition, cardiac surgery involves a period of cardiac I/R, as well as the induction of systemic inflammatory responses due to surgical tissue trauma and cardiopulmonary bypass (CPB) exposure, all of which can impact mitochondrial function.

The inflammatory response to CPB includes activation of both humoral and cellular components in early and late phases, attributed to blood interaction with nonendothelial bypass circuit surfaces and I/R injury, respectively. The result is a cascading release of cytokines, enzymes, and other vasoactive substances, which manifests as a systemic inflammatory response syndrome picture.[28] The impact of systemic inflammatory states on mitochondrial function can be substantial.[29] Generally, mitochondrial respiration is impaired by inflammation, a response that is conserved across a variety of inflammatory states and organisms, suggesting that energetic conservation may confer adaptive advantages as long as the response is temporary.[30] Inflammation can also activate mitochondrial quality control and antioxidant programs to facilitate recovery. However, if inflammation is severe, cellular (including mitochondrial) components can be damaged, which further interferes with energy production and may lead to cell death. As such, the level of inflammatory response due to surgical tissue trauma and exposure to CPB would be expected to correlate with the degree of mitochondrial dysfunction and cell death in cardiac surgical patients.

Furthermore, mitochondrial dysfunction and damage can itself exacerbate the inflammatory response. Certain pathways of cell death can result in the extracellular release of intracellular products, which are then known as damage-associated molecular patterns (DAMPs). DAMPs interact with pattern recognition receptors to upregulate proinflammatory or anti-inflammatory responses[31-33] and inflammasome activation.[34] DAMPs of mitochondrial origin include mtDNA, cytochrome c, mitochondrial transcription factor A (mtTFA), ATP, and high-mobility group box 1 (HMGB1). Intracellularly, mitochondrial dysfunction causes translocation of mtDNA into the cytoplasm, where it upregulates proinflammatory signaling through nuclear factor kappa-light-chain-enhancer of activated B cells (NF-kB) and inflammasome activation.

Fortunately, there is some capacity for recovery after mitochondrial injury (**Fig. 1**). Recovery is facilitated through the induction of a group of mitochondrial quality control (MQC) mechanisms that separate and degrade unhealthy mitochondria and mitochondrial components while retaining healthy elements (through the processes of fission, fusion, and mitophagy), and generate new mitochondrial components (biogenesis). The actions of these processes are at once oppositional and complementary; as such, they must be tightly regulated by a complex machinery both at baseline and in response to stress to maintain an optimally functioning mitochondrial network. Indeed, proteins that regulate mitochondrial fission and fusion are the targets of signaling pathways activated in normal development, exercise/metabolic demand, or by heart failure, diabetes, cardiomyopathy, or I/R, among other pathologies.[35] Similarly, mitophagy is upregulated through several different pathways depending on the stimulus (eg, the Parkin-PINK1 pathway for decreased membrane potential and I/R and Fundc1 in hypoxic stress), and proteins that are well-known as regulators of mitochondrial biogenesis are also impacted by elements of the Parkin mitophagy pathway.[36] MQC processes are of obvious interest due to their potential to improve cardiac recovery in a variety of clinical settings and have recently been extensively reviewed.[37]

Given the variety of perturbations that may impact mitochondrial function in the perioperative period, what is the evidence that mitochondrial dysfunction is clinically relevant for cardiac surgical patients? First, in adults undergoing coronary artery bypass or valve surgery on CPB, mitophagy, mitochondrial biogenesis, and mtDNA damage (strand breaks) immediately post-CPB are increased compared with pre-CPB in atrial tissue.[38] The upregulation in mitochondrial biogenesis, in particular, seems to be

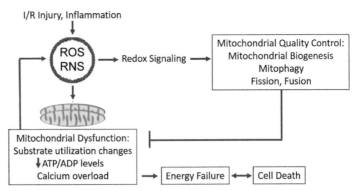

Fig. 1. Perioperative I/R and inflammation induce oxidative stress (reactive oxygen and nitrogen species), which modulate MQC programs through redox signaling. Excessive oxidative stress may also contribute to mitochondrial dysfunction, resulting in energetic failure and cell death. RNS, reactive nitrogen species.

driven by post-transcriptional mechanisms, highlighting those mechanisms as potential therapeutic targets.

Cardiac surgical patients are also at high risk for atrial fibrillation (AF), which is associated with increased morbidity and mortality. The risk of developing AF may be increased by inflammation or changes in calcium signaling,[39] both of which are central features of mitochondrial dysfunction and I/R injury. Recent studies have demonstrated that high levels of mtDNA in peripheral blood before cardiac surgery,[40] or significant increases from precardiac to postcardiac surgery (indicating tissue injury)[41] are predictive of developing new-onset postoperative AF. In addition, cardiac surgery patients with preexisting mitochondrial dysfunction (decreased respiration and increased sensitivity to MPTP opening with calcium) in right atrial tissue also had a higher incidence of new-onset postoperative AF,[42] and in patients with preexisting AF, mitochondrial ETC activity is lower and oxidative stress higher than in those without AF before cardiac surgery.[43]

SPECIFIC CARDIAC SURGICAL PATIENT POPULATIONS AND MITOCHONDRIAL DYSFUNCTION

As previously discussed, mitochondrial dysfunction also plays a role in the pathogenesis of heart failure[3,6,7]; long-term mechanical unloading with a left ventricular assist device may improve mitochondrial function[44] and ultrastructural remodeling, particularly in ischemic cardiomyopathy patients.[45] For heart failure patients who progress to heart transplantation, mitochondrial dysfunction can occur in the donor heart, increasing the risk of early graft failure (formally defined as primary graft dysfunction when significant inotropic or mechanical circulatory assistance are required for failure without other discernible cause within 24 hours posttransplant[46]). Donor factors that may contribute to donor heart mitochondrial dysfunction include increased catecholamine exposure and cytosolic calcium, as well as decreased hormone levels following brain death. Contributing procedural factors are primarily the cold and warm ischemic times for organ transport and implantation, and the duration of CPB (unlike in other cardiac surgical procedures, graft ischemic time and recipient CPB time may be mutually exclusive). Recipient factors that may contribute to mitochondrial dysfunction include high pulmonary vascular resistance, which increases myocardial afterload, and the systemic inflammatory response to intraprocedure CPB and any preoperative exposure to mechanical circulatory support.

Finally, apart from the comorbidities already discussed (heart failure, diabetes), 2 other conditions that may predispose to mitochondrial dysfunction in cardiac surgical patients are worth discussion: aging and cardiomyopathies. With aging, oxidative phosphorylation is increasingly disrupted,[47,48] which plays a part in declining organ functional reserve; this observed decreased energetic capacity may be explained by increases in mtDNA deletions in cardiac tissue from aging patients (**Fig. 2**).[49] Conversely, ROS production is progressively elevated with age.[50] These changes may increase the propensity for injury after cardiac I/R with aging, which has been shown in both rats and human patients.[51,52] Cardiomyopathies can reflect a wide variety of underlying disease processes, some with a notable component of mitochondrial dysfunction. Viral[53] or bacterial infections (particularly sepsis[54]) can cause myocarditis and/or a systemic inflammatory response, and thereby contribute to perioperative cardiac mitochondrial dysfunction. A number of mitochondrial diseases are associated with cardiomyopathies (**Table 1**).[55] These are important to consider for 2 reasons: (1) because the heart has a relatively high energy requirement, cardiac dysfunction may be the only

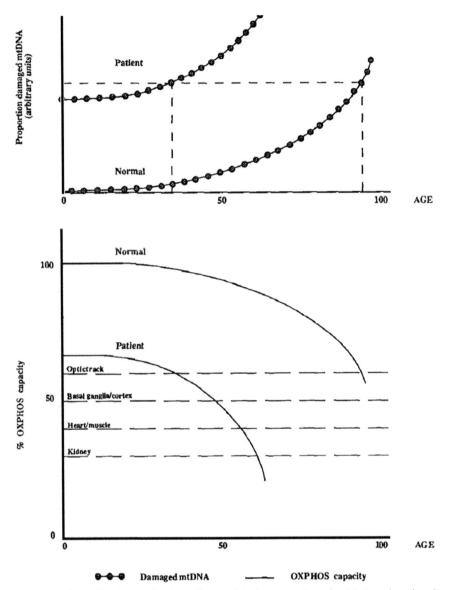

Fig. 2. Hypothesis for the mechanism of age-related progression of oxidative phosphorylation (OXPHOS) diseases. The upper panel shows the proposed accumulation of somatic mtDNA mutations with age.[47,48] Patients are born with a certain percentage of mutant mtDNAs, some patients with more than others. The dashed lines indicate the relative ages when sufficient mutations accumulate to cause disease. The lower panel shows the decline of OXPHOS capacity of healthy individuals and patients with underlying mtDNA mutations. Different tissues have different minimum energy thresholds, below which dysfunction is clinically apparent, shown by dashed lines. OXPHOS declines for both healthy individuals and patients, consistent with the accumulation of somatic mtDNA damage. However, because of the inherited mtDNA mutation, patients start with a lower initial OXPHOS capacity and thus drop below the expression thresholds much earlier than normal individuals. (*From* Wallace DC. Diseases of the mitochondrial DNA. Annu Rev Biochem 1992;61:1175-212; with permission.)

Table 1
Mitochondrial diseases associated with cardiomyopathies or other cardiac disease

Mitochondrial Disease	Cardiac Manifestations	Other System Manifestations
ETC complex deficiencies		
Complex I deficiency	Hypertrophic cardiomyopathy	Growth failure, developmental delay, epilepsy, ataxia, weakness, spasticity, leukoencephalopathy, macrocephaly, sensorineural deafness, hepatic dysfunction, lactic acidosis, hypoglycemia
Complex II deficiency	Hypertrophic, dilated, and noncompaction cardiomyopathies	Growth failure, developmental delay, weakness, spasticity, ataxia, epilepsy, leukodystrophy, contractures, ophthalmoplegia, pigmentary retinopathy, optic atrophy, lactic acidosis
Complex III deficiency	Hypertrophic, dilated, and histiocytoid cardiomyopathies	Growth failure, exercise intolerance, optic atrophy, strokelike episodes, epilepsy, lactic acidosis, hypoglycemia
Complex IV deficiency	Dilated, hypertrophic, and histioctyoid cardiomyopathies	Growth failure, developmental delay, ataxia, epilepsy, hypotonia, sensorineural hearing loss, optic atrophy, pigmentary retinopathy, liver dysfunction, renal tubulopathy, lactic acidosis
Leigh syndrome	Cardiomyopathy and arrhythmias	Respiratory failure, dysphagia, hypotonia, dystonia, ataxia, peripheral neuropathy, ophthalmoparesis, nystagmus, optic atrophy
Mitochondrial tRNA genes		
MERRF (myoclonic epilepsy with ragged red fibers) syndrome	Dilated and histiocytoid cardiomyopathy	Epilepsy, ataxia, weakness, sensorineural hearing loss, short stature, lactic acidosis
MELAS (mitochondrial encephalomyopathy, lactic acidosis, and strokelike episodes) syndrome	Hypertrophic cardiomyopathy	Muscle weakness, strokelike episodes, dementia, epilepsy, sensorineural hearing loss, lactic acidosis, diabetes, short stature
Mitochondrial DNA depletion		
Mitochondrial neurogastrointestinal encephalopathy syndrome (MNGIE)	Hypertrophic cardiomyopathy	Gastrointestinal dysmotility, cachexia, ptosis, ophthalmoplegia, hearing loss, peripheral neuropathy, leukoencephalopathy

(continued on next page)

Table 1 (continued)		
Mitochondrial Disease	**Cardiac Manifestations**	**Other System Manifestations**
CoQ10 deficiency		
Coenzyme Q10 deficiency	Hypertrophic cardiomyopathy	Growth failure, developmental delay, weakness, epilepsy, ataxia, pigmentary retinopathy, sensorineural hearing loss, liver dysfunction, renal impairment, pancytopenia, lactic acidosis
3-Methylglutaconic acidurias		
3-Methylglutaconic aciduria type II (Barth syndrome)	Noncompaction, dilated, and hypertrophic cardiomyopathies	Growth failure, weakness, arrhythmias, neutropenia
3-Methylglutaconic aciduria, type V (dilated cardiomyopathy and ataxia syndrome)	Dilated and noncompaction cardiomyopathies	Growth failure, ataxia, testicular dysgenesis, anemia
Mitochondrial complex V deficiency	Hypertrophic cardiomyopathy	Growth failure, developmental delay, hypotonia, ataxia, epilepsy, leukodystrophy distinctive facial features, lactic acidosis, hyperammonemia
Sengers syndrome	Hypertrophic cardiomyopathy	Growth failure, cataracts, hypotonia, weakness, lactic acidosis
Defects in iron–sulfur cluster		
Friedreich ataxia	Hypertrophic cardiomyopathy	Ataxia, dysarthria, peripheral sensory neuropathy, diabetes mellitus
Multiple deletions		
Kearns-Sayre syndrome	Arrhythmias	Progressive external ophthalmoplegia, pigmentary retinopathy, ataxia, weakness, deafness, renal insufficiency, dementia, short stature, diabetes

Abbreviations: ETC, electron transport chain; tRNA, transfer RNA.

Adapted from El-Hattab AW, Scaglia F. Mitochondrial Cardiomyopathies. Front Cardiovasc Med 2016;3:25; and Meyers DE, Basha HI, Koenig MK. Mitochondrial cardiomyopathy: pathophysiology, diagnosis, and management. Tex Heart Inst J 2013;40(4):389.

clinical manifestation of mitochondrial dysfunction that is as yet sub-clinical in other organ systems, and (2) cardiomyopathies (or other organ dysfunctions) in these patients can be precipitated by stressors including febrile illness or surgery, with metabolic decompensation and/or acute heart failure. One important cardiomyopathy subset that is regularly encountered in the perioperative space is hypertrophic cardiomyopathy (HCM). Although a variety of genetic mutations cause the HCM phenotype, it is thought that common features are excessive sarcomeric energy use, mitochondrial dysfunction and morphologic disorganization, and overall myocardial remodeling.[56] The clinical impact of myocardial bioenergetics deficits and reduced metabolic reserve has not been described specifically for patients with HCM in the context of cardiac surgery, but should be considered when there is otherwise unexplained poor perioperative cardiac function.

OPPORTUNITIES FOR INTERVENTION

Mitochondrial dysfunction is clearly pervasive in the cardiac surgical patient population. The mechanisms discussed previously naturally prompt consideration of opportunities for intervention to prevent or modulate damage, or encourage repair after mitochondrial injury. A brief categorical overview follows here, but a detailed discussion of evidence for (or against) these strategies is beyond the scope of this work; recent reviews are referenced in each section.

First, a number of physiologic, anesthetic, and surgical factors can be modulated in the perioperative period to protect mitochondrial function. Hyperglycemia in the perioperative setting has several detrimental effects, including increased oxidative stress and I/R injury in cardiac tissue.[57] In adult cardiac surgery patients, acute hyperglycemia is particularly common during CPB, even in nondiabetic patients. As might be expected, there is a well-established association with hyperglycemia during CPB and increased morbidity and mortality.[58,59] As such, intraoperative glycemic control, perhaps particularly during the I/R phase, is recommended for diabetic and nondiabetic patients alike, although there is some debate over treatment thresholds due to the increased risk of hypoglycemia with aggressive treatment.[60]

Hypercalcemia at the time of I/R and inflammatory stress would also be expected to exacerbate mitochondrial injury due to intracellular calcium overload and increased activation of cell death. It is common practice, however, for calcium supplementation to given at the time of separation from CPB (after cross-clamp removal and some period of reperfusion has elapsed), with the goals of augmenting myocardial contractility and systemic vascular resistance. In considering the competing risk of injury versus augmented contractility, calcium supplementation should be judicious with regard to magnitude, administration (avoiding large, rapid boluses), and timing. A phase 4 clinical trial investigating the clinical efficacy of calcium administration at the time of separation from CPB (ICARUS Trial) is registered in ClinicalTrials.gov at the time of this writing.[61]

Perioperative anesthetic administration may also have an impact on mitochondrial function. Propofol is known to have antioxidant effects due to a structural similarity to vitamin E, and demonstrates myocardial mitochondrial preservation in preclinical studies. Outcomes in studies with cardiac surgical patients have been mixed.[62–64] Somewhat confusingly, there is also clinical evidence that inhalational agents may confer a preconditioning effect, and provide enhanced cardioprotection when compared with propofol[65,66]; the results of these studies have not yet overwhelmingly impacted clinical practice in favor of either inhalational agent or propofol infusion as the preferred anesthetic technique in cardiac surgery.

The impact of I/R injury on mitochondria can be limited by minimizing ischemic time, cooling of myocardial tissue, and induction of diastolic electromechanical arrest to lower metabolic requirements, through the administration of cardioplegia. The protective effects of cardioplegia depend first on distribution in the myocardium; patients with coronary pathology or other microvascular abnormalities may benefit from retrograde administration. Although there is wide variation in practice, cardioplegia solutions are typically either crystalloid or blood-based, and most contain a high concentration of potassium to induce cardiac arrest. The previously mentioned flexibility in myocardial substrate metabolism results in increased carbohydrate metabolism in the immediate reperfusion phase after aortic cross-clamp and removal.[67] Such transient perioperative changes in substrate use, as well as preexisting alterations in myocardial metabolism due to prior ischemia or other comorbid conditions point to the potential for therapeutic adjustments of substrate supply during cardiac surgery.[3] A number of cardioplegia and organ preservation solutions incorporate components to facilitate substrate utilization, such as glycolytic substrates, amino acids, and specifically ketoglutarate in histidine-tryptophan-ketoglutarate (HTK) cardioplegia.[68,69] More generally, the addition or adjustment of several other cardioplegia components have been studied, including potassium, calcium, sodium, histidine, tryptophan, adenosine, magnesium, and lidocaine (**Table 2**). These have shown promise in animal studies, but variable impact on outcomes in clinical studies.[70,71] Some of these elements are components of so-called "long-acting" cardioplegia solutions, which are given less frequently during surgery to minimize surgical interruption, shortening ischemic times for long or complex procedures; despite this, clinical studies have not reliably shown an improvement in myocardial injury.[72] Overall, there is not yet clear *clinical* evidence for one specific cardioplegia solution or strategy that is most advantageous for myocardial protection.[73]

Similarly, strategies to optimize the composition and conditions of reperfusion at the end of ischemia have also been investigated in efforts to minimize reperfusion injury, and may be of particular use in settings of prolonged ischemia or hypoxia (heart or lung transplants, or cyanotic pediatric cardiac surgery).[74] Administration of warm cardioplegia before cross-clamp removal (terminal warm induction or "hot shot") is meant to allow washout of ischemic metabolic byproducts and augment aerobic metabolism while continued electromechanical arrest minimizes energy demand. Clinical evidence is limited: some small studies show improvements in biochemical markers of I/R injury and/or hemodynamic parameters, but none have demonstrated outcome differences.[75] Finally, perioperative infusions of glucose, insulin, and potassium (GIK) also have been used to support metabolism during cardiac surgery, with mixed results for different outcomes in clinical studies.[76]

The application of antioxidant therapies is an intuitive approach to counteracting the damaging effect of increased oxidative stress in tissues secondary to I/R injury, inflammation, and/or mitochondrial dysfunction.[62] It is common practice for free-radical scavenging drugs like mannitol to be included in CPB circuit priming fluid[77] or in cardioplegia solutions (eg, HTK, del Nido).[78] Beyond this, clinical outcomes with experimental antioxidant therapies have not been promising. This is perhaps not surprising when we consider oxidative stress by the following definition: "an imbalance between oxidants and antioxidants in favor of the oxidants, leading to a disruption of redox signaling and control and/or molecular damage."[79] With this view, it becomes clear that the most fundamental concern in broadly applied or poorly timed antioxidant treatment is the potential to mask or prevent critical intracellular ROS signaling mechanisms, and interfere with cellular stress response pathways. Targeted approaches that take these issues into consideration through improved precision of delivery and dosing, such as synthetic mitochondrial antioxidants (eg, MitoQ or MitoVit-E), have been tested but have not yet translated into widespread clinical application.[80]

On the other side of the oxidant:antioxidant balance lies the potential for therapeutic manipulation of ROS signaling, on which the concept of ischemic conditioning relies. Pre, post, and remote ischemic conditioning have all been investigated widely in several settings,[81] and generally involve the application of short cycles of ischemia

Table 2

Categories of cardioplegia strategies used for cardioprotection, with example solutions, representative component concentrations, and additives for each category

Cardioplegia Type	Example Solutions and Concentrations	Na⁺, mM/L	K⁺, mM/L	Mg²⁺, mM/L	Mannitol	Ca²⁺, mM/L	HTK, mM/L	Glucose, mM/L	Lidocaine	Adenosine	NaHCO₃	Modifications
Crystalloid-based												
Intracellular	Custodiol, HTK, Bretschneider's, University of Wisconsin Solution	15	9	4	x	0.015	198/2/1					Glutamate, aspartate
Extracellular	Plegisol, Celsior, St Thomas, Stanford solution	110–120	16–26	32	x	2.4						Glutamate, aspartate
Blood-based (includes endogenous oxygen carrying, substrates, buffers, antioxidants, oncotic pressure, inflammatory factors)												
4:1 Blood:crystalloid	Buckberg	140	20–10 (i-m)	13–9 (i-m)				6	260 mg/L (induction)			Glutamate, aspartate, CPD, tromethamine
1:4 Blood:crystalloid, long-acting	del Nido (in 1 L Plasma-Lyte A)	26 meq Plasma-Lyte A		2 mg	3.2 g				130 mg		13 meq	Glutamate, aspartate
Microplegia (blood-based cardioplegia principles apply; with relatively less edema, increased neutrophil accumulation and endothelial dysfunction)												
Various additive and concentration options	ALM with insulin (8 mL additive:l L blood)	30–8 meq/L (i-m)		2 g/20 mL					25 mg/l mL	6 mg/2 mL		2.5 IU Insulin added to ALM volume

Abbreviations: ALM, adenosine and lidocaine with magnesium; CPD, citrate-phosphate-dextrose; HTK, histidine, tryptophan, ketoglutarate; i-m, concentrations for induction or maintenance of cardioplegia; Plasma-lyte A concentrations/L (Baxter), 140 mEq sodium, 5 mEq potassium, 3 mEq magnesium, 98 mEq chloride, 27 mEq acetate, and 23 mEq gluconate; x, may be added as a modifier.

Component and additive concentration information is for reference and comparison between solutions only; not for clinical use.

Data from Refs.[87–90]

and reperfusion (directly to the tissue at risk, or to a remote tissue in the case of remote ischemic preconditioning), with the goal of increasing ischemic tolerance and minimizing I/R injury. The complex and fascinating mechanisms of these conditioning phenomena converge on a number of subcellular targets, notably including mitochondria; these pathways have been intensely studied and reviewed.[82] As is also the case for many of the therapies and approaches already discussed, cardiac surgery represents an appealing platform for application of these strategies, because the timing of perioperative stress and potential tissue injury can be anticipated, and along with it the timing of therapy. Clinical studies of both preconditioning and postconditioning in adult and pediatric cardiac surgery demonstrate promising results, but adoption has not been robust due to the requirement for repeated clamping and unclamping of the aorta. Remote (limb) conditioning has obvious practical advantages, and has been promising in preclinical and small clinical trials, but recently failed to demonstrate protective effects in 3 large multicenter trials in cardiac surgical patients.[83] This was likely due to several factors, including limited additional advantage over the multitude of cardioprotective strategies already in place in the perioperative period, and the impact of patient comorbidities and medications (including the use of propofol, which has a free-radical scavenging role, as discussed previously).

Finally, strategies that would enhance recovery in the setting of chronic pathology or after acute injury are also intuitive and appealing. As outlined briefly previously, MQC mechanisms work in concert to clear defective mitochondrial components and generate new ones, maintaining a functional mitochondrial network. There is documented evidence of MQC dysregulation in several pathologies and stressors that are highly relevant to cardiac surgical patients, including diabetes, heart failure, aging, and I/R injury.[35,37,84] As such, interest exists in targeting elements of the MQC pathways. However, MQC mechanisms can have both pathologic or beneficial effects, depending on the conditions under which they are applied; for example, overexpression of peroxisome proliferator-activated receptor gamma coactivator 1-alpha (PGC-1a), a transcriptional regulator of mitochondrial biogenesis and antioxidant defense mechanisms, results in cardiac hypertrophy and heart failure, but with PGC-1a knockdown and impaired biogenesis upregulation, mice also develop heart failure in response to increased afterload, and increased tissue damage in sepsis.[85,86] Similarly dichotomous results have been observed for mitophagy and mitochondrial dynamics pathways,[84] suggesting that perhaps even more so than in the case of antioxidant therapies, highly specific application of MQC therapies (patient selection, dosing, timing, precision of treatment at the subtissue level) will be the key to their effective use.

SUMMARY

In summary, mitochondria are key to the cellular response to energetic demand, but are also vital to ROS signaling, calcium hemostasis, and regulation of apoptosis and necrosis pathways in cell death. Mitochondrial dysfunction and disruption of any of these vital processes can lead to chronic or acute pathology, particularly in tissues with high metabolic demand and mitochondrial content, such as the heart. In cardiac surgery, several perioperative factors can impact mitochondrial function, including I/R injury and an increased systemic inflammatory response due to exposure to CPB and surgical tissue trauma. Patients with diabetes, heart failure, advanced age, or cardiomyopathies may have underlying mitochondrial dysfunction or be more sensitive to perioperative injury. Mitochondrial dysfunction most immediately impacts postoperative myocardial contractility, but also predisposes to arrhythmias. A multitude of strategies to minimize the impact of perioperative factors on mitochondrial function have been incorporated into routine clinical care (hypothermia, avoidance of hypergly-cemia or hypercalcemia, substrate and other additions to cardioplegia solutions, anesthetic choice), whereas other more targeted therapies (antioxidants, ischemic conditioning, modulators of MQC mechanisms), remain under investigation or are in development for use in selected settings.

REFERENCES

1. Westerhof N. Cardiac work and efficiency. Cardiovasc Res 2000;48(1):4–7.
2. Schaper J, Meiser E, Stammler G. Ultrastructural morphometric analysis of myocardium from dogs, rats, hamsters, mice, and from human hearts. Circ Res 1985;56(3):377–91.
3. Stanley WC, Recchia FA, Lopaschuk GD. Myocardial substrate metabolism in the normal and failing heart. Physiol Rev 2005;85(3):1093–129.
4. Wentz AE, d'Avignon DA, Weber ML, et al. Adaptation of myocardial substrate metabolism to a ketogenic nutrient environment. J Biol Chem 2010;285(32): 24447–56.
5. Razeghi P, Young ME, Alcorn JL, et al. Metabolic gene expression in fetal and failing human heart. Circulation 2001;104(24):2923–31.
6. Neubauer S, Horn M, Cramer M, et al. Myocardial phosphocreatine-to-ATP ratio is a predictor of mortality in patients with dilated cardiomyopathy. Circulation 1997; 96(7):2190–6.
7. Kolwicz SC Jr, Purohit S, Tian R. Cardiac metabolism and its interactions with contraction, growth, and survival of cardiomyocytes. Circ Res 2013;113(5): 603–16.
8. Montaigne D, Marechal X, Coisne A, et al. Myocardial contractile dysfunction is associated with impaired mitochondrial function and dynamics in type 2 diabetic but not in obese patients. Circulation 2014;130(7):554–64.
9. Croston TL, Thapa D, Holden AA, et al. Functional deficiencies of subsarcolem-mal mitochondria in the type 2 diabetic human heart. Am J Physiol Heart Circ Physiol 2014;307(1):H54–65.
10. Song J, Yang R, Yang J, et al. Mitochondrial dysfunction-associated arrhythmo-genic substrates in diabetes mellitus. Front Physiol 2018;9:1670.
11. Frank A, Bonney M, Bonney S, et al. Myocardial ischemia reperfusion injury: from basic science to clinical bedside. Semin Cardiothorac Vasc Anesth 2012;16(3): 123–32.
12. Crompton M, Andreeva L. On the involvement of a mitochondrial pore in reperfu-sion injury. Basic Res Cardiol 1993;88(5):513–23.
13. Griffiths EJ, Halestrap AP. Protection by cyclosporin A of ischemia/reperfusion-induced damage in isolated rat hearts. J Mol Cell Cardiol 1993;25(12):1461–9.
14. Schieber M, Chandel NS. ROS function in redox signaling and oxidative stress. Curr Biol 2014;24(10):R453–62.
15. Schreck R, Rieber P, Baeuerle PA. Reactive oxygen intermediates as apparently widely used messengers in the activation of the NF-kappa B transcription factor and HIV-1. EMBO J 1991;10(8):2247–58.
16. Chen W, Gabel S, Steenbergen C, et al. A redox-based mechanism for cardiopro-tection induced by ischemic preconditioning in perfused rat heart. Circ Res 1995; 77(2):424–9.
17. Penna C, Rastaldo R, Mancardi D, et al. Post-conditioning induced cardioprotec-tion requires signaling through a redox-sensitive mechanism, mitochondrial ATP-

sensitive K+ channel and protein kinase C activation. Basic Res Cardiol 2006; 101(2):180–9.

18. Weinbrenner C, Schulze F, Sarvary L, et al. Remote preconditioning by infrarenal aortic occlusion is operative via delta1-opioid receptors and free radicals in vivo in the rat heart. Cardiovasc Res 2004;61(3):591–9.

19. Chen YR, Zweier JL. Cardiac mitochondria and reactive oxygen species generation. Circ Res 2014;114(3):524–37.

20. Granger DN, Kvietys PR. Reperfusion injury and reactive oxygen species: the evolution of a concept. Redox Biol 2015;6:524–51.

21. Mammucari C, Raffaello A, Vecellio Reane D, et al. Mitochondrial calcium uptake in organ physiology: from molecular mechanism to animal models. Pflugers Arch 2018;470(8):1165–79.

22. Bliksoen M, Baysa A, Eide L, et al. Mitochondrial DNA damage and repair during ischemia-reperfusion injury of the heart. J Mol Cell Cardiol 2015;78:9–22.

23. Keith M, Geranmayegan A, Sole MJ, et al. Increased oxidative stress in patients with congestive heart failure. J Am Coll Cardiol 1998;31(6):1352–6.

24. Maack C, Kartes T, Kilter H, et al. Oxygen free radical release in human failing myocardium is associated with increased activity of rac1-GTPase and represents a target for statin treatment. Circulation 2003;108(13):1567–74.

25. Green DR, Galluzzi L, Kroemer G. Cell biology. Metabolic control of cell death. Science 2014;345(6203):1250256.

26. Zhang J, Liu D, Zhang M, et al. Programmed necrosis in cardiomyocytes: mitochondria, death receptors and beyond. Br J Pharmacol 2018. [Epub ahead of print].

27. Chistiakov DA, Shkurat TP, Melnichenko AA, et al. The role of mitochondrial dysfunction in cardiovascular disease: a brief review. Ann Med 2018;50(2):121–7.

28. Warren OJ, Smith AJ, Alexiou C, et al. The inflammatory response to cardiopulmonary bypass: part 1–mechanisms of pathogenesis. J Cardiothorac Vasc Anesth 2009;23(2):223–31.

29. Cherry AD, Piantadosi CA. Regulation of mitochondrial biogenesis and its intersection with inflammatory responses. Antioxid Redox Signal 2015;22(12):965–76.

30. Singer M. Mitochondrial function in sepsis: acute phase versus multiple organ failure. Crit Care Med 2007;35(9 Suppl):S441–8.

31. Matzinger P. Tolerance, danger, and the extended family. Annu Rev Immunol 1994;12:991–1045.

32. Seong SY, Matzinger P. Hydrophobicity: an ancient damage-associated molecular pattern that initiates innate immune responses. Nat Rev Immunol 2004;4(6): 469–78.

33. Zhang Q, Raoof M, Chen Y, et al. Circulating mitochondrial DAMPs cause inflammatory responses to injury. Nature 2010;464(7285):104–7.

34. Shimada K, Crother TR, Karlin J, et al. Oxidized mitochondrial DNA activates the NLRP3 inflammasome during apoptosis. Immunity 2012;36(3):401–14.

35. Nan J, Zhu W, Rahman MS, et al. Molecular regulation of mitochondrial dynamics in cardiac disease. Biochim Biophys Acta Mol Cell Res 2017;1864(7):1260–73.

36. Gottlieb RA, Thomas A. Mitophagy and mitochondrial quality control mechanisms in the heart. Curr Pathobiol Rep 2017;5(2):161–9.

37. Tahrir FG, Langford D, Amini S, et al. Mitochondrial quality control in cardiac cells: mechanisms and role in cardiac cell injury and disease. J Cell Physiol 2019; 234(6):8122–33.

38. Andres AM, Tucker KC, Thomas A, et al. Mitophagy and mitochondrial biogenesis in atrial tissue of patients undergoing heart surgery with cardiopulmonary bypass. JCI Insight 2017;2(4):e89303.
39. Denham NC, Pearman CM, Caldwell JL, et al. Calcium in the Pathophysiology of Atrial Fibrillation and Heart Failure. Front Physiol 2018;9:1380.
40. Zhang J, Xu S, Xu Y, et al. Relation of mitochondrial DNA copy number in peripheral blood to postoperative atrial fibrillation after isolated off-pump coronary artery bypass grafting. Am J Cardiol 2017;119(3):473–7.
41. Sandler N, Kaczmarek E, Itagaki K, et al. Mitochondrial DAMPs are released during cardiopulmonary bypass surgery and are associated with postoperative atrial fibrillation. Heart Lung Circ 2018;27(1):122–9.
42. Montaigne D, Marechal X, Lefebvre P, et al. Mitochondrial dysfunction as an arrhythmogenic substrate: a translational proof-of-concept study in patients with metabolic syndrome in whom post-operative atrial fibrillation develops. J Am Coll Cardiol 2013;62(16):1466–73.
43. Emelyanova I, Ashary Z, Cosic M, et al. Selective downregulation of mitochondrial electron transport chain activity and increased oxidative stress in human atrial fibrillation. Am J Physiol Heart Circ Physiol 2016;311(1):H54–63.
44. Lee SH, Doliba N, Osbakken M, et al. Improvement of myocardial mitochondrial function after hemodynamic support with left ventricular assist devices in patients with heart failure. J Thorac Cardiovasc Surg 1998;116(2):344–9.
45. Heerdt PM, Schlame M, Jehle R, et al. Disease-specific remodeling of cardiac mitochondria after a left ventricular assist device. Ann Thorac Surg 2002;73(4):1216–21.
46. Kobashigawa J, Zuckermann A, Macdonald P, et al. Report from a consensus conference on primary graft dysfunction after cardiac transplantation. J Heart Lung Transplant 2014;33(4):327–40.
47. Lesnefsky EJ, Chen Q, Hoppel CL. Mitochondrial metabolism in aging heart. Circ Res 2016;118(10):1593–611.
48. Linnane AW, Marzuki S, Ozawa T, et al. Mitochondrial DNA mutations as an important contributor to ageing and degenerative diseases. Lancet 1989;1(8639):642–5.
49. Sugiyama S, Hattori K, Hayakawa M, et al. Quantitative analysis of age-associated accumulation of mitochondrial DNA with deletion in human hearts. Biochem Biophys Res Commun 1991;180(2):894–9.
50. Judge S, Jang YM, Smith A, et al. Age-associated increases in oxidative stress and antioxidant enzyme activities in cardiac interfibrillar mitochondria: implications for the mitochondrial theory of aging. FASEB J 2005;19(3):419–21.
51. Lesnefsky EJ, Lundergan CF, Hodgson JM, et al. Increased left ventricular dysfunction in elderly patients despite successful thrombolysis: the GUSTO-I angiographic experience. J Am Coll Cardiol 1996;28(2):331–7.
52. Lesnefsky EJ, He D, Moghaddas S, et al. Reversal of mitochondrial defects before ischemia protects the aged heart. FASEB J 2006;20(9):1543–5.
53. Wei J, Gao DF, Wang H, et al. Impairment of myocardial mitochondria in viral myocardial disease and its reflective window in peripheral cells. PLoS One 2014;9(12):e116239.
54. Watts JA, Kline JA, Thornton LR, et al. Metabolic dysfunction and depletion of mitochondria in hearts of septic rats. J Mol Cell Cardiol 2004;36(1):141–50.
55. El-Hattab AW, Scaglia F. Mitochondrial cardiomyopathies. Front Cardiovasc Med 2016;3:25.

56. Vakrou S, Abraham MR. Hypertrophic cardiomyopathy: a heart in need of an energy bar? Front Physiol 2014;5:309.
57. Yang Z, Laubach VE, French BA, et al. Acute hyperglycemia enhances oxidative stress and exacerbates myocardial infarction by activating nicotinamide adenine dinucleotide phosphate oxidase during reperfusion. J Thorac Cardiovasc Surg 2009;137(3):723–9.
58. Doenst T, Wijeysundera D, Karkouti K, et al. Hyperglycemia during cardiopulmonary bypass is an independent risk factor for mortality in patients undergoing cardiac surgery. J Thorac Cardiovasc Surg 2005;130(4):1144.
59. Navaratnarajah M, Rea R, Evans R, et al. Effect of glycaemic control on complications following cardiac surgery: literature review. J Cardiothorac Surg 2018; 13(1):10.
60. Girish G, Agarwal S, Satsangi DK, et al. Glycemic control in cardiac surgery: rationale and current evidence. Ann Card Anaesth 2014;17(3):222–8.
61. Lomivorotov V. Calcium administration in patients undergoing cardiac surgery under cardiopulmonary bypass (ICARUS Trial): prospective randomized, double-blind placebo-controlled superiority trial. 2019. NCT Number: NCT03772990. Available at: https://clinicaltrials.gov/ct2/show/NCT03772990. Accessed January 15, 2019.
62. Zakkar M, Guida G, Suleiman MS, et al. Cardiopulmonary bypass and oxidative stress. Oxid Med Cell Longev 2015;2015:189863.
63. Rogers CA, Bryan AJ, Nash R, et al. Propofol cardioplegia: a single-center, placebo-controlled, randomized controlled trial. J Thorac Cardiovasc Surg 2015; 150(6):1610–9.e13.
64. Ansley DM, Raedschelders K, Choi PT, et al. Propofol cardioprotection for on-pump aortocoronary bypass surgery in patients with type 2 diabetes mellitus (PRO-TECT II): a phase 2 randomized-controlled trial. Can J Anaesth 2016; 63(4):442–53.
65. Li F, Yuan Y. Meta-analysis of the cardioprotective effect of sevoflurane versus propofol during cardiac surgery. BMC Anesthesiol 2015;15:128.
66. Yang XL, Wang D, Zhang GY, et al. Comparison of the myocardial protective effect of sevoflurane versus propofol in patients undergoing heart valve replacement surgery with cardiopulmonary bypass. BMC Anesthesiol 2017;17(1):37.
67. Pietersen HG, Langenberg CJ, Geskes G, et al. Myocardial substrate uptake and oxidation during and after routine cardiac surgery. J Thorac Cardiovasc Surg 1999;118(1):71–80.
68. Rosenkranz ER. Substrate enhancement of cardioplegic solution: experimental studies and clinical evaluation. Ann Thorac Surg 1995;60(3):797–800.
69. Ali JM, Miles LF, Abu-Omar Y, et al. Global cardioplegia practices: results from the global cardiopulmonary bypass survey. J Extra Corpor Technol 2018;50(2): 83–93.
70. Siddiqi S, Blackstone EH, Bakaeen FG. Bretschneider and del Nido solutions: are they safe for coronary artery bypass grafting? If so, how should we use them? J Card Surg 2018;33(5):229–34.
71. Dobson GP, Faggian G, Onorati F, et al. Hyperkalemic cardioplegia for adult and pediatric surgery: end of an era? Front Physiol 2013;4:228.
72. Hoyer A, Lehmann S, Mende M, et al. Custodiol versus cold Calafiore for elective cardiac arrest in isolated aortic valve replacement: a propensity-matched analysis of 7263 patients. Eur J Cardiothorac Surg 2017;52(2):303–9.
73. Ferguson ZG, Yarborough DE, Jarvis BL, et al. Evidence-based medicine and myocardial protection–where is the evidence? Perfusion 2015;30(5):415–22.

74. Beyersdorf F. The use of controlled reperfusion strategies in cardiac surgery to minimize ischaemia/reperfusion damage. Cardiovasc Res 2009;83(2):262–8.
75. Volpi S, Ali JM, De Silva R. Does the use of a hot-shot lead to improved outcomes following adult cardiac surgery? Interact Cardiovasc Thorac Surg 2019;28(3): 473–7.
76. Fan Y, Zhang AM, Xiao YB, et al. Glucose-insulin-potassium therapy in adult patients undergoing cardiac surgery: a meta-analysis. Eur J Cardiothorac Surg 2011;40(1):192–9.
77. Miles LF, Coulson TG, Galhardo C, et al. Pump priming practices and anticoagulation in cardiac surgery: results from the global cardiopulmonary bypass survey. Anesth Analg 2017;125(6):1871–7.
78. Larsen M, Webb G, Kennington S, et al. Mannitol in cardioplegia as an oxygen free radical scavenger measured by malondialdehyde. Perfusion 2002; 17(1):51–5.
79. Jones DP. Redefining oxidative stress. Antioxid Redox Signal 2006;8(9–10): 1865–79.
80. Muntean DM, Sturza A, Dănilă MD, et al. The role of mitochondrial reactive oxygen species in cardiovascular injury and protective strategies. Oxid Med Cell Longev 2016;2016:8254942.
81. Sprick JD, Mallet RT, Przyklenk K, et al. Ischaemic and hypoxic conditioning: potential for protection of vital organs. Exp Physiol 2019;104(3):278–94.
82. Heusch G. Molecular basis of cardioprotection: signal transduction in ischemic pre-, post-, and remote conditioning. Circ Res 2015;116(4):674–99.
83. Candilio L, Hausenloy D. Is there a role for ischaemic conditioning in cardiac surgery? F1000Res 2017;6:563.
84. Picca A, Mankowski RT, Burman JL, et al. Mitochondrial quality control mechanisms as molecular targets in cardiac ageing. Nat Rev Cardiol 2018;15(9): 543–54.
85. Rowe GC, Jiang A, Arany Z. PGC-1 coactivators in cardiac development and disease. Circ Res 2010;107(7):825–38.
86. Cherry AD, Suliman HB, Bartz RB, et al. Peroxisome proliferator-activated receptor gamma co-activator 1 alpha as a critical co-activator of the murine hepatic oxidative stress response and mitochondrial biogenesis in *S. aureus* sepsis. J Biol Chem 2014;289(1):41–52.
87. Habertheuer A, Kocher A, Laufer G, et al. Cardioprotection: a review of current practice in global ischemia and future translational perspective. Biomed Res Int 2014;2014:325725.
88. Kim K, Ball C, Grady P, et al. Use of del Nido cardioplegia for adult cardiac surgery at the Cleveland Clinic: perfusion implications. J Extra Corpor Technol 2014; 46(4):317–23.
89. Onorati F, Santini F, Dandale R, et al. "Polarizing" microplegia improves cardiac cycle efficiency after CABG for unstable angina. Int J Cardiol 2013;167(6): 2739–46.
90. Vinten-Johansen J. Whole blood cardioplegia: do we still need to dilute? J Extra Corpor Technol 2016;48(2):P9–14.

Cardiac Surgery and the Blood-Brain Barrier

Ayman Hendy, MB BCh, FRCPC[a],*, Richard Hall, MD, FRCPC[a,b,c]

KEYWORDS

- Blood-brain barrier • Cardiac surgery • Postoperative cognitive dysfunction
- Brain biomarkers

KEY POINTS

- The interface between the brain tissue and the cerebral vessels is called the blood-brain barrier (BBB).
- BBB properties are primarily determined by junctional complexes between the cerebral vascular endothelial cells.
- Some degree of brain injury is likely to occur during cardiac surgery because of the nature of the surgery (hypothermia, cardiopulmonary bypass [CPB] use, hypoperfusion of the brain, possible microembolic showers to cerebral circulation, and activation of the systemic inflammatory response).
- Currently assessment of BBB disruption after cardiac surgery falls into three categories: neurocognitive tests, laboratory measurement of brain biomarkers in the blood and the cerebrospinal fluid, and brain imaging (MRI).
- BBB disruption after cardiac surgery occurs; the magnitude and duration of the alterations is uncertain but likely transient in most patients and limited to the immediate perioperative period.

INTRODUCTION
Historic Background

The concept of a barrier between the peripheral circulation and central nervous system (CNS) was first developed as a result of the pioneer work of Paul Ehrlich, a German physiologist, in 1885. He was the first to observe that injecting a dye into the peripheral circulation would accumulate in the peripheral tissues at a much higher concentration than that observed in the CNS. His explanation was that the CNS had less affinity for

Disclosure Statement: There are no commercial or financial conflicts of interest and no funding sources for all authors.
[a] Department of Anesthesia, Pain Management and Perioperative Medicine, Dalhousie University, Halifax, Nova Scotia, Canada; [b] Department of Critical Care Medicine, Dalhousie University, Halifax, Nova Scotia, Canada; [c] Department of Anesthesia, Halifax Infirmary Hospital, Room 5452, 1796 Summer Street, Halifax, Nova Scotia B3H 3A7, Canada
* Corresponding author. Department of Anesthesia, Halifax Infirmary Hospital, Room 5452, 1796 Summer Street, Halifax, Nova Scotia B3H 3A7, Canada.
E-mail address: aymanhendy@gmail.com

the dye compared with other tissues. However, his student Edwin Goldmann (in 1905) performed an interesting reverse experiment where he injected the dye into cerebrospinal fluid (CSF), and found that its concentration was much higher in the CNS tissues compared with peripheral tissues. Their work demonstrated that there is a barrier or a structure that separates the CNS from the peripheral circulation.[1-3] Lina Stern was the first to call it the blood-brain barrier (BBB).[4] The exact location and structure of the BBB was definitively described as a result of using an electron microscope and injections of biovesicles in 1967 by Thomas Reese and Morris Karnovsky and their colleagues.[5]

ANATOMY OF BLOOD-BRAIN BARRIER

The BBB is a highly regulated and maintained interface that separates the peripheral circulation and CNS. The primary component of the BBB is the highly specialized monolayer of endothelial cells that line the cerebral capillaries. A more dynamic and functional definition includes the description of other components of BBB anatomy, such as astrocytes, pericytes, neurons, and the extracellular matrix. The term neurovascular unit rather than BBB is used to more correctly describe this collective structure essential for providing the protection and maintenance of homeostasis of the CNS (**Fig. 1**).[6]

Brain Endothelial Cells

Endothelial cells lining the cerebral capillaries are considered the most important component of the BBB. These highly specialized endothelial cells differ from other endothelial cells found elsewhere in the body in the following instances[7,8]:

- Absence of fenestrations
- More extensive tight junctions (TJs)
- Sparse pinocytic vesicular transport
- Presence of specific cellular transporters (endothelial transporters) for moving ions, nutrients, and other substances including drugs between blood and CNS

BBB properties are primarily determined by junctional complexes between the cerebral endothelial cells. The most important junctions are TJs and adherens junctions (AJs).

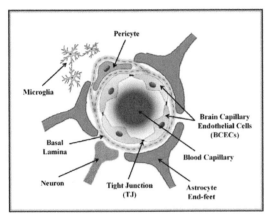

Fig. 1. Schematic diagram of BBB. (*From* Sarkar A, Fatima I, Jamal QMS, et al. Nanoparticles as a Carrier System for Drug Delivery across Blood Brain Barrier. Curr Drug Metab 2017;18(2):129-137; with permission.)

Endothelial cell TJs limit the paracellular flux of hydrophilic molecules across the BBB. In contrast, small lipophilic substances, such as oxygen (O_2) and carbon dioxide (CO_2), move freely according to their concentration gradient. Nutrients including glucose and amino acids enter the brain via specific carriers, whereas receptor-mediated endocytosis mediates the uptake of larger molecules including insulin, leptin, and iron transferrin.[9,10]

Tight junctions

TJs are series of intramembranous strands that span the intercellular clefts between adjacent vascular endothelial cells (see **Fig. 1**).[11] These TJ strands consist of three integral membrane proteins: (1) claudin, (2) occludin, and (3) junctional adhesion molecules. Several cytoplasmic proteins have been described that associate with TJ (transmembrane proteins) and contribute to TJ integrity in epithelial and brain endothelial cells. Among these transmembrane proteins are zonula occludens (ZO) proteins ZO-1, ZO-2, ZO-3, cingulin, and others. Cytoplasmic proteins link membrane proteins to actin, which is the primary cytoskeleton protein for the maintenance of the structural and functional integrity of the endothelium.

Adherens junctions

The AJs mediate the adhesion of endothelial cells to each other and regulate paracellular permeability.[12] They also play a role in cell maturation, maintenance, plasticity, and regulation of tensile forces.

AJs are composed of a cadherin–catenin complex and its associated proteins. Formation of TJs generally requires the existence of AJs, and central to the organization of those two dynamic junctions is the continuous crosstalk between AJs and TJs.

Endothelial transporters

At the brain endothelial cell surface there exists influx transporters (which move a substance from blood to CNS thus increasing CNS concentrations) and efflux transporters (which move a substance from brain to blood thus preventing CNS accumulation).[13] A variety of efflux and influx transporter systems have been identified, including ATP-binding cassette transporters, organic anion and organic cation transporters, peptide transporters, nucleoside transporters, and monocarboxylate transporters (**Table 1**).

Astrocytes

Astrocytes are the star-shaped cellular elements of the neuroglia (literally nerve glue or nerve cement), which is the nonneuronal supporting tissue of the CNS.[14] They have an important role in the development and function of the BBB through astrocyte-endothelial cell interaction. Astrocytes also have a direct influence on the dynamic control of the brain microcirculation. Dilatation of arterioles triggered by neuronal activity is dependent on intracellular calcium responses within the astrocyte network.

Table 1	
Carrier-mediated transporters at the blood-brain barrier	
Influx Transporters (to CNS)	**Efflux Transporters (from CNS)**
Organic anion transporting polypeptides (OATPs in humans),	P-glycoprotein (P-gp)
Organic cation transporters (OCTs in humans),	Breast cancer resistance protein (BCRP)
Nucleoside transporters,	Multidrug-resistance proteins (MRPs)
Monocarboxylate transporters (MCTs in humans),	
Putative transport systems for peptide transport.	

Neuron-astrocytes signaling is necessary for regulating the energy supply to support neuronal function.

Pericytes

Pericytes are cells present at intervals along the walls of capillaries (and postcapillary venules).[15] In the CNS, they are important for blood vessel formation, maintenance of the BBB, regulation of immune cell entry to the CNS, and control of brain blood flow. Pericytes are the least studied cellular component of the BBB but seem to play a key role in angiogenesis, structural integrity and differentiation of the vessel, and formation of endothelial TJs.

Brain Structures Lacking a Blood-Brain Barrier

The BBB is present in all brain regions, except for the circumventricular organs including area postrema, median eminence, neurohypophysis, pineal gland, subfornical organ, and lamina terminalis.[16] Blood vessels in these areas of the brain have fenestrations that permit diffusion of blood-borne molecules across the vessel wall. These unprotected areas of the brain regulate the autonomic nervous system and endocrine glands of the body.

TRANSFER OF MATERIALS BETWEEN BLOOD AND THE NERVOUS TISSUE

Transfer of materials (including drugs) occurs through one of the following four methods[14,17,18]:

Passive Diffusion

Passive diffusion involves the movement of solutes across BBB along their concentration gradient without expenditure of energy or involvement of a carrier protein. Several factors influence a substance's ability to passively diffuse: lipid solubility, polarity, molecular size, concentration in blood, and surface area available for diffusion. In general, polar and hydrophilic substances are more difficult to diffuse across the BBB compared with lipophilic substances. Molecular size is less important than lipid solubility in determining which compounds cross the BBB. Examples of drugs that can passively diffuse across biologic membranes include opioids (ie, morphine, heroin), diphenhydramine, and steroids.

Carrier-Mediated Transport

Carrier-mediated transport involves interactions of a substrate with a transport/carrier protein, providing a route for diffusion of substances across a membrane with the direction of transport dictated by the solute concentration gradient. Such transport systems are used for the transport of essential nutrients (ie, glucose) into the brain and the elimination of metabolic waste. A classic example of carrier-mediated transport is the GLUT-1 transporter responsible for transport of glucose, which is localized to the luminal (facing blood) and abluminal (facing nervous tissue) borders of the brain endothelial cells.

CNS drugs may also be transported via carrier-mediated transport. For example, the sodium-independent large neutral amino acid transporter (LAT-1) mediates transport of L-dopa, used for treatment of Parkinson disease.

Endocytosis

Another important mechanism of transport across the BBB is endocytosis. Endocytosis occurs to a limited degree in the endothelial cells of the brain vasculature; however, specific types of endocytosis including receptor-mediated endocytosis and absorptive-mediated endocytosis provide a means for selective uptake of macromolecules into the CNS. Insulin is transported into brain cells by receptor-mediated endocytosis.

Active Transport

Active transport of substrates across the BBB is energy dependent and usually requires ATP as the energy source. Such processes enable movement of substances against their concentration gradient. The CNS transport of the opioid analgesic morphine and its metabolites exemplifies the transport mechanisms involved in drug handling at the BBB interface (**Fig. 2**).

BLOOD-BRAIN BARRIER INTEGRITY

Several diseases and CNS insults are capable of affecting BBB integrity.[14] Examples include traumatic brain injury, intracerebral hemorrhage, primary and metastatic neoplasms, inflammatory diseases (meningitis, ventriculitis, and cerebral abscess), and severe toxic–metabolic derangements (encephalopathy). The BBB is disrupted during periods of ischemia, anoxia, sudden hypertension, seizures, inflammation, and administration of hyperosmolar solutions. A final common pathway of enhanced BBB permeability and loss of BBB integrity is seen in all of the previously mentioned insults.

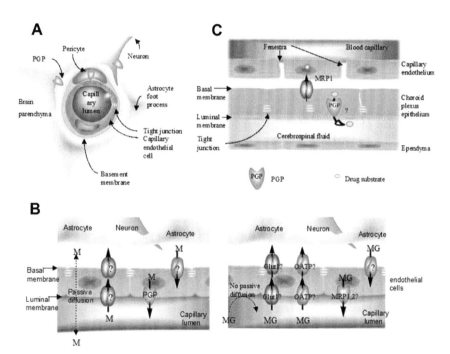

Fig. 2. Transfer of morphine and its metabolites across BBB. (*A, C*) Morphine (M) and morphine-3 and 6-glucuronide (MG) transport across the BBB. (*B*) Morphine uptake from the circulation to the brain extracellular fluid is by passive transport and an unknown saturable carrier-mediated processes. MRP, multidrug-resistance proteins; OATP, organic anion transporting polypeptides; PGP, P-glycoprotein. (*From* Roberts DJ, Goralski KB. A critical overview of the influence of inflammation and infection on P-glycoprotein expression and activity in the brain. Expert Opin Drug Metab Toxicol 2008;4(10):1245-64; with permission.)

Reversible Opening of Blood-Brain Barrier

The diverse nature of diseases and conditions affecting BBB integrity stimulated the research to find ways for reversibly opening BBB for delivering medications to the CNS. Several techniques have been used (eg, antibacterial antibodies, ultrasound bursts, shock wave).[19,20] Currently, rapid intra-arterial infusion of mannitol is the safest method in humans. This is used in delivering chemotherapy to brain tumors in certain neurosurgical centers.

Assessment of Blood-Brain Barrier Integrity

At present the assessment of the BBB integrity after CNS insult falls into one of the following three categories: (1) clinical assessment (mainly neurocognitive tests), (2) imaging studies (mainly MRI with dye injection), and (3) laboratory testing (mainly use of brain biomarkers).[21]

The neurocognitive tests

These are noninvasive ways to measure important aspects of cognition: attention, memory, language, reaction time, and perception.[22,23] They usually are performed using paper and pencil tests or computerized tests.

Tests have been developed to examine each function of cognition previously mentioned. The CogState computerized testing tool was comparable with neuroimaging in some studies done on patients with Alzheimer disease for detection of abnormal cognition.

Imaging studies

Most imaging studies use MRI with gadolinium-containing dye to assess the integrity of the BBB because computed tomography scanning is less sensitive.[24] Studies examining MRI in cardiac surgery patients usually use MRI at different time points to examine baseline status (before cardiac surgery) and again in the postoperative period. Dye leak or CSF enhancement is considered a positive sign for BBB disruption. In the context of cardiac surgery, the difficulty in performing these studies is the frequency with which the examinations can be performed and the timing of the examinations. It is likely that BBB dysfunction is transient and most prevalent in the intraoperative to immediate postoperative time points and for logistical reasons it is difficult to perform timely MRI studies at critical time points. This means that the timing of the insult may be missed using this technique for BBB examination.

Brain biomarkers

Until recently the neurologic function and hence the integrity of the BBB relied mainly on clinical examination and imaging studies. However, the need for an easier and more quantitative method for assessing neuronal function has led to the search for rapid and reliable blood tests that can be followed overtime (brain biomarkers).[25] Different brain biomarkers have been investigated and their clinical application in medicine started with traumatic brain injury but rapidly found its way into other clinical conditions including: Alzheimer disease, Parkinson disease, neurologic infections, and cardiac surgery. The biomarkers that seem to be indicative of brain injury severity are:

- Glial tissue markers (S100B protein, glial fibrillary acidic protein)
- Neuronal tissue markers (tau protein, neuron-specific enolase)
- Albumin

S100B is an astrocyte-specific protein that can spill from injured cells and enter the extracellular space or bloodstream. Serum levels of S100B increase in patients during the acute phase of brain damage. An increase in S100B has been observed immediately after traumatic or nontraumatic BBB disruption because of raised synthesis and release from an injury activated glial tissue. However, its specificity for detecting brain injury during cardiac surgery is controversial.[26] In a study by Jönsson and colleagues,[27] where they tried to find a relationship between S100B levels and cognitive dysfunction, S100B level was measured at different time points (hourly for the first 6 hours, and then at 8, 10, 15, 24, and 48 hours after surgery). No significant relationship between S100B levels and neuropsychological outcome was observed. S100B levels 1 hour after cardiac surgery seemed to be the most informative. The same group followed patients for 40 months and found that even slightly elevated S100B values in blood 2 days after cardiac operation implied a bad prognosis for outcome, and especially so in combination with any CNS complication.[28]

Tau proteins are microtubular binding proteins localized in the axonal compartment of neurons that binds tubulin and promotes microtubule assembly and stability. Brain injury from different mechanisms including BBB disruption releases cleaved Tau proteins (C-tau) into the extracellular space where they are transported to the CSF. CSF levels of C-tau reflect axonal damage after CNS insult. The increased serum C-tau levels in patients with severe head injury are associated with a compromised BBB function. Tau seems to be more specific than other biomarkers because it is only found in the CNS.[29]

Albumin, as a naturally occurring protein with a molecular weight of 65,000 to 70,000 Da, is an optimal candidate for measurement of BBB function because it is synthesized peripherally, not catabolized within the CNS, and does not readily diffuse across an intact BBB. The CSF to serum albumin quotient (Q_A) requires the measurement of albumin in CSF and serum collected contemporaneously. The limitation of this method is that once albumin has entered the extracellular space of the brain it continues to diffuse and therefore it may not be a reliable index of the duration or progression of the leak across BBB.[30] The requirement for repeated CSF albumin measurement is a further limitation to this technique.

CARDIAC SURGERY AND THE BLOOD-BRAIN BARRIER

Some degree of brain injury is likely to occur during cardiac surgery because of the nature of the surgery (hypothermia, cardiopulmonary bypass [CPB] use, hypoperfusion of the brain, possible microembolic showers to cerebral circulation, and activation of the systemic inflammatory response).[31] It is hypothesized that BBB disruption is the underlying mechanism for most of the subtle CNS effects seen after cardiac surgery. In the first two decades of open heart surgery the main CNS events of concern were stroke and acute confusional states "pump brain."[32] Although highly prevalent, the exact incidence and magnitude of BBB dysfunction after cardiac surgery remains to date undetermined. This is likely a result of the many covariants that may contribute to the insult and the difficulty of studying the degree of BBB dysfunction occurring over time in humans in vivo.

The occurrence of BBB disruption after CPB has been definitively shown in animal models using invasive methods. This has been achieved by demonstrating albumin migration from blood into CSF, extravasations of Evans blue dye through the BBB into the brain, and increased inducible transcription factor gene expression in BBB cells exposed to neutrophils of patients undergoing cardiac operations.[33]

Aggravation of Blood-Brain Barrier Disruption in Cardiac Surgery

The effects of deep hypothermia and cerebral venous congestion have been investigated in humans and animals to determine their effect on BBB disruption in

Table 2
Important studies in humans that have examined BBB integrity during cardiac surgery

Author, Published Year	Study Question	Method	Findings
Wang et al,[36] 2017	Does systemic inflammatory response induced by CPB affect morphine and its metabolites distribution in blood and CSF in patients having descending thoracic aortic aneurysm repair? Markers measured included CSF/plasma albumin ratio measured at repeated intervals during surgery and in the CVICU	Observational study sample size 33 patients (18 open repair and 15 endovascular repair)	Plasma and CSF interleukin-6 concentrations increased postoperatively and reflected the magnitude of the surgical insult CSF/plasma albumin changes suggesting some disruption of BBB integrity Morphine distribution into the CSF was not significantly altered suggesting that BBB P-gp function may not be affected by the perioperative inflammatory response Metabolite disposition was altered indicating dysfunction of an unknown transporter function
Kok et al,[37] 2017	Can brain biomarkers predict cognitive dysfunction after cardiac surgery? (CABG with and without CPB)	Cognitive function assessment using CogState computerized test at 3 and 15 mo after surgery (sample size 57 patients) Blood samples were obtained preoperatively, after sternal closure and at 6 h and 24 h postoperatively Markers measured included: Brain fatty acid binding protein, NSE, and S100B	Brain fatty acid binding protein was already significantly higher before surgery in patients who developed POCD At 3 mo after surgery high levels of plasma free hemoglobin at sternal closure were associated with negative influence on cognitive performance High baseline scores on neurocognitive tests and higher level of education proved to beneficially influence cognitive outcome Neuronal injury related biomarkers were of no clear prognostic value

Study	Objective	Methods	Findings
Abrahamov et al,[38] 2017	BBB disruption after cardiac surgery (diagnosis and correlation to cognition)	Observational study, sample size 7 patients undergoing CABG with CPB were assigned to serial cerebral MRI evaluations, preoperatively and on POD 1 and 5 Examinations were analyzed for BBB disruption and microemboli load using dynamic contrast enhancement MRI and diffusion-weighted imaging methods, respectively Neuropsychologic tests were performed 1 day preoperatively and on POD 5	The location of BBB disruption was most prominent in the frontal lobes MRI evidence of microembolization was demonstrated in 14% of patients (1 out of 7) BBB disruption as defined by MRI enhancement was evident in 71% of patients (5 out of 7) The location and intensity of the BBB disruption, rather than the microembolic load, correlated with postoperative neurocognitive dysfunction
Hernández-García et al,[39] 2016	Brain injury biomarkers in the setting of cardiac surgery	Literature review	Brain biomarkers S100B, NSE, GFAP, and Tau protein seem to be indicators of global brain dysfunction at the cellular level To date there is no biomarker entirely suitable for detection of brain injury after cardiac surgery
Patel et al,[40] 2015	The presence of new MRI lesions and cognitive decline after cardiac surgery	Systematic review of relevant literature	Acute cerebral injury is common and often more extensive than clinical symptoms would suggest Atheromatous disease of the aorta may be an important factor in predicting the risk of new MRI lesions
Shi-Min,[41] 2014	Biomarkers of cerebral injury in cardiac surgery Meta-analysis	Quantitative data of S100, S100B, and NSE	The biomarkers appeared earlier and lasted longer in the CSF than in serum All 3 biomarkers exhibited a similar kinetic trend in the bloodstream reaching a peak value at the end of CPB Cardiac operations may lead to cerebral damage and BBB changes as a consequence of CPB and low core temperature

(continued on next page)

**Table 2
(continued)**

Author, Published Year	Study Question	Method	Findings
Maekawa, et al,[42] 2014	Relationship of brain gray matter loss to POCD Prospective observational study	Sample size 28 patients who had MRI and neurocognitive tests completed before and after surgery POCD was defined as an individual decrease in more than 2 tests of at least 1 standard deviation from the group baseline mean for that test The degree of gray matter loss in the MTL of each patient was calculated	Patients who experienced POCD within 2 wk after cardiac surgery had significantly greater loss of gray matter in the MTL than patients who did not experience POCD The pathogenesis of gray matter loss of MTL may reflect a combination of neuronal degeneration and ischemic pathologies
Reinsfelt et al,[43] 2012	Are biomarkers of brain injury in the setting of cardiac surgery (aortic valve replacement) more accurately measured in CSF than plasma to avoid extraneuronal sources of the biomarkers?	Prospective, descriptive study 10 patients for aortic valve replacement CSF was obtained the day before surgery and 24 h after surgery for measuring CSF levels of: albumin and brain biomarkers (NSE, Tau protein, S-100B, and GFAP)	The 2 CSF markers of glial cell injury, S-100B and GFAP, increased by 35% and 25%, respectively CSF albumin increased by 13%, whereas serum albumin decreased by 27%; thus, the CSF to serum albumin ratio increased by 61% indicating disruption of the BBB The structural integrity of the BBB was impaired as evidenced by increased CSF albumin and an increase in the CSF to serum albumin ratio The increase in CSF S-100B and GFAP, the 2 biomarkers of astrocyte damage could suggest that astrocyte injury may be involved in the cardiac surgery-induced impaired integrity of the BBB

Abbreviations: CABG, coronary artery bypass graft; GFAP, glial fibrillary acidic protein; MTL, medial temporal lobe; NSE, neuron-specific enolase; POCD, postoperative cognitive dysfunction; POD, postoperative day.

cardiac surgery. The effect of deep hypothermic circulatory arrest (DHCA) was studied in an animal model of CPB by Bartels and colleagues.[34] They performed a pilot randomized controlled study where one group of animals (rats) were subjected to CPB for 30 minutes and then DHCA (pericranial temperature of 16°C–18°C for 60 minutes), whereas the other group were subjected sham surgery (no CPB) for 90 minutes. Both groups had MRI 24 hours after surgery and they used intravenous gadobutrol contrast agent as a marker for disruption. Gadobutrol is approved for use in humans and it has low molecular weight allowing for the detection of minor BBB disruption. Their results indicated that MRI successfully detected increased brain capillary permeability to gadobutrol, but no significant quantitative changes in select proteins relevant for BBB.

In a study by Dabrowski and colleagues,[35] the effect of raised cerebral venous pressure (measured by retrograde cannulation of the right jugular vein bulb) on the release of brain biomarkers was investigated in 128 patients undergoing CABG with CPB. Blood samples were collected during surgery and in the early postoperative period for measurement of plasma concentration of glial fibrillary acidic protein, tau protein, arteriovenous lactate, and jugular vein oxygen saturation. All were analyzed in relation to jugular venous bulb pressure (JVBP). They found that CPB increased JVBP and an increased JVBP more than 12 mm Hg intensified the release of brain biomarker concentrations. Clinical correlation using cognitive testing showed that those patients with higher JVBP had worse cognitive outcome.

Table 2 lists studies that have examined alternations/disruption in the BBB function/integrity because of cardiac surgery in humans using any of the three methods for assessing BBB integrity during cardiac surgery: (1) clinical, (2) imaging studies, and (3) laboratory. We chose to limit studies to the previous 15 years to account for changes in the conduct of cardiac surgery as it has evolved overtime.

As can be seen from our review of the studies, BBB disruption after cardiac surgery occurs. The magnitude and duration of the alterations is uncertain but likely transient in most patients and limited to the immediate perioperative period. The role of BBB disruption in drug handling has received only limited attention. The influence of BBB disruption on the development of cognitive dysfunction is still uncertain. The role of biomarkers in establishing BBB disruption is unresolved and current evidence does not support routine use in the clinical arena.

SUMMARY

Neurologic abnormality after cardiac surgery is common. Up to 50% of patients show some evidence of neurologic dysfunction as evidenced by studies of neurocognitive function, MRI imaging, and brain biomarker laboratory testing. BBB disruption/malfunction may be the underlying cause for some of the neurologic abnormality seen in postoperative cardiac patients. The cause of BBB disruption is multifactorial including: ischemia, anoxia, systemic inflammation, and embolic events. Several inherent technical procedures during cardiac surgery are detrimental to BBB function. These include cerebral venous congestion caused by cannula placement in the superior vena cava and DHCA. To date there is no single test or measure that can predict BBB disruption in cardiac surgery.

REFERENCES

1. Chow BW, GU C. The molecular constituents of the blood-brain barrier. Trends Neurosci 2015;38(10):598–608.

2. Pramod Dash, blood brain barrier and cerebral metabolism. 1997-present. Available at: https://nba.uth.tmc.edu/neuroscience/m/s4/chapter11.html. Accessed April 15, 2018.
3. Serlin Y, Shelef I, Knyazer B, et al. Anatomy and physiology of the blood-brain barrier. Semin Cell Dev Biol 2015;38:2–6.
4. Vein A. Science and fate: Lina Stern (1878–1968), a neurophysiologist and biochemist. J Hist Neurosci 2008;(17):195–206.
5. Bonetta L. Endothelial tight junctions form the blood–brain barrier. J Cell Biol 2005;169(3):378–9.
6. Obermeier B, Daneman R, Ransohoff RM. Development, maintenance and disruption of the blood-brain barrier. Nat Med 2013;19(12):1584–96.
7. Sarkar A, Fatima I, Jamal QMS, et al. Nanoparticles as a carrier system for drug delivery across blood brain barrier". Curr Drug Metab 2017;18(2): 129–37.
8. Rajani RM, Williams A. Endothelial cell–oligodendrocyte interactions in small vessel disease and aging. Clin Sci (Lond) 2017;131(5):369–79.
9. Stamatovic S, Keep RF, Andjelkovic A. Brain endothelial cell-cell junctions: how to "open" the blood brain barrier. Curr Neuropharmacol 2008;6(3):179–92.
10. Barar J, Rafi MA, Pourseif MM, et al. Blood-brain barrier transport machineries and targeted therapy of brain diseases. Bioimpacts 2016;6(4):225–48.
11. Luissint AC, Artus C, Glacial F, et al. Tight junctions at the blood brain barrier: physiological architecture and disease-associated dysregulation. Fluids Barriers CNS 2012;9:23.
12. Hartsock A, Nelson WJ. Adherens and tight junctions: structure, function and connections to the actin cytoskeleton. Biochim Biophys Acta 2008;1778(3): 660–9.
13. Uneno M, Nakagawa T, Wu B, et al. Transporters in the brain endothelial barrier. Curr Med Chem 2010;17(12):1125–38.
14. Lawther B, Kumar S, Krovvidi H. Blood-brain barrier. Cont Educ Anaesth Crit Care Pain 2011;11(4):128–32.
15. Attwell D, Mishra A, Hall CN, et al. What is a pericyte? J Cereb Blood Flow Metab 2016;36(2):451–5.
16. Smith H, weerakkody Y, et al. Blood brain barrier. Available at: https://radiopaedia.org/articles/blood-brain-barrier-3. Accessed June 28, 2018.
17. Hladky SB, Barrand MA. Fluid and ion transfer across the blood-brain and blood-cerebrospinal fluid barriers; a comparative account of mechanisms and roles. Fluids Barriers CNS 2016;13(1):19.
18. Pardridge WM. Drug transport across the blood–brain barrier. J Cereb Blood flow Metab 2012;32:1959–72.
19. Stanley I. Rapoport osmotic opening of the blood–brain barrier: principles, mechanism, and therapeutic applications. Cell Mol Neurobiol 2000;20(No. 2): 217–30.
20. Chen Y, Liu L. Modern methods for delivery of drugs across the blood–brain barrier. Adv Drug Deliv Rev 2012;64:640–65.
21. Winblad B, Palmer K, Kivipelto M, et al. Mild cognitive impairment beyond controversies: report of the International Working Group on Mild Cognitive Impairment. J Intern Med 2004;256:240–6.
22. Marques-Costa C, Almiro PA, Simões MR. Computerized cognitive tests in elderly: a psychometric review. Eur Rev Appl Psychol 2018;68:61–8.

23. De Jager CA, Hogervorst E, Combrinck M, et al. Sensitivity and specificity of neuropsychological tests for mild cognitive impairment, vascular cognitive impairment and Alzheimer's disease. Psychol Med 2003;33(6):1039–50.

24. Wityk RJ, Goldsborough MA, Hillis A, et al. Diffusion- and perfusion-weighted brain magnetic resonance imaging in patients with neurologic complications after cardiac surgery. Arch Neurol 2001;58(4):571–6.

25. Smith C. Biomarkers on the brain: putting biomarkers together for a better understanding of the nervous system Dec. 7, 2017. Available at: https://www.sciencemag.org/features/2017/12/biomarkers-brain-putting-biomarkers-together-better-understanding-nervous-system. Accessed June 28, 2018.

26. Koh SX, Lee JK. S100B as a marker for brain damage and blood-brain barrier disruption following exercise. Sports Med 2014;44(3):369–85.

27. Jönsson H, Johnsson P, Bäckström M, et al. Controversial significance of early S100B levels after cardiac surgery. BMC Neurol 2004;4(1):24.

28. Johnsson P, Bäckström M, Bergh C, et al. Increased S100B in blood after cardiac surgery is a powerful predictor of late mortality. Ann Thorac Surg 2003;75(1):162–8.

29. Guo T, Noble W, Hanger D. Roles of Tau protein in health and disease. Acta Neuropathol 2017;133:665–704.

30. Blyth BJ, Farhavar A, Gee C, et al. Validation of serum markers for blood-brain barrier disruption in traumatic brain injury. J Neurotrauma 2009;26(9):1497–507.

31. Hogue C, Gottesman RF, Stearns J. Mechanisms of cerebral injury from cardiac surgery. Crit Care Clin 2008;24(1):83–94.

32. Scott DA, Evered LA, Silbert BS. Cardiac surgery, the brain, and inflammation. J Extra Corpor Technol 2014;46(1):15–22.

33. Saunders NR, Dziegielewska KM, Møllgard K, et al. Markers for blood-brain barrier integrity: how appropriate is Evans blue in the twenty-first century and what are the alternatives? Front Neurosci 2015;29(9):385.

34. Bartels K, Ma Q, Talaignair N, et al. Effects of deep hypothermic circulatory arrest on the blood brain barrier in a cardiopulmonary bypass model: a pilot study. Heart Lung Circ 2014;23(10):981–4.

35. Dabrowski W, Kotlinska E, Rzecki Z, et al. Raised jugular venous pressure intensifies release of brain injury biomarkers in patients undergoing cardiac surgery. J Cardiothorac Vasc Anesth 2012;26(6):999–1006.

36. Wang Y, Goralski KB, Roberts DJ, et al. An observational study examining the effects of a surgically induced inflammatory response on the distribution of morphine and its metabolites into cerebrospinal fluid. Can J Anaesth 2017;64:1009–22.

37. Kok EF, Koerts J, Tucha O, et al. Neuronal damage biomarkers in the identification of patients at risk of long-term postoperative cognitive dysfunction after cardiac surgery. Anaesthesia 2017;72:359–69.

38. Abrahamov D, Levran O, Naparstek S, et al. Blood–brain barrier disruption after cardiopulmonary bypass: diagnosis and correlation to cognition. Ann Thorac Surg 2017;104:161–9.

39. Hernández-García C, Rodríguez A, Egea-Guerrero JJ. Brain injury biomarkers in the setting of cardiac surgery: still a world to explore. Brain Inj 2016;30(1):10–7.

40. Patel N, Minhas JS, Chung EM. The presence of new MRI lesions and cognitive decline after cardiac surgery: a systematic review. J Card Surg 2015;30(11):808–12.

41. Shi-Min Y. Biomarkers of cerebral injury in cardiac surgery. Anadolu Kardiyol Derg 2014;14(7):638–45.
42. Maekawa K, Baba K, Otomo S, et al. Low pre-existing gray matter volume in the medial temporal lobe and white matter lesions are associated with post-operative cognitive dysfunction after cardiac surgery. PLoS One 2014;9(1): e87375.
43. Reinsfelt B, Ricksten SE, Zetterberg H, et al. Cerebrospinal fluid markers of brain injury, inflammation, and blood-brain barrier dysfunction in cardiac surgery. Ann Thorac Surg 2012;94:549–55.

The Future Directions of Research in Cardiac Anesthesiology

Jessica Spence, MD, FRCPC[a,b], C. David Mazer, MD, FRCPC[c,d],*

KEYWORDS

- Cardiothoracic anesthesia • Research • Trial design • Future

KEY POINTS

- Advances in cardiac anesthesia have led to the identification of new knowledge gaps that need to be addressed.
- In addressing these knowledge gaps, researchers need to expand their focus beyond the intraoperative period to broader and longer term outcomes of high importance to patients.
- The process of doing so requires new approaches to the conduct of research in anesthesia, through the use of changing types of data, novel analytical techniques, and innovative methodologic approaches, which will ultimately benefit our patients.

Cardiac anesthesia is relatively new, first described less than 100 years ago for patients undergoing mitral commissurotomy.[1] Since that time, both cardiac surgery and cardiac anesthesia have evolved rapidly, with the development of cardiopulmonary bypass (CPB), pharmacologic and mechanical support techniques, minimally invasive surgery, antifibrinolytics, transesophageal echocardiography, and intraoperative processed electroencephalographic monitoring, among other advances. These advances have occurred in the setting of a changing scientific milieu, with the shift from expertise-based to evidence-based clinical practice,[2] resulting in a need for clinical research to support the use of interventions. With this, cardiac anesthesiology research, which historically focused on intraoperative and immediate postoperative

Disclosure Statement: None.
^a Departments of Anesthesia and Critical Care and Health Research Methods, Evaluation, and Impact, McMaster University, HSC 2V9 - 1280 Main Street West, Hamilton, ON L8S 4K1, Canada; ^b Population Health Research Institute (PHRI), C3-7B David Braley Cardiac, Vascular and Stroke Research Institute (DBCVSRI), 237 Barton Street East, Hamilton, ON L8L 2X2, Canada; ^c Department of Anesthesia, Li Ka Shing Knowledge Institute of St. Michael's Hospital, 30 Bond Street, Toronto, ON M5B 1W8, Canada; ^d Departments of Anesthesia and Physiology, University of Toronto, Toronto, ON, Canada
* Corresponding author. Department of Anesthesia, St. Michael's Hospital, 30 Bond Street, Toronto, Ontario M5B 1W8, Canada.
E-mail address: david.mazer@unityhealth.to

physiologic phenomena,[3] has recently begun to examine the short- and long-term effects of perioperative interventions on outcomes of greater importance to patients, including major morbidity and mortality.

Although risk-adjusted perioperative mortality associated with cardiac surgery has been significantly decreased,[4] there remains an important need to improve the quality of recovery, particularly in light of the older and sicker population being referred for cardiac surgery. Current knowledge gaps include interventions that mitigate the adverse effects of CPB, improve the diagnosis and management of perioperative myocardial infarction (MI) in cardiac surgical patients, prevent postoperative neurologic decline, and optimize outcomes after valve replacement surgery. Finally, because many aspects of routine practice in anesthesiology lack a strong evidence base, and the results of randomized controlled trials (RCTs) are sometimes difficult to extrapolate to everyday clinical practice, there is a need to study not only the efficacy of interventions (or how they work in ideal circumstances), but also their effectiveness (or how they work in the real world of clinical practice). However, with these new areas of inquiry comes a need for larger trials, in an era where there is limited availability of public funding to support clinical research. Given this tension, researchers in cardiac anesthesia need to rethink how clinical research is designed and conducted as they investigate the following areas.

KNOWLEDGE GAPS THAT NEED TO BE ADDRESSED
Mitigating the Inflammatory Effects of Cardiopulmonary Bypass

The invention of CPB revolutionized the conduct of cardiac surgery, allowing for open heart and other procedures requiring cardiac arrest. However, the contact of blood with the nonendothelial surfaces of the CPB circuit is associated with an intense inflammatory response, which results in platelet aggregation and thrombocytopenia, activation of the coagulation cascade, and decreased circulating coagulation factors.[5–7] The release of inflammatory mediators from endothelial cells and leukocytes causes capillary leakage and vasodilation.[6,8] Common issues that arise in patients while weaning from CPB and during the immediate postoperative period, including myocardial dysfunction, vasoplegia, and bleeding, are attributed to this inflammatory response.[6,8] Studies have evaluated the impact of a variety of approaches to attenuating the systemic inflammatory response to CPB, including complete avoidance of CPB,[9] use of biocompatible circuits,[10] and pharmacologic agents targeting different steps in the inflammatory cascade.[11,12]

Steroids are an intervention of particular interest, as demonstrated by the 56 RCTs included in one recent systematic review.[13] They are appealing because of their consistent anti-inflammatory effect, low cost, and widespread availability. However, a recent meta-analysis demonstrated an unclear impact on postoperative mortality, with a relative risk of 0.85 (95% confidence interval, 0.71–1.01; $P = .07$; $I^2 = 0\%$).[13] Subgroup analyses of the 2 largest trials examining the use of steroids in cardiac surgery have demonstrated great variability in the response to steroids, with some patients (particularly those in older age groups) more likely to experience harm from steroid administration and others, who may have been at greater risk of developing a severe systemic inflammatory response, more likely to benefit.[14] Given this variability in interindividual response to steroids, future research in cardiac anesthesia needs to identify the phenotype associated with severe inflammatory responses to CPB and evaluate targeted therapies in this population, including steroids and other interventions that circumvent the inflammatory pathway.

Diagnosis and Management of Perioperative Myocardial Infarction after Cardiac Surgery

MI is among the most common and prognostically important complications after cardiac surgery.[9,15] MIs in cardiac surgical patients are currently diagnosed through the measurement of troponin values. The degree to which this biomarker is elevated in the 24 hours after surgery is the only identified independent predictor—beyond age—of 30-day mortality after coronary artery bypass surgery.[14] However, the troponin values normally used for the diagnosis of MI are common after cardiac surgical procedures because of manipulation of the myocardium. The extent of elevation can be attributed to multiple factors beyond ischemia, including the quality of myocardial preservation on CPB and magnitude of direct myocardial tissue trauma.[16] As such, the 4th Universal Definition for MI after cardiac surgery (ie, type 5 MI) includes a troponin value that is more than 10 times the 99th percentile of the upper range limit of normal.[16] There is, however, limited evidence to support this choice of biomarker threshold, particularly given that troponin elevation varies according to the type of surgery, with procedures that involve less myocardial tissue trauma (eg, minimally invasive or coronary artery bypass grafting) associated with a lower range of normal values.[17,18] It is also unclear that troponin elevations below this cut-point are not of prognostic importance. In addition, there is limited evidence as to the optimal management of type 5 MIs, particularly those associated with nonobstructive etiologies.[16] Finally, most laboratories now use high-sensitivity troponin assays, rather than the older generation troponin assays that have been previously been used in studies evaluating the epidemiology of MI after cardiac surgery. Thus, there is a need to determine high-sensitivity troponin threshold (or that of other bioassays) associated with prognostically important myocardial injury after cardiac surgery.

Neurologic Outcomes of Cardiac Surgery

Stemming from their association with functional decline and subsequent long-term care placement,[19,20] postoperative neurologic injuries are a highly feared complication of cardiac surgery. Stroke and transient ischemic attack are classified as type 1 neurologic injuries whereas delirium and postoperative cognitive dysfunction are classified as type 2 injuries.[21] The reported incidence of type 1 neurologic injuries, which are thought to stem from atheroembolic events or hypoperfusion, ranges from 1% to 10%.[22] Type 2 neurologic injuries are more common and less well-understood. In addition, because of the inconsistent way in which postoperative cognitive dysfunction is defined and measured, its incidence ranges from 3% to 79%.[19,20] Whether postoperative cognitive dysfunction reflects age-related cognitive decline or an adverse effect of anesthesia or surgery on cognitive function remains unclear, and there is conflicting evidence regarding the cognitive trajectories of patients undergoing cardiac surgery when compared with nonsurgical controls.[20] Determining the role that patient and procedural factors play in its development is an area that requires further investigation.

Multiple trials have evaluated interventions to decrease the incidence of neurologic injuries after cardiac surgery. Various pharmacologic agents with neuromodulatory effects, including ketamine, magnesium, lidocaine, dexamethasone, and piracetam, have been evaluated but none has demonstrated a beneficial effect.[22] Interventions that focus on the prevention of atheroembolism or hypoperfusion have yielded more promising results. A recent network meta-analysis found that surgical approaches that minimize aortic manipulation (which is thought to be a major source of atheroembolism) may decrease the incidence of postoperative stroke,[23] although off-pump approaches alone seem to have no effect.[9] A number of studies have found that higher mean arterial pressure targets while on CPB are associated with a decreased risk of stroke after cardiac surgery,[22] although this evidence is limited by the fact that it is mostly observational. One promising strategy is the use of intraoperative monitoring techniques—most commonly near-infrared spectroscopy—to identify and allow anesthesiologists to minimize cerebral hypoperfusion. Low quality evidence from small, mostly observational studies, has suggested a relationship of decreased in cerebral oxygen saturation—detected using intraoperative near-infrared spectroscopy—with postoperative cognitive decline.[24] However, no randomized studies have demonstrated that measures to reverse cerebral desaturation lead to improved cognitive outcomes after cardiac surgery. A recent multicenter pilot study demonstrated that it was, in fact, feasible to reverse cerebral desaturations through a protocolized approach.[25] However, whether this translates to improvements in important clinical outcomes remains unknown, and needs to be evaluated in a large, multicenter RCT.

Postoperative delirium an acute change in mental status characterized by confusion and inattention[26] is a factor that is, associated with both short- and long-term postoperative cognitive dysfunction.[27] It has also been associated with increases in intensive care and hospital length of stay, institutional discharge, and death.[26] Delirium is common among cardiac surgery patients, with an estimated incidence that ranges from 3% to 78%, with the wide range attributable to type of surgery, diagnostic criteria, and the approach to case identification.[28] Compared with the general population of hospitalized elderly, cardiac surgery patients are among those at greatest risk of delirium, with a relative risk of 8.3 when compared with patients undergoing noncardiac surgery.[26] Observational studies have identified nonmodifiable risk factors for delirium that include age, preoperative cognitive impairment, hearing or vision impairment, and severity of illness.[26–28] Modifiable risk factors include perioperative medication type and dose, sleep disturbance, hydration status, and immobility or use of physical restraints.[26–28] Despite the recognition of risk factors, the etiology of postoperative delirium remains unclear, and seems to be multifactorial.[28] Several studies have identified a relationship with biomarker elevations,[22] whereas others have noted a relationship with the presence of subclinical ischemic insults (covert strokes) on MRI.[29] The limited studies conducted thus far have explored the role of different anesthetic techniques in preventing postoperative delirium. Intraoperative monitoring of electroencephalography to titrate the depth of anesthesia has demonstrated preliminary benefit in decreasing the incidence of delirium in noncardiac surgery populations,[30] but has not been studied in patients undergoing cardiac surgery. Dexmedetomidine, used intraoperatively for anesthesia and postoperatively for sedation, has been shown to decrease the incidence of delirium in a number of small studies in the cardiac surgical population.[31] Larger clinical trials are required to demonstrate robust evidence, and establish the optimal dose and timing of dexmedetomidine administration.

Postoperative delirium is often attributed to common anesthetic medications,[28] but no studies have evaluated the effect of alternate anesthetic regimes for cardiac surgery. Several RCTs have compared benzodiazepines to dexmedetomidine for sedation after cardiac surgery in the intensive care unit and have demonstrated a trend toward increased delirium with benzodiazepine sedation, with a relative risk of 1.23 (95% confidence interval, 0.93–1.67).[32] This evidence has led to recommendations from the American Geriatric Society[33] and Society for Critical Care Medicine[32] that benzodiazepine use be minimized in elderly and patients in the intensive care unit. As a result, except in special circumstances, benzodiazepines for sedation after cardiac surgery is no longer considered consistent with the standard of care. This strategy is not true for benzodiazepine use during cardiac surgery, where the practice remains common.[34] Benzodiazepine use remains common during cardiac surgery because of the favorable hemodynamic and anxiolytic properties of these medications, as well a belief that they decrease the risk of intraoperative awareness. Although 1 study has identified higher doses of intraoperative benzodiazepines as a risk factor for postoperative delirium,[35] no studies have evaluated the effect of a benzodiazepine-free anesthetic regime on delirium after cardiac surgery. However, good alternatives to benzodiazepines exist, and there is now uncertainty as to whether or not benzodiazepines should be used during surgery, as demonstrated by the large variation in clinical practice.[34] Whether benzodiazepines should be avoided during cardiac surgery in most patients is a question that needs to be answered.

Transfusion Strategies in Cardiac Surgery

Cardiac surgery is associated with a high incidence of perioperative bleeding and transfusion of allogeneic blood products. Although the TRICS III trial and subsequent meta-analyses have demonstrated that restrictive red blood cell transfusion is safe and noninferior to liberal transfusion in moderate- to high-risk cardiac surgical patients, in hypothesis-generating subgroup analyses, there was a paradoxic and significant interaction between transfusion threshold and age, where the restrictive strategy seemed to be superior to the liberal strategy in patients 75 years or older.[36,37] Given this finding, there is an important need to determine whether a restrictive strategy is indeed superior to liberal strategy in elderly patients. In addition, there is a need to explore individualized approaches to transfusion using non–hemoglobin-based triggers. Furthermore, the role of anemia prevention using erythropoietic strategies including intravenous iron and erythropoietin requires further evaluation. Finally, the optimal approaches to hemostatic therapy and transfusion of non–red blood cell products need to be rigorously assessed.

Optimizing the Long-Term Outcomes of Patients after Valve Surgery

Severe valvulopathy requires surgical valve replacement, which may be done using either a mechanical or a bioprosthetic valve. Mechanical valves are recommended for younger patients, because they are associated with less structural degeneration and resultant need for reoperation.[38] However, mechanical valves are also at increased risk of thromboembolic events, necessitating lifelong anticoagulation and its associated bleeding risk.[38] As a result, the expected lifespan after mechanical valve replacement in nonelderly adults when compared with age- and sex-matched counterparts is approximately halved.[39]

For patients who require aortic valve replacement, the Ross procedure, which replaces a patient's diseased aortic valve with their own pulmonary valve and places a homograft in the pulmonary position,[40] offers a promising alternative. Proponents of the procedure suggest that the operation is superior to conventional valve replacement because the pulmonary autograft is a living, dynamic structure providing superior hemodynamics, a lower risk of thromboembolism (with no long-term anticoagulation requirement), and a lower risk of endocarditis. Low-quality evidence suggests that the Ross procedure is associated with a lower incidence of thromboembolism, bleeding, or valve-related events compared with conventional aortic valve replacement.[41] Given the significant lifespan deficit that occurs after valve replacement, further research is required to evaluate whether the Ross procedure is a superior option for aortic valve replacement.

Beyond alternative approaches to surgery, information is required as to the optimal approach to anticoagulation after valve surgery. Much of the morbidity stemming from valve replacement is related to thrombotic complications and, when anticoagulation is used to prevent them, bleeding. Current guidelines recommend anticoagulation with a vitamin K antagonist after mechanical valve replacement, although the target international normalized ratio varies across guideline agencies.[42] These recommendations are based on very low-quality observational evidence, and even bioprosthetic valves are not without thrombotic risk.[42] There are multiple knowledge gaps with respect to anticoagulation after valve replacement that need to be addressed in the coming years, specifically, whether antiplatelet or anticoagulant medications are preferred to mitigate the risk of thrombosis after bioprosthetic valve replacement, particularly in the first 3 months after implantation, when these valves are at the highest risk.[43] Finally, despite guideline recommendations for specific international normalized ratio targets after mechanical valve replacement, the optimal international normalized ratio target that balances thrombotic with bleeding risk is unknown, and robust data from large RCTs comparing high with low international normalized ratio targets are required.

NEW APPROACHES TO RESEARCH IN CARDIAC ANESTHESIA

There are 4 factors that, in most situations, determine the sample size requirement for an RCT:

i. The threshold statistical significance level,
ii. The desired statistical power (ie, the probability that a test of significance will pick up on an effect that is present),
iii. The incidence of the outcome of interest in the population being studied, and
iv. The anticipated treatment effect size.

The first 2 of these factors are arbitrary and determined mostly by convention, although because of issues related to reproducibility, it has been suggested that more conservative approaches such as lowering the P value threshold and increasing the statistical power be adopted.[44,45] The incidence of the outcome in the population is usually estimated from available data. Patient-important outcomes including major morbidity and mortality are less common and mediated by multiple causal pathways.[46] Thus, interventions that typically target 1 causal mechanism and are directed toward improving patient-important outcomes will optimistically have a modest (ie, ≤25%) treatment effect size. The combination of low incidence and modest effect sizes lead to the need for a large sample size for a trial to be adequately powered to evaluate the impact of an intervention on a patient-important outcome. For example, assuming threshold level of statistical significance of .05, a statistical power of 0.80, and an incidence of 30-day mortality after cardiac surgery of 5%, an intervention that was anticipated to have a 25% relative risk reduction (ie, to reduce mortality to 3.75%) would require a total sample size of 8404 patients, without taking into account loss to follow-up. Given the multiple possible interventions, the many questions in anesthesia that need to be answered, and the current limitations in available research funding, researchers need to pursue new approaches to answering these questions.

Novel Analytical Techniques

One approach involves the use of what has been called "big data." This term was coined in 2001 to describe "data that contains greater variety arriving in increasing volumes with ever-higher velocity."[47] In other words, big data involves datasets that are too large and complex to be analyzed using conventional analytical software. As anesthesia groups increasingly adopt electronic charting, and health care institutions and governments transition to electronic health records and databases, there is an enormous amount of health care information available for analysis. This provides the opportunity for perioperative research derived from very large populations. Important hypotheses and associations can be generated through the evaluation of this big data, but the statistical expertise required to do so is well beyond the abilities of most clinician-researchers. In addition, there is the issue of data quality and inaccuracy that is inherent in large administrative databases. However, this "noise" can be overcome through the use of massive (on the order of multiple terabytes) datasets and analytical techniques that are iterative and branching (as opposed to the traditional linear approach used in most statistical analyses). This emerging approach to data analysis, which automates analytical model building, is known as machine learning.[48] In doing so, computers consider innumerable variables and build an analytical model that describes the intricate and branching relationships between them, rather than execute explicit programming.

Machine learning techniques or at least knowledge derived using them will be coming soon to an operating room near you. Recently described examples of the use of machine learning in anesthesia include the use of arterial waveform parameters to predict postinduction hypotension (with a sensitivity and specificity of 88% and 87%, respectively) 15 minutes before it occurred,[49] an algorithm developed using 796 preoperative variables to predict postoperative pain,[50] and the use of propofol and remifentanil dosing histories and demographic data to predict bispectral index during target-controlled infusion.[51] However, machine learning data analytical techniques have some shortcomings, not the least of which is a complexity that exceeds human understanding.[48] Machine learning predictive models by definition do not require human comprehension to work, existing in a metaphoric black box. As such, guidelines for developing and reporting machine learning predictive models in biomedical research have been developed to ensure transparency and methodologic rigor.[52] In addition, as with any predictive model developed using a very large dataset, machine learning models are vulnerable to overfitting,[48] which may result in them describing noise rather than clinically important relationships between variables. It is important that models be stringently tested and validated, with their findings interpreted through a clinical lens. Finally, despite their ability to account for numerous confounders and describe complex interrelationships, machine learning models remain limited by the datasets they are derived from. Unmeasured confounders not included in an administrative dataset will not be accounted for by a machine learning model. Until this shortcoming is overcome, randomized clinical trials, with their ability to ensure balanced risk factors and prognosis between intervention arms, will remain the gold standard for causal inference. Thus, although machine learning may generate management algorithms to predict things such as postinduction hypotension, the implementation of these algorithms into clinical practice should await prospective evaluation using RCT methodology so that clinicians can be confident that they improve patient-important outcomes.

Pragmatic Trials

The traditional individual patient RCT is useful to establish the efficacy of an intervention among a carefully selected population under optimal conditions following detailed protocols. In contrast, pragmatic trials address the clinical effectiveness of interventions, that is, whether it works when used in every day clinical care when applied to broad populations. Given the wide variability in practice across individual anesthesiologists,[53] and the uncertainty as to what constitutes best practice in many clinical scenarios, pragmatic trials in cardiac anesthesia are required. Examples of the variations in routine practice that need to be studied include withholding or giving home medications on the day of surgery, mean arterial pressure targets on CPB, and liberal versus conservative oxygenation. The most appropriate way to evaluate broad-based approaches to cardiac anesthesia care, like algorithm-based approaches or institutional cardiac anesthesia policies, is to assess their impact on a population, under the same conditions as would be present in actual practice. Historically, researchers have done this by randomizing interventions at the level of a group of patients (or cluster), rather than at the level of the individual patient, as in traditional RCTs. The main challenge of a cluster-randomized trial is the substantial loss of statistical power that occurs as a result of clustering (ie, individuals within a cluster are usually more similar than individuals across clusters, which needs to be accounted for within sample size calculations).[54] The use of a crossover between intervention arms within the cluster after a set period of time (ie, a crossover period) partly overcomes this issue, as each cluster acts as its own control (**Fig. 1**A). This is known as a randomized cluster crossover trial. Every time a cluster crosses over some of statistical power lost because of clustering is regained, provided there are no carry-over effects.[55] In situations where they may be a carry-over effect (ie, where it may be difficult to resume the "control" intervention after the intervention of interest has been in place) an alternate design, the stepped wedge trial, may be used. In the stepped wedge design each cluster crosses over from the control to the intervention arm at a time point determined at random but does not cross back to the control arm (see **Fig. 1**B).

Other pragmatic designs have incorporated randomization into cohort studies or registries, such that patient data and outcomes are collected from trial and administrative databases, rather than contemporaneous assessment by research staff. The trials within cohorts design recruits and randomizes eligible subjects from an existing cohort to an intervention, with comparison outcome data being obtained from the ongoing cohort database. The advantages of the design are that the cohort provides pool from which patients can be recruited, multiple interventions can be tested simultaneously, and control arm outcomes can be extracted.[56] Similarly, registry-based randomized trials use registries as a platform for case records, data collection, randomization, and follow-up, resulting in improved efficiency and cost.[57]

Adaptive Trial Designs

Pragmatic trials are not well-suited to answering questions of clinical efficacy. This is because the noise introduced by the broad inclusion of patients who cannot benefit from the intervention will diminish the signal of effect that would otherwise be seen under in a selected population and controlled conditions. Bayesian or adaptive designs are an innovation in individual patient RCT design developed to improve the economic efficiency and speed of RCT completion, as well as the likelihood that trial results will be scientifically or clinically relevant.[58] Adaptive designs are different from traditional RCTs in that they allow continual modifications to key aspects of the trial design while the trial is ongoing. As patients are enrolled in a trial using an adaptive design, information accumulates about their outcomes, which reduces the uncertainty regarding the true efficacy of the intervention being studied. Adaptive clinical trials take advantage of this accumulating information by modifying key trial parameters based on data as it is collected and according to a priori rules. Key characteristics that can be modified include sample size, randomization ratio, number of treatment groups, treatment administered or treatment dose, number and frequency of interim analyses, and the patient subpopulation being considered (such that those identified as being most likely

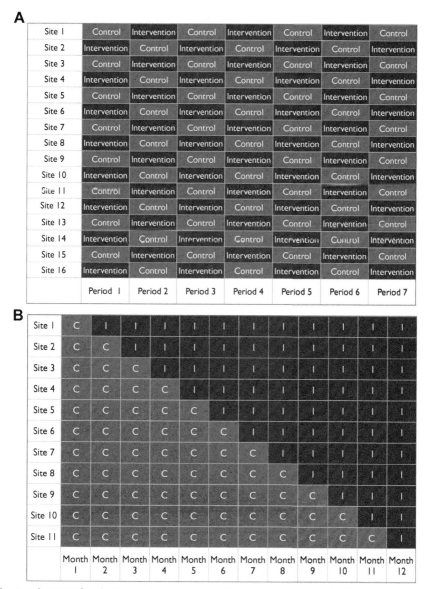

Fig. 1. Schematic for cluster randomized trials. (*A*) Sample site randomization schedule for a cluster crossover trial including 16 sites (clusters) with 7 crossover periods. (*B*) Schematic for a stepped wedge trial that includes 11 sites that randomly cross from control (C) to intervention (I) arms over 12 one-month periods.

to benefit can be selectively recruited).[58] Platform trials are a type of adaptive design that evaluates multiple treatments simultaneously, based on the assumption that populations of patients with a disease are heterogenous, and thus may respond differently to the same intervention.[59]

Compared with a traditional RCT, the design phase of an adaptive trial is longer, because understanding the performance characteristics of the trial requires extensive statistical simulation using a variety of possible treatment effects and population response characteristics. In addition, unless clinical decision rules are clearly defined a priori, there is a risk of introducing bias when making practical adaptations ad hoc. Finally, the complexity of the study design and conduct requires advanced training in methodology and statistics, which can also make it difficult to explain the trial concepts to funding agencies and peer reviewers. Nonetheless, adaptive designs have remarkable potential to speed up, shorten, or otherwise improve clinical trials. Going forward, adaptive designs will become increasingly common, and less the exclusive territory of statisticians.

SUMMARY

Cardiac anesthesia has come a long way since its origins and has firmly established itself as a subspecialty group that has unique skills, training, and expertise. Several noteworthy advances in the practice of cardiac anesthesia have been made in recent years, although these have also led to the identification of new knowledge gaps. Moving forward, the specialty of cardiac anesthesia needs to address these gaps and, in doing so, expand its focus beyond the intraoperative period to broader and longer-term outcomes that are of high importance to patients. In doing so, there is a need to adapt the conduct of research in anesthesia, through the use of changing types of data, novel analytical techniques, and innovative methodologic approaches that will ultimately benefit our patients.

ACKNOWLEDGMENTS

CDM is supported by a Merit Award from the University of Toronto Department of Anesthesia and grants from the Canadian Institutes of Health Research (301852; 421703).

REFERENCES

1. Wynands JE. The contribution of Canadian anaesthetists to the evolution of cardiac surgery. Can J Anaesth 1996;43(5 Pt 1):518–34.
2. Smith R, Rennie D. Evidence-based medicine–an oral history. JAMA 2014;311(4): 365–7.
3. Sessler DI. Long-term consequences of anesthetic management. Anesthesiology 2009;111(1):1–4.
4. D'Agostino RS, Jacobs JP, Badhwar V, et al. The Society of Thoracic Surgeons adult cardiac surgery database: 2018 update on outcomes and quality. Ann Thorac Surg 2018;105(1):15–23.
5. Barry AE, Chaney MA, London MJ. Anesthetic management during cardiopulmonary bypass: a systematic review. Anesth Analg 2015;120(4):749–69.
6. Warren OJ, Smith AJ, Alexiou C, et al. The inflammatory response to cardiopulmonary bypass: part 1–mechanisms of pathogenesis. J Cardiothorac Vasc Anesth 2009;23(2):223–31.
7. Wan S, LeClerc JL, Vincent JL. Inflammatory response to cardiopulmonary bypass: mechanisms involved and possible therapeutic strategies. Chest 1997; 112(3):676–92.
8. Ahlgren SC, Wang JF, Levine JD. C-fiber mechanical stimulus-response functions are different in inflammatory versus neuropathic hyperalgesia in the rat. Neuroscience 1997;76(1):285–90.

9. Lamy A, Devereaux PJ, Prabhakaran D, et al. Off-pump or on-pump coronary-artery bypass grafting at 30 days. N Engl J Med 2012;366(16):1489–97.
10. Rubens FD, Mesana T. The inflammatory response to cardiopulmonary bypass: a therapeutic overview. Perfusion 2004;19(Suppl 1):S5–12.
11. Verrier ED, Shernan SK, Taylor KM, et al. Terminal complement blockade with pexelizumab during coronary artery bypass graft surgery requiring cardiopulmonary bypass: a randomized trial. JAMA 2004;291(19):2319–27.
12. Mahaffey KW, Van de Werf F, Shernan SK, et al. Effect of pexelizumab on mortality in patients with acute myocardial infarction or undergoing coronary artery bypass surgery: a systematic overview. Am Heart J 2006;152(2):291–6.
13. Dvirnik N, Belley-Cote EP, Hanif H, et al. Steroids in cardiac surgery: a systematic review and meta-analysis. Br J Anaesth 2018;120(4):657–67.
14. Dieleman JM, van Dijk D. Corticosteroids for cardiac surgery: a summary of two large randomised trials. Neth J Crit Care 2016;24(5):6–10.
15. Domanski MJ, Mahaffey K, Hasselblad V, et al. Association of myocardial enzyme elevation and survival following coronary artery bypass graft surgery. JAMA 2011;305(6):585–91.
16. Thygesen K, Alpert JS, Jaffe AS, et al. Fourth universal definition of myocardial infarction (2018). Circulation 2018;138(20):e618–51.
17. Sinning JM, Hammerstingl C, Schueler R, et al. The prognostic value of acute and chronic troponin elevation after transcatheter aortic valve implantation. EuroIntervention 2016;11(13):1522–9.
18. Lurati Buse GA, Koller MT, Grapow M, et al. The prognostic value of troponin release after adult cardiac surgery - a meta-analysis. Eur J Cardiothorac Surg 2010;37(2):399–406.
19. Roach GW, Kanchuger M, Mangano CM, et al. Adverse cerebral outcomes after coronary bypass surgery. N Engl J Med 1996;335(25):1857–63.
20. Selnes OA, Gottesman RF, Grega MA, et al. Cognitive and neurologic outcomes after coronary-artery bypass surgery. N Engl J Med 2012;366(3):250–7.
21. Eagle KA, Guyton RA, Davidoff R, et al. ACC/AHA guidelines for coronary artery bypass graft surgery: a report of the American College of Cardiology/American Heart Association Task Force on Practice Guidelines. Circulation 1999;100(13):1464–80.
22. McDonagh DL, Berger M, Mathew JP, et al. Neurological complications of cardiac surgery. Lancet Neurol 2014;13(5):490–502.
23. Zhao DF, Edelman JJ, Seco M, et al. Coronary artery bypass grafting with and without manipulation of the ascending aorta: a network meta-analysis. J Am Coll Cardiol 2017;69(8):924–36.
24. Zheng F, Sheinberg R, Yee MS, et al. Cerebral near-infrared spectroscopy monitoring and neurologic outcomes in adult cardiac surgery patients: a systematic review. Anesth Analg 2013;116(3):663–76.
25. Deschamps A, Hall R, Grocott H, et al. Cerebral oximetry monitoring to maintain normal cerebral oxygen saturation during high-risk cardiac surgery: a randomized controlled feasibility trial. Anesthesiology 2016;124(4):826–36.
26. Inouye SK, Westendorp RG, Saczynski JS. Delirium in elderly people. Lancet 2014;383(9920):911–22.
27. Saczynski JS, Marcantonio ER, Quach L, et al. Cognitive trajectories after postoperative delirium. N Engl J Med 2012;367(1):30–9.
28. Arora RC, Djaiani G, Rudolph JL. Detection, prevention, and management of delirium in the critically ill cardiac patient and patients who undergo cardiac procedures. Can J Cardiol 2017;33(1):80–7.

29. Hatano Y, Narumoto J, Shibata K, et al. White-matter hyperintensities predict delirium after cardiac surgery. Am J Geriatr Psychiatry 2013;21(10):938–45.
30. Whitlock EL, Torres BA, Lin N, et al. Postoperative delirium in a substudy of cardiothoracic surgical patients in the BAG-RECALL clinical trial. Anesth Analg 2014;118(4):809–17.
31. Wu M, Liang Y, Dai Z, et al. Perioperative dexmedetomidine reduces delirium after cardiac surgery: a meta-analysis of randomized controlled trials. J Clin Anesth 2018;50:33–42.
32. Devlin JW, Skrobik Y, Gelinas C, et al. Clinical practice guidelines for the prevention and management of pain, agitation/sedation, delirium, immobility, and sleep disruption in adult patients in the ICU. Crit Care Med 2018;46(9):e825–73.
33. American Geriatrics Society expert panel on postoperative delirium in older adults. Postoperative delirium in older adults: best practice statement from the American Geriatrics Society. J Am Coll Surg 2015;220(2):136–48.e1.
34. Spence J, Belley-Cote E, Devereaux PJ, et al. Benzodiazepine administration during adult cardiac surgery: a survey of current practice among Canadian anesthesiologists working in academic centres. Can J Anaesth 2018;65(3):263–71.
35. Kazmierski J, Kowman M, Banach M, et al. Incidence and predictors of delirium after cardiac surgery: results from The IPDACS Study. J Psychosom Res 2010; 69(2):179–85.
36. Mazer CD, Whitlock RP, Fergusson DA, et al. Six-month outcomes after restrictive or liberal transfusion for cardiac surgery. N Engl J Med 2018;379(13):1224–33.
37. Mazer CD, Whitlock RP, Shehata N. Restrictive versus liberal transfusion for cardiac surgery. N Engl J Med 2018;379(26):2576–7.
38. Baumgartner H, Falk V, Bax JJ, et al. 2017 ESC/EACTS guidelines for the management of valvular heart disease. Eur Heart J 2017;38(36):2739–91.
39. Concha M, Aranda PJ, Casares J, et al. The Ross procedure. J Card Surg 2004; 19(5):401–9.
40. Ross DN. Homograft replacement of the aortic valve. Lancet 1962;2(7254):487.
41. McClure GR, Belley-Cote EP, Um K, et al. The Ross procedure versus prosthetic and homograft aortic valve replacement: a systematic review and meta-analysis. Eur J Cardiothorac Surg 2019;55(2):247–55.
42. Gupta S, Belley-Cote EP, Sarkaria A, et al. International normalized ratio targets for left-sided mechanical valve replacement. Thromb Haemost 2018;118(5):906–13.
43. Holbrook A, Schulman S, Witt DM, et al. Evidence-based management of anticoagulant therapy: antithrombotic therapy and prevention of thrombosis, 9th ed: American College of Chest Physicians Evidence-Based Clinical Practice Guidelines. Chest 2012;141:e152S–84S.
44. Ioannidis JPA. The proposal to lower P value thresholds to .005. JAMA 2018; 319(14):1429–30.
45. Lamberink HJ, Otte WM, Sinke MRT, et al. Statistical power of clinical trials increased while effect size remained stable: an empirical analysis of 136,212 clinical trials between 1975 and 2014. J Clin Epidemiol 2018;102:123–8.
46. Lurati Buse GA, Devereaux PJ. Anesthesia needs large international clinical trials. HSR Proc Intensive Care Cardiovasc Anesth 2010;2(3):153–5.
47. Laney D. Management-controlling-data-volume-velocity-and-variety.pdf. 2001. Available at: http://blogs.gartner.com/doug-laney/files/2012/01/ad949-3D-Data-. Accessed December 19, 2018.
48. Mathis MR, Kheterpal S, Najarian K. Artificial intelligence for anesthesia: what the practicing clinician needs to know: more than black magic for the art of the dark. Anesthesiology 2018;129(4):619–22.

49. Hatib F, Jian Z, Buddi S, et al. Machine-learning algorithm to predict hypotension based on high-fidelity arterial pressure waveform analysis. Anesthesiology 2018; 129(4):663–74.

50. Tighe PJ, Harle CA, Hurley RW, et al. Teaching a machine to feel postoperative pain: combining high-dimensional clinical data with machine learning algorithms to forecast acute postoperative pain. Pain Med 2015;16(7):1386–401.

51. Lee HC, Ryu HG, Chung EJ, et al. Prediction of bispectral index during target-controlled infusion of propofol and remifentanil: a deep learning approach. Anesthesiology 2018;128(3):492–501.

52. Luo W, Phung D, Tran T, et al. Guidelines for developing and reporting machine learning predictive models in biomedical research: a multidisciplinary view. J Med Internet Res 2016;18(12):e323.

53. Duggan A, Koff E, Marshall V. Clinical variation: why it matters. Med J Aust 2016; 205(10):S3–4.

54. Arnup SJ, Forbes AB, Kahan BC, et al. Appropriate statistical methods were infrequently used in cluster-randomized crossover trials. J Clin Epidemiol 2016;74: 40–50.

55. Connolly SJ, Philippon F, Longtin Y, et al. Randomized cluster crossover trials for reliable, efficient, comparative effectiveness testing: design of the Prevention of Arrhythmia Device Infection Trial (PADIT). Can J Cardiol 2013;29(6):652–8.

56. Relton C, Torgerson D, O'Cathain A, et al. Rethinking pragmatic randomised controlled trials: introducing the "cohort multiple randomised controlled trial" design. BMJ 2010;340:c1066.

57. Li G, Sajobi TT, Menon BK, et al. Registry-based randomized controlled trials-what are the advantages, challenges, and areas for future research? J Clin Epidemiol 2016;80:16–24.

58. Pallmann P, Bedding AW, Choodari-Oskooei B, et al. Adaptive designs in clinical trials: why use them, and how to run and report them. BMC Med 2018;16(1):29.

59. Berry SM, Connor JT, Lewis RJ. The platform trial: an efficient strategy for evaluating multiple treatments. JAMA 2015;313(16):1619–20.

UNITED STATES POSTAL SERVICE®
Statement of Ownership, Management, and Circulation
(All Periodicals Publications Except Requester Publications)

1. Publication Title	2. Publication Number	3. Filing Date
ANESTHESIOLOGY CLINICS	000 – 277	9/18/2019

4. Issue Frequency	5. Number of Issues Published Annually	6. Annual Subscription Price
MAR, JUN, SEP, DEC	4	$360.00

7. Complete Mailing Address of Known Office of Publication *(Not printer) (Street, city, county, state, and ZIP+4®)*

ELSEVIER INC.
230 Park Avenue, Suite 800
New York, NY 10169

Contact Person
STEPHEN R. BUSHING

Telephone *(Include area code)*
215-239-3688

8. Complete Mailing Address of Headquarters or General Business Office of Publisher *(Not printer)*

ELSEVIER INC.
230 Park Avenue, Suite 800
New York, NY 10169

9. Full Names and Complete Mailing Addresses of Publisher, Editor, and Managing Editor *(Do not leave blank)*

Publisher *(Name and complete mailing address)*

TAYLOR BALL, ELSEVIER INC.
1600 JOHN F KENNEDY BLVD. SUITE 1800
PHILADELPHIA, PA 19103-2899

Editor *(Name and complete mailing address)*

COLLEEN DIETZLER, ELSEVIER INC.
1600 JOHN F KENNEDY BLVD. SUITE 1800
PHILADELPHIA, PA 19103-2899

Managing Editor *(Name and complete mailing address)*

PATRICK MANLEY, ELSEVIER INC.
1600 JOHN F KENNEDY BLVD. SUITE 1800
PHILADELPHIA, PA 19103-2899

10. Owner *(Do not leave blank. If the publication is owned by a corporation, give the name and address of the corporation immediately followed by the names and addresses of all stockholders owning or holding 1 percent or more of the total amount of stock. If not owned by a corporation, give the names and addresses of the individual owners. If owned by a partnership or other unincorporated firm, give its name and address as well as those of each individual owner. If the publication is published by a nonprofit organization, give its name and address.)*

Full Name	Complete Mailing Address
WHOLLY OWNED SUBSIDIARY OF REED/ELSEVIER, US HOLDINGS	1600 JOHN F KENNEDY BLVD. SUITE 1800 PHILADELPHIA, PA 19103-2899

11. Known Bondholders, Mortgagees, and Other Security Holders Owning or Holding 1 Percent or More of Total Amount of Bonds, Mortgages, or Other Securities. If none, check box. ▶ ☐ None

Full Name	Complete Mailing Address
N/A	

12. Tax Status *(For completion by nonprofit organizations authorized to mail at nonprofit rates) (Check one)*
The purpose, function, and nonprofit status of this organization and the exempt status for federal income tax purposes:
☒ Has Not Changed During Preceding 12 Months
☐ Has Changed During Preceding 12 Months *(Publisher must submit explanation of change with this statement)*

PS Form **3526**, July 2014 *[Page 1 of 4 (see instructions page 4)]* PSN: 7530-01-000-9931   PRIVACY NOTICE: See our privacy policy on www.usps.com

---

13. Publication Title	14. Issue Date for Circulation Data Below
ANESTHESIOLOGY CLINICS	JUNE 2019

15. Extent and Nature of Circulation			Average No. Copies Each Issue During Preceding 12 Months	No. Copies of Single Issue Published Nearest to Filing Date
a. Total Number of Copies *(Net press run)*			208	220
b. Paid Circulation *(By Mail and Outside the Mail)*	(1)	Mailed Outside-County Paid Subscriptions Stated on PS Form 3541 *(Include paid distribution above nominal rate, advertiser's proof copies, and exchange copies)*	68	79
	(2)	Mailed In-County Paid Subscriptions Stated on PS Form 3541 *(Include paid distribution above nominal rate, advertiser's proof copies, and exchange copies)*	0	0
	(3)	Paid Distribution Outside the Mails Including Sales Through Dealers and Carriers, Street Vendors, Counter Sales, and Other Paid Distribution Outside USPS®	79	97
	(4)	Paid Distribution by Other Classes of Mail Through the USPS *(e.g. First-Class Mail®)*	0	0
c. Total Paid Distribution *(Sum of 15b (1), (2), (3), and (4))*			147	176
d. Free or Nominal Rate Distribution *(By Mail and Outside the Mail)*	(1)	Free or Nominal Rate Outside-County Copies included on PS Form 3541	45	25
	(2)	Free or Nominal Rate In-County Copies included on PS Form 3541	0	0
	(3)	Free or Nominal Rate Copies Mailed at Other Classes Through the USPS *(e.g. First-Class Mail)*	0	0
	(4)	Free or Nominal Rate Distribution Outside the Mail *(Carriers or other means)*	0	0
e. Total Free or Nominal Rate Distribution *(Sum of 15d (1), (2), (3) and (4))*			45	25
f. Total Distribution *(Sum of 15c and 15e)*			192	201
g. Copies not Distributed *(See Instructions to Publishers #4 (page #3))*			16	19
h. Total *(Sum of 15f and g)*			208	220
i. Percent Paid *(15c divided by 15f times 100)*			76.56%	87.56%

* If you are claiming electronic copies, go to line 16 on page 3. If you are not claiming electronic copies, skip to line 17 on page 3.

PS Form **3526**, July 2014 *(Page 2 of 4)*

16. Electronic Copy Circulation	Average No. Copies Each Issue During Preceding 12 Months	No. Copies of Single Issue Published Nearest to Filing Date
a. Paid Electronic Copies ▶		
b. Total Paid Print Copies (Line 15c) + Paid Electronic Copies (Line 16a) ▶		
c. Total Print Distribution (Line 15f) + Paid Electronic Copies (Line 16a) ▶		
d. Percent Paid (Both Print & Electronic Copies) (16b divided by 16c × 100) ▶		

☒ I certify that 50% of all my distributed copies (electronic and print) are paid above a nominal price.

17. Publication of Statement of Ownership

☒ If the publication is a general publication, publication of this statement is required. Will be printed
in the DECEMBER 2019 issue of this publication.

☐ Publication not required.

18. Signature and Title of Editor, Publisher, Business Manager, or Owner

STEPHEN R. BUSHING - INVENTORY DISTRIBUTION CONTROL MANAGER

Stephen R. Bushing

Date 9/18/2019

I certify that all information furnished on this form is true and complete. I understand that anyone who furnishes false or misleading information on this form or who omits material or information requested on the form may be subject to criminal sanctions (including fines and imprisonment) and/or civil sanctions (including civil penalties).

PS Form **3526**, July 2014 *(Page 3 of 4)*   PRIVACY NOTICE: See our privacy policy on www.usps.com

Moving?

Make sure your subscription moves with you!

To notify us of your new address, find your **Clinics Account Number** (located on your mailing label above your name), and contact customer service at:

Email: **journalscustomerservice-usa@elsevier.com**

800-654-2452 (subscribers in the U.S. & Canada)
314-447-8871 (subscribers outside of the U.S. & Canada)

Fax number: 314-447-8029

Elsevier Health Sciences Division
Subscription Customer Service
3251 Riverport Lane
Maryland Heights, MO 63043

*To ensure uninterrupted delivery of your subscription, please notify us at least 4 weeks in advance of move.

Printed and bound by CPI Group (UK) Ltd, Croydon, CR0 4YY

08/05/2025

01864747-0001